12-25-2009

For Harvey Blumenthal, M.D.

Just imagine, how fortunate we were to be allowed to study the human brain, the crown jewel of God's Creation!

With love and admiration,

John A. Coates

THE DIVINE BANQUET OF THE BRAIN
AND OTHER ESSAYS

The Divine Banquet of the Brain
and Other Essays

Macdonald Critchley, C.B.E., M.D., F.R.C.P., hon. F.A.C.P.

The National Hospital
Queen Square
London, England

Raven Press • New York

Raven Press, 1140 Avenue of the Americas, New York, New York 10036

Made in the United States of America

International Standard Book Number 0-89004-348-5
Library of Congress Catalog Card Number 78-2461

Library of Congress Cataloging in Publication Data

Critchley, Macdonald.
 The divine banquet of the brain and other essays.

 Bibliography: p.
 1. Brain—Addresses, essays, lectures. 2. Neurology—Addresses, essays, lectures. I. Title.
QP376.C74   612′.8   78-2461
ISBN 0-89004-348-5

Fifth Printing, July 1986

Preface

"Scribble, scribble, scribble, eh Mister Gibbon; another fat book, eh Mister Gibbon?", as King George III remarked to the historian. What justification can there be for these continual additions to the mountain of print? Does it not suggest that one is intruding into a library without first knocking at the door?

Whosoever ventures to compile a miscellany of essays risks displeasing critics both serious and good humoured. And yet, as every columnist knows well, curious pleasures attend this particular medium. These are probably more evident to the perpetrator than to the recipient. Even so, as Louis Nizer in his wisdom made clear, a collection of articles of diversity has the advantage that a loose jointed structure need not maintain a continuous thought. One can open the book at any chapter and fare as well reading backwards as forwards.

For an author there is another attraction. Some of his minor and ephemeral efforts may have been at the time modest *jeus d'esprit* written with zeal and respect, only to remain buried in some obscure volume dedicated to a senior colleague, or revered teacher or friend. Re-reading these pieces and polishing them anew evokes a mood of nostalgia and serves as a veritable *recherche du temps perdu*. Thus the essay on "The idea of a presence" recalls to me as in a flash, memories of 6½ war-years in the Royal Navy. This was a period that familiarized me with the horrendous experiences of hundreds of shipwrecked sailors who had survived days or even weeks in some frail craft exposed to the rigours of the North Atlantic or the torturing heat and thirst on tropical seas.

The article on Phrenology was my valedictory lecture to the Staff and students of the National Hospital, Queen Square. In a less serious vein it also culls up the memory of a contretemps with Customs officials when told I was bringing into England one of Gall's original skulls.

What memories are conjured up by reopening the unlikely topic of calculating idiots. Precious weeks in Moscow working in harmonious collaboration with my old friend Professor Luria, come back to mind. Likewise are revived memories of happy days and nights in prewar Budapest—then the most glittering star in the galaxy of the Austro-Hungarian empire. At one time this paper appeared in a *Festschrift* to my dear friend—grandson of the famous Semmelweiss—Tibor de Lehoczky, with whom I so often shared the gastronomic delights of the *Kakuk* and the Imperial Tokay, and also the seductive gipsy music. Alas, that restaurant was obliterated by shellfire in 1945, never to be restored.

Rewriting the story of Broca takes one back to the little walled town of Sommières, nestling in the vineyards between Arles and Montpellier. The distinction of unveiling a plaque honouring the two doctors Dax was a solemn yet riotous occasion. It resembled nothing so much as a chapter out of Chevalier's *Clochemerle*. A gargantuan repast in the Mairie, followed by a procession through the decorated streets, preceded by the Band of the Fire Brigade, were but the fantastic preliminaries.

Adopting a more serious tone, I submit that this volume is justified if only because it contains a hitherto unpublished tribute to the greatest neurologist of his time, Gordon Holmes. There has never before appeared in print a personal account of Holmes, the man himself. Others to come will doubtless write weighty records of his contributions to neurology, but no one else living can speak or write of the human aspects of this great notability. If for no other reason, I trust that "The Divine Banquet of the Brain" will bring enjoyment to readers and participants.

Santa Fé,　　　　　　　　　　　　　　　*Macdonald Critchley*
N.M. 1979

Contents

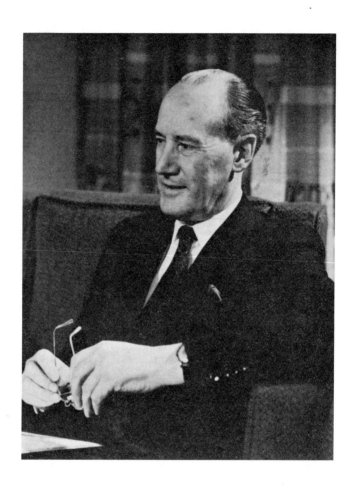

Macdonald Critchley, M.D., F.R.C.P., Hon. F.A.C.P., Hon. M.D., Hon. D. en M., received his medical degree with first class honours from Bristol University. At the present time, he is a consulting physician to the National Hospital, and the consulting neurologist to King's College Hospital.

Critchley was appointed Goulstonian Lecturer at the Royal College of Physicians in 1930, Long Fox Lecturer at the University of Bristol in 1935, and a Hunterian Professor at the Royal College of Surgeons in 1935. In 1942 and 1945, respectively, he delivered the Bradshaw and Croonian Lectures at the Royal College of Physicians. He served from 1965–1973 as president of the World Federation of Neurology. In the past, he has also held positions as Vice-President of the Royal College of Physicians; Dean at the Institute of Neurology, President of the International League against Epilepsy, and President of the Association of British Neurologists from 1965 to 1973.

Macdonald Critchley has received many honours and awards, including: The Victor Horsley Gold Medal in 1964; the Gowers Medal award in 1965; the Hughlings Jackson Gold Medal and Memorial Lectureship in 1966; the Veraguth Gold Medal award at Bern in 1968, and the Samuel T. Orton award in 1974. Critchley was an Arthur Hall Memorial Lecturer at the University of Sheffield in 1969; a Rickman Godlee Lecturer at the University of London in 1970, and a Cavendish Lecturer at the West London Medical Chirurgical Society in 1976.

For many years, he has devoted special attention to disorders of higher nervous activity and in particular to aphasiology and other disorders of language. He is also a well known pioneer in the field of Developmental Dyslexia in children, upon which subject he has written extensively and has also been the recipient of the Samuel T. Orton award for his contributions within this field.

The Idea of a Presence

The purpose of this article is to describe a rather unusual mental experience which may occur in some psychotics, rarely in epileptics as an aura, and even in normal persons in certain circumstances. Scarcely any clear-cut account of this phenomenon exist in neuro-psychiatric writings, in the English language at any rate, though it has been alluded to in the literature of divinity and of occultism. Almost alone among psychiatrists, Jaspers in 1913 has given an adequate description. Certainly it finds a place in fiction, but this fact is not necessarily a disadvantage, for, as Dupré used to teach ". . . *voulez-vous pénétrer les secrets de la psychiatrie? Lisez les poètes et les romanciers.*" The phenomenon in question comprises a feeling, or an impression—sometimes amounting to a veritable delusion—that the person concerned is "not alone." Or, if it should be that he is actually in the company of others, that there is also some other being present, when really this is not so. The experience is often vague, intangible, and elusive, for the visitant can neither be seen, heard, nor felt. In other words the phenomenon is an extracampine one, to employ the terminology used by Bleuler.

Sometimes the idea is vivid; sometimes it is subtle and ephemeral. In duration it may be either sustained or transient. Or, yet again, it may repeatedly come and go, wax and wane. The identity of the visitant or "presence" is but rarely established. Usually the feeling merely entails the belief that there is "someone" in the vicinity. Or, the impression may not amount to anything more than an intangible feeling "as if" one were not alone. The "someone" in question may possess either a beneficent or a sinister quality—either protective or menacing. At other times there is no emotional accompaniment: the visitant in these cases is neutral, colourless, and devoid of personal significance (though realisation of the fallaciousness of the belief may engender its own emotions of awe, wonder, bewilderment, or fear).

This "idea of a presence" may be illustrated by a couple of examples which came to one's notice while serving with the Royal Navy during the war.

A sailor, whose ship had been torpedoed, was adrift in a life-boat with a few other ratings. Rations were minimal, consisting of a biscuit and a few ounces of water a day for each man. No protection existed against the cold and wet, and, as the frail craft was tossed about on the mountainous seas, hopes of survival vanished. Indeed the actuarial chances of being rescued

1

were very slender. As physical exhaustion and mental distress increased, the sensorium of the shipwrecked sailors became more and more cloudy. My patient now began to experience a curious phenomenon. There kept recurring in his mind the notion that immediately astern of the life-boat a rescue-vessel was under way, with boom lowered, ready to pick up survivors. Each time this idea arose, he would eagerly look around and scan the ocean, but time and again his hopes were shattered, for no trace of any vessel in fact existed.

This was the first instance which came to my attention, and it was actually atypical in that the "presence" entailed not a person but an inanimate object, namely a rescue-ship. The sailor, be it noted, was not alone at the time. He was one of a little band of survivors, and hence he formed a unit within a small and isolated community, which itself could be regarded as very much "alone". Whether his other shipmates also experienced this idea of a presence—similar or dissimilar in type—is not known. Because of the great suggestibility of members of a shipwrecked community and their tendency towards mass hallucinosis and mass confabulation, we need not be astonished if his idea of a presence was not also shared.

Shortly after this particular rating had been interviewed, another shipwreck-survivor was met with who also had suffered a comparable mental experience. A Fleet Air Arm pilot, who had crashed into the sea during the *Bismarck* action, described to me how he and his observer, while adrift in a rubber dinghy, kept imagining that there was a third person along with the two of them.

Here again the circumstances were comparable. Severe physical discomfort had been present, going on to utter collapse. There had been exposure to bitter cold and wet; and intense thirst and lack of food had led to a dangerous degree of dehydration and inanition. Prospects of rescue were remote, and though from time to time hopes would soar in an extravagant and unwarranted fashion, they would soon be dashed again with realisation of their tragic plight.

In a post-war account of a raft which was adrift for weeks in the Straits of Malacca, two men, a Swede and a Finn, were involved. The former was attacked and devoured by sharks. The other sailor, who was eventually rescued, afterwards wrote ". . . for the whole voyage I'd had the strange feeling that someone else was with me, watching over me, and keeping me safe from harm. . . . It was as if there were sometimes three people on the raft, not two. With Ericsson dead I felt it more strongly than ever." (Tiira, *Raft of Despair*).

A similar mental phenomenon has also been recorded among Antarctic explorers, as for example in the case of Shackleton and his companion. After struggling across the island of South Georgia against the hazards of a violent blizzard, they eventually reached the shelter and fellowship of their base camp. Recalling this adventure Shackleton said, "I had a curious feeling on the march that there was another person with us." It intrigues us to learn that at this point his comrade interpolated that he too had been aware of some similar experience, but that he had hitherto hesitated to mention the fact.

When discussing this phenomenon as involving normal persons exposed to severe peril, privation, or exhaustion, I have occasionally been told of other similar cases. It has been described to me in mountaineers immobilised by bad weather at great heights, as well as in prisoners on a cruel march from one German concentration camp to another. An explorer scaling Mount Everest developed this same trick of the imagination, probably from anoxia rather than exhaustion. During his solitary voyage around the world in a tiny sailing vessel, Slocum at times had the fancy that he had a companion with him.

Something akin may also occur in association with organic neurological states. Being purely subjective experiences they are not always conspicuous. The patient may be reluctant to volunteer the information; the neurologist in his ignorance may neglect to inquire for it, or to record it if mentioned. Consequently we are apt to regard it as a rare phenomenon, though perhaps unjustifiably so.

Thus an epileptic may develop the idea of a presence as part of the aura. A number of examples may be given:

(a) An epileptic woman of 24 had had fits for seven years. Before each of her attacks she used to get a horrible frightening feeling that someone (or something) was behind her, and was pushing her forwards.

(b) An epileptic female of 72 years was prone to curious, transient attacks of compulsive immobility with loss of vision to the right side. Her right hand would then seem to her to swell to twice its size and to appear "ugly and spiteful". This illusion might continue for hours. At these times she might also have an intangible sensation as if someone sinister ("a bad spirit") were standing behind her left shoulder.

In the next case an hallucinatory element was also present of a primitive kind. By acting as a *point de repère* it was elaborated by the patient into a quasi-delusional state.

(c) A boy of 15 was taking coffee in an open-air café. He suddenly imagined he saw something glistening far over to his right. His mind immediately leapt to the conclusion that someone was standing behind him and to the right, trying to hypnotise him by shining a light into his eyes. In alarm he turned his head and eyes to the right, and then lost consciousness.

In the following case it is uncertain whether the phenomenon was hallucinatory or not.

(d) A male epileptic of 26 who had suffered from fits for ten years, developed a terrifying idea that an unfamiliar and unprepossessing face was lurking behind his right shoulder. At times his head felt swollen to twice its size. There were clinical and encephalographic data to show that in this patient the epilepsy was symptomatic of some progressive but chronic diffuse encephalitic process.

In cases like these, the epileptic patient, believing that someone stands in the rear, may turn the head and body in an effort to bring the being into view, and then almost immediately he falls unconscious. Perhaps some of the common cases of versive (or adversive) epilepsy really belong here, the preliminary turning movements being not so much an involuntary rotation as a willed and purposeful act of inspection.

The idea of a presence may also occur as a symptom in narcoleptics, especially during the stage of predormital unease. Hypnagogic hallucinations are apt to appear to such patients, but as a preliminary to these, there may be a brief period of quasi-hallucinosis, where the presence of an intruder in the room is imagined intellectually rather than perceived as a sense-datum. The following case-report illustrates this point. M. H., a female narcoleptic patient, was a victim of very disturbed sleep at nighttime. She might wake in the night with such a vivid impression that some intruder was in her room that she would switch on the light. In her more elaborate interdormital delirious episodes she would be hallucinated, especially in the tactile and auditory spheres.

It may be that the third narcoleptic described by Lord Brain was also a victim of this idea of a presence, occurring during the night, though the possibility of actual hallucinations cannot be excluded. The patient at times would wake in the darkness to find himself out of bed and in a state of fear, believing that someone was in the room creeping towards him. In his panic he would scream; twice he broke windows, and once he kicked a hole in the door.

Among the vague and curious anomalies of corporeal awareness (or body-image) occurring with lesions of the subordinate parietal lobe, an idea of a "presence" may intrude.

Hoff and Engerth reported on a patient who showed a left-sided hemiparesis and a hemianopia. The patient declared that the left half of the body did not belong to him. Sometimes while walking he got the notion that behind him and to his left he was being followed by someone, namely his double. Whenever this idea developed he would lose the feeling of strangeness which affected the left half of his body.

A well-known poet told me that during a childhood illness he developed a curious feeling as if someone (actually a mere acquaintance) had entered his body. Thus he became a composite being with this other person sharing his pains and discomfort. This impression lasted some days and so vivid was it that he naturally believed that the doctors and nurses in attendance knew all about it too.

Here we have a modification of the idea of a presence, the visitant taking up a position not in an extrapersonal spatial relationship, but within the subject's own body. In some ways this forms an antithesis of depersonalization. This patient of course had no parietal lesion. Some other cases are even more complicated in character. A man of 53 with temporal lobe epilepsy (kindly shown me by Dr. Denis Williams) on one occasion sustained an attack which was preceded by the curious notion that his bodily self had grown to one and one-sixteenth of its original size. So vivid was this belief that he was in great fear in case his personality should permanently enter the sixteenth fraction and then separate from the remainder. He could hear himself exclaiming: "Yes, please; yes, please . . . ."

Zillig's patient (suffering from parietal injury) developed a fantastic confusional state in which he believed that he consisted of nothing but a head and neck severed from the rest of the body. He imagined he lay in a basket, as a torn-off head among a ghastly collection of other such heads. Outside the basket, decapitated men walked back and forth. This belief was not based upon any hallucinatory experience, but was a sort of dream-state of great complexity.

Elsewhere I have reported the case of a woman with biparietal atrophy who, among other numerous symptoms, would often wake in the night with a trenchant feeling that someone was in the room—a person whom she knew very well indeed. Sometimes it would dawn upon her that this visitant was none other than herself. The *alter ego* seemed always to be located out of sight, behind her and to her left. So poignant at times was this feeling that she might be impelled to get out of bed and go on tiptoe from room to room with the object of surprising this interloper.

That neurological patients whose sensorium is clear are reluctant to confess to such bizarre and macabre experiences is not surprising. This intangible feeling perhaps amounting to a firm belief but subsequently proving to be erroneous or delusional is so unexpected, incongruous, and uncanny, as to disturb the victim. Like the amputee and his phantom limb, he may well prefer not to mention it.

The idea of a presence is all the more upsetting to the layman for it is a theme which has been not infrequently touched upon by poets and by romantic writers. The conception of the haunted malefactor is not far removed. As an example of literary allusions belonging more or less to this category we may mention T. S. Eliot's "The Waste Land" It has been mentioned by Flaubert (". . . He has the feeling that some monstrosity is floating around him—the horror of a crime about to be perpetrated"—"Temptation of Saint Anthony"); by Maupassant ("The Horla"); by H. G. Wells (". . . . I woke with a start, and with an odd fancy that some greyish animal had just rushed out of the chamber"—"The Time Machine"); and by Denis Wheatley ("The Haunting of Toby Jug").

The symptom may accordingly possess an unsavoury connotation, particularly when the unseen presence seems to threaten rather than to sustain.

But this is not always the case. There is a weighty theological tradition, if not a literature, too, which implies a protective companionship, the conception indeed of a guardian angel. Thus in Roman Catholic communities the notion of an *angelo custode* is a common teaching and is depicted in religious art as an angel with a wide wingspan standing as an unseen protector behind a little child. A special prayer illustrates this belief: *"Angele Dei, qui custodes es mei, me tibi commitium pietate superna, hodie illumina custodi rege et guberna."*

In similar vein, Satan may at times be depicted in symbolic form crouching beneath the feet of the child. But in Muslim doctrine, the good angel stands behind the right shoulder while the devil is behind the left (hence the superstition of the left hand as being unclean, unlucky, sinister, and not "right").

It is not surprising therefore to find that a supernatural or theistic interpretation is adduced by the religious as the obvious explanation of the idea of a presence, especially in the case of distressed and exhausted shipwrecked seamen. The "Guardian Angel" motif is inescapable to those with strong beliefs. As Tiira said of his experiences while adrift, ". . . . perhaps it was my mother's prayers for me in Finland. She was always anxious for my safety. Maybe this strong bond between us came to my mental rescue at this time."

How far is this phenomenon a commonplace among normal children? Doubtless it occurs more often than is often realised. Something comparable may lie behind the "invisible playmate" theme of the lonely child, the orphan, or the evacuee; or those who are homeless, unwanted, or hungry for sympathy and love. In states of putative danger, or illness, or in uneasy solitude, the idea of a presence may be particularly vivid, and may be confidently associated by the child with its belief in a celestial protecting agency or companion.

Similar affective factors may also be mirrored in adults between whom a deep love and understanding form a strong though intangible bond. Though actually separated, they may seem to be together in spirit if not in reality. This is shown in some of the moving *lettres d'amour* which are available to the public eye. Thus, despite its artificiality and flamboyance, we read a suggestion of this phenomenon in a letter from Oscar Wilde to his wife: ". . . The messages of the gods to each other travel not by pen and ink, and indeed your bodily presence here would not make you more real: for I feel your fingers in my hair and your cheek brushing mine. The air is full of the music of your voice, my soul and body seem no longer mine, but mingled in some exquisite ecstasy with yours."

In theological literature we find the most explicit references to this phenomenon. Under the term "the sense of present reality" William James described a feeling of objective presence, a perception of "something there", more deep and more general than any of the special and particular "senses" by which current psychology supposes existent realities to be originally revealed. James spoke of it as a hallucination which is imperfectly developed. He quoted the experience of a close friend of his: "I have several times within the past few years felt the so-called 'consciousness of a presence'. . . . After I had got into bed and blown out the candle, I lay awake thinking—when suddenly I *felt* something come into the room and stay close to my bed. It remained only a minute or two. I did not recognise it by any ordinary sense, and yet there was a horribly unpleasant "sensation" connected with it. It stirred something more at the roots of my being than any ordinary perception. . . . I was conscious of its departure as of its coming. . . . The certainty that there in outer space stood *something* was indescribably stronger than the ordinary certainty of companionship when we are in the close presence of ordinary living people. The something seemed close to me, and intensely more real than any ordinary perception."

This witness was described by James as being endowed with one of the keenest intellects he knew. In this person too, hypnagogic hallucinations of a tactile kind also occurred from time to time. The malefic and unpleasant associations of the visitant are noteworthy. But apparently on other occasions the idea of a presence may entail a quality of joyful elation.

"There was not a mere consciousness of something there, but fused in the central happiness of it, a startling awareness of some ineffable good. Not vague either, not like the emotional effect of some poem, or scene, or blossom, or music, but the sure knowledge of the close presence of a sort of mighty person." James went on to quote a writer in the *Journal of Psychial Research* who proclaimed: ". . . suddenly, without a moment's warning my whole being seemed roused to the highest state of tension or aliveness, and I was aware, with an intenseness not easily imagined by those who never experienced it, that another being or presence was not only in the room, but quite close to me."

This writer identified the visitant with a particular person—a friend of his. He was imagined as standing out of sight, behind and to the left. By slowly turning his eyes to the side, the writer could then see and recognise the gray-blue material of his trousers which appeared "semi-transparent, like tobacco-smoke in consistency". In other words, the idea of a presence had now given place to a visual hallucination.

Another instance was given by James. "Quite early in the night I was awakened. . . . I then turned on my side to go to sleep again, and immediately felt a consciousness of a presence in the room, and singular to state, it was not the consciousness of a live person, but of a spiritual presence. . . . I felt also at the same time a strong feeling of superstitious dread, as if something strange and fearful were about to happen."

James also quoted the testimony of a friend of Flournoy who wrote: "Whenever I practise automatic writing, what makes me feel that it is not due to a subconscious self is the feeling I always have of a foreign presence, external to my body. It is sometimes so definitely characterised that I could point to its exact position. This impression of presence is impossible to describe. It varies in intensity and clearness according to the personality from whom the writing professes to come. If it is someone whom I love, I feel it immediately, before any writing has come."

Finally James described an example occurring in a very intelligent blind subject. He was liable to the fancy that a gray-bearded man clad in a pepper and salt suit would squeeze himself under the crack of the door, and then cross the room towards a sofa. This would appear to have been merely an abstract conceit for the blind man possessed no vivid visual imagery, and no other special sense was involved in this idea of a presence.

In *Phantasms of the Living*—that extraordinary sourcebook by Gurney, Myers, and Podmore—certain paragraphs are appropriate to our subject. The authors referred to what they call hallucinations of the lowest or most rudimentary grade. These consist in vague impressions of sense data without any actual stimulus being perceived. For example, they described cases where auditory hallucinations occur and yet no spectral words are actually heard in the ordinary meaning of the word. The voices seem to be formed and spoken within the chest, or the voices are regarded as being "soundless". Phenomena of this kind were equated by these authors with the "psychic hallucinations" described by Baillarger, in contra-distinction to ordinary psycho-sensorial hallucinations. In the visual sphere psychic hallucinations may reveal themselves as a type of delusion or potential hallucination which consists in the sense of a presence. An example was given where a normal person woke in the night with a curious feeling that his great friend, who was in India at the time, was in his room. He had an impulse to call out his name and although by now he was wide awake it took him some moments to realise that his friend could not possibly be there in the room. On yet another occasion the same person went to sleep having been thinking a good deal about his brother in America. In the middle of the night he woke up once again with the feeling that his brother was in the room and had been speaking to him. Yet another case was quoted where a subject had the feeling on many occasions that her sister was in the room. Sometimes the feeling was so strong that she would get up and wander round the house looking for her sister.

Still upon the subject of religious mysticism and ecstacy, we may quote Janet, who observed the same phenomenon in his extraordinary patient Madeleine. Under the term *sentiment de présence* Janet described—none too lucidly—an intangible feeling of the all-pervading presence of the deity. Unfortunately, Janet did not discuss the phenomenon further and in simple language.

In works of a purely religious character, certain mystical experiences are often described, though it is usually difficult to distinguish between actual visions and less tangible mental and spiritual impressions of a presence. The phenomena detailed by Saint Teresa of Jesus (1515–1582) in her autobiography illustrate this difficulty. She was prey to diverse visions of which at least three types were identified, the bodily, the imaginary, and the intellectual. The last-named were the purest and loftiest of them all, and conform to our mundane ideas of an extracampine hallucination. ". . . I was in prayer one day . . . when I saw Christ close by me, or, to speak more correctly, felt Him; for I saw nothing with the eyes of the body, nothing with the eyes of the soul. . . . I went to my confessor in great distress, to tell him of it. He asked in what form I saw our Lord. I told him I saw no form. He then said: 'How did you know that it was Christ?' I replied that I did not know how I knew it, but I could not help knowing that He was close beside me. . . . For if I say that I see Him neither with the eyes of the body, nor with those of the soul . . . how is it that I can understand and maintain that He stands beside me, and be more certain of it than if I saw Him? If it be supposed that it is as if a person were blind, or in the dark, and therefore unable to see another who is close to him, the comparison is not exact."

The writings of Brother Lawrence of the Resurrection (1591–1611) upon "The Practice of the Presence of God" are also relevant. "The presence of God is an applying of our spirit to Him, or a realisation of His presence which can be brought about either by the imagination or the understanding.

"I know of one who, for forty years, has practised the presence of God intellectually, and he gives it several other names . . . he calls it . . . an impression or a loving gaze or a sense of God. . . . He says, however, that all these expressions for the presence of God are synonyms, they express the same thing, the presence which has come to be natural to him, in this way: By repeated acts and by frequently recalling his mind to God he has developed such a habit that, so soon as he is free from external occupations, and even while he is still busy, his very soul, without any forethought on his part, is lifted above all earthly things. . . . It is this which he calls the actual presence of God which includes all other kinds and much more besides, so that he lives now as if there were only God and himself in the world: conversing always with Him, entreating Him at need and rejoicing with Him in a thousand ways."

Lhermitte, in his monograph *Mystiques et faux mystiques* (1952), also briefly referred to this phenomenon as *le sentiment de présence*. He quoted two cases which may or may not be strictly relevant to our present series. The clinical history of his first patient makes dramatic reading. "Some years ago", wrote Lhermitte, "I received a visit from a man whose arrival was unusual, to say the least. To the maid who opened the door, he exclaimed: 'Don't come near me. . . . *He* is there!' *He* was the devil." The patient who was a man of great learning submitted a long written narrative of his state of demoniacal possession. But on reading the text closely it seems probable that this patient was actually hallucinating, some of the time at least. Lhermitte's second patient was a lady who was secretary to a most important personage. For more than twenty years she had been attended by an imaginary handsome cavalier upon a magnificent horse. This phenomenon first appeared abruptly while she was walking down the Avenue des Champs-Elysées. The rider was always on her right-hand side. She could always see him but not clearly . . . the vision was more like a glistening shadow. It was almost but not quite constant; being more vivid when she was lonely, and absent if she was walking out of doors with someone else. It seems definite that this case was not so much an example of an idea of a presence, as an actual *hallucination d'un compagnon*. Lhermitte regarded the vision as a symbol of desires of trends which she did not dare declare.

Finally we may mention the idea of a presence as occurring in psychotics and more especially in schizophrenics. This topic formed the basis of the original paper written by Jaspers. Here the author described six cases of dementia praecox. The first patient said "I had the feeling that someone was inside me and then stepped out, perhaps out of the side or somehow. . . . I felt as if someone constantly walked by my side." The second patient would feel as if his father were in the room behind him. The third patient had the impression that someone was one or two yards behind her propelling her forwards—though actually she felt no touch to her body. The fourth patient was more complex. When listening to music he was in the habit of making rhythmic movements. On occasions he would have the idea that his fiancée was standing behind him, back to back, making synchronous and similar movements. His fifth patient wrote, ". . . I felt as though there were someone behind the bed who was writing down all my words." Jasper's sixth patient constantly felt as though someone were present, whom she could not see and who was watching her. The author quoted a patient of Forel's who had the notion that he was receiving messages though they were inaudible. The autobiography of Strindberg was also quoted. ". . . I sensed the presence of someone who had come there during my absence. I could not see him but I felt his presence."

Discussion

The problem of the idea of a presence offers an interesting contribution to the study of sense-deception as a whole. It is strikingly evident from a scrutiny of the case-records and protocols, that the "idea" of a presence ordinarily constitutes a sort of rudimentary hallucination. There is every gradation between a feeling "as if" a presence were in the vicinity; through an intermediate stage of confident belief in the existence of an invisible, inaudible, and intangible entity; up to finally an actual visual, auditory, or tactile hallucination.

It is obvious that recourse to medical literature is poorly rewarding in a study of this phenomenon. Verbal discussion has, however, often raised other phenomena which are allied, to say the least, to this "idea" of a presence and which bear if not a relationship then at least a superficial resemblance. For example, when the idea of a presence entails the identification of the visitant as an *alter ego,* or one's other self, then we encroach immediately upon the territory of the *Doppelgänger.* Thus, closest in nature, is the "bipartition fantasy" or the phenomenon of the "emancipation of the Ego" encountered in a variety of psychotic states. For example, an intelligent post-encephalitic psychopath began to develop at the age of 41 years the illusion of being two people. He could not actually see, hear, or touch his other self, but he would imagine it occupying a definite position in space, to the side of but slightly behind the real body and out of sight. His *alter ego* would seem to urge him to do silly things. Urquhart's subject developed this same idea of doubling of the personality (the *alter ego* being imperceptible) under the influence of hashish. As he himself put it, ". . . the impression was that of wandering out of myself. I had two beings."

When the belief of duality becomes elaborated, and proceeds to a veritable hallucination, we attain the *heautoscopy* described by Lhermitte, or, as it used to be called, "specular hallucinosis". Not infrequently the idea of a presence is equated with Capgras' syndrome. But strictly speaking the term Capgras' syndrome should be confined to the mental phenomenon also called the "illusion of doubles" or—more usually—*l'illusion des sosies.* This refers to the non-recognition of familiar persons, with the postulation of imaginary differences and the further expressed belief that the real person has been replaced by a double. The factor of distinction is sometimes spoken of as the "negative double", the imaginary resemblances constituting the "positive double".

Using strictly these defining terms it is obvious that Capgras' syndrome bears no real relationship to the phenomenon which forms the topic of this paper. The same applies to the syndrome of Fregoli, or *le delire d'inter-metamorphose.** Though sometimes confused, this condition is quite different from the idea of a presence, being really a variant of Capgras' syndrome.

At times the idea of a presence can be looked upon as being almost the opposite phenomenon to the more common illusory states of unreality which may develop alongside the depersonalisations. It is not without interest that the same types of morbid condition—temporal epilepsy, con-

---

* The term *syndrome de Fregoli* needs explanation. Leopoldo Fregoli was an Italian actor, born in Rome in 1867, who excelled as a mimic. He was able to switch rapidly from one role to another with such success that he could produce single-handed a complete play, undertaking the roles of every character in the piece, male or female.

fusional states, exhaustion, anoxia, narcolepsy, parietal lesions, ecstasy, hypnagogic twilight states—may be attended either by the symptoms of unreality (derealisation) or by its opposite, namely the idea of a presence. This paradoxical experience, whereby a given symptom may stem from diametrically opposite pathologies, and moreover that diametrically contradictory clinical manifestations may develop with the very same type of lesion—is by no means rare in neurology, and deserves closer attention than it has received to date.

I have been at fault in detaining you so long, having been carried away by the intangible forces which prevented me from adhering to my usual poverty of speech. May I conclude with a quotation from T. S. Eliot which crystallises most of what I have been trying to express?

> Who is the third who walks always beside you?
> When I count there are only you and I together,
> But when I look ahead up the white road
> There is always another one walking beside you,
> Gliding, wrapt in a brown mantle, hooded
> I do not know whether a man or a woman
> —But who *is* that on the other side of you?

The Evolution of Man's Capacity for Language

The spate of criticism which followed the publication a hundred years ago of the *Origin of Species* often included the protest that Darwin in his argument had ignored man's higher mental faculties. This was perhaps true in fact, though captious in spirit. A recent critic, Leslie Paul, has written: "There is therefore through the invention of speech the entry into and the exploration of a new dimension of human activity. I think it was rather provincial and dull-witted of Darwin not to have shown a glimmer of interest in all this." In any event the gap was filled four years later when his geological colleague, Lyell, devoted a chapter in his classical *Antiquity of Man* to a comparison between the origin and growth of languages and of species. Schleicher, a botanist as well as a professional philologist, had called attention, three years before ever reading Darwin's book, to the struggle for existence among words, the disappearance of primitive forms, and the immense expansion and differentiation which may be produced by ordinary causes in a single family of speech. He looked upon languages as natural organisms, which, according to definite physical influences and independently of human will, take origin and mature, grow old and die, and therefore manifest the series of phenomena to which are given the name of "life." In 1863, Schleicher issued his pamphlet *Die Darwinsche Theorie und die Sprachwissenschaft,* which was the expansion of a letter he had written to Professor Häckel acknowledging a copy of the *Origin of Species.* Herein he argued that the inception of species is notably paralleled in the genealogy of language, and particularly of the Aryan and Semitic tongues. Analogous with the struggle for life among the more or less favoured species in the animal and vegetable kingdoms, a struggle for survival occurs among individual languages.

This analogy between the evolution of species and of language was discussed in contemporary scientific literature. F. W. Farrar believed that comparative philology supported Darwin's hypotheses in two important respects, viz., the effect of infinitesimal modifications in gradually bringing about great changes; and the preservation of the best and strongest elements in the struggle for existence. Just as very many primordial cells, closely resembling each other, may have been the earliest rudiments of all living organisms, so in philology different linguistic families may have sprung from multitudes of "speech cells" or "sound cells," that is, the fundamental roots of language. Like an extinct species, a language—once extinct—can never reappear. Intermediate linguistic forms also die out. Thus external factors disturb the primitive relationship of languages, and consequently one may find radically different languages existing side by side. Farrar said, "All this, as every naturalist is well aware, represents a condition of things precisely similar to that which prevails in animated nature."

Darwin's contemporary, Max Müller, who occupied the Chair of Comparative Philology at Oxford, was also interested in this parallelism between the struggle for existence in the biological sense and in the case of languages. He laid stress on an important difference, however. It is not on account of inherent defects that languages gradually become extinct, but rather because of external causes; that is to say, the physical, moral, and political weaknesses of those who speak the languages concerned. Müller considered that a much more pertinent linguistic analogy with Darwinism lay in the struggle for survival among words and grammatical forms which is constantly going on in every language, whereby shorter and easier forms gain the upper hand.

Views of this kind were of topical interest a century ago, but since then philologists, with the possible exception of Jespersen, have been largely out of sympathy with the application of Darwinian ideas to their own subject.

In 1871 Darwin himself dealt in some detail with the human faculties which he had rightly omitted from his earlier monograph; in *Descent of Man* the problem of speech was specifically discussed. The faculty of articulate speech, he wrote, in itself offers no insuperable objection to the belief that man had evolved from some lower form. The mental powers in some early progenitor of man must have been more highly developed than in any existing ape, before even the most imperfect form of speech could have come about. The continued advancement of this power would have reacted on the mind itself, by enabling and encouraging it to pursue long trains of thought. Complex reflection can no more be carried on without the aid of words, whether spoken or silent, than can a long abstraction without the use of figures or algebra.

Darwinian theories and ideas pervaded every aspect of scientific and philosophic thought, and Max Müller was also caught up in the current excitement. Leaving aside his purely linguistic considerations, we may examine his views upon the evolution of the speech faculties in man. After detailing *seriatim* the characters of mind and body which are shared by man and animal, he went on to enquire in 1861:

> Where, then, is the difference between brute and man? What is it that man can do, and of which we find no signs, no rudiments, in the whole brute world? I answer without hesitation: the one great barrier

between the brute and man is *language*. Man speaks, and no brute has ever uttered a word. Language is our Rubicon, and no brute will dare to cross it. This is our matter-of-fact answer to those who speak of development, who think they discover the rudiments at least of all human faculties in apes, and who would fain keep open the possibility that man is only a more favoured beast, the triumphant conqueror in the primeval struggle for life. Language is something more palpable than a fold of the brain or an angle of the skull. It admits of no cavilling, and no process of natural selection will ever distil significant words out of the notes of birds or the cries of beasts.

Professor Müller's views were, on the whole, opposed to those of Darwin, and their differences of opinion were studied and discussed at length by the German linguist Noiré. Strongly critical of "Darwinian foibles, incompleteness and one-sidedness," Noiré proclaimed in 1879 that Max Müller was the only equal, not to say superior, antagonist who had entered the arena against Darwin. "Here is reason, here language, here humanity. None shall pass here; none penetrate into the sanctuary who cannot tell me first how reason, how speech, was born. And the shouting bands of the assailants were struck dumb, for they could give no answer."

Although Professor Müller was, in the main, out of sympathy with Darwin, nevertheless he proclaimed in 1873: "In language, I was a Darwinian before Darwin." As early as 1861 he was trying to reconcile Darwin's doctrines with linguistic phenomena. He compared Darwin with Epicurus, and he spoke of the origins of language in terms of natural selection, or—as he preferred to call it—natural elimination.

Anatomical Basis for Language

Any discussion of the evolution of man's capacity for language must entail an enquiry, not only into the appropriate intellectual equipment, but also into the necessary and actual anatomical substratum. This latter is a twofold problem. In the first place, a physiological cerebral mechanism exists peculiar to man. In addition, the faculty of speech requires certain peripheral instrumentalities, which can fulfil a complex co-ordinated activity of the lips, palate, tongue, pharynx, larynx, and respiratory apparatus. Herein lies the structural basis for the achievement of an audible motor-skill of the utmost delicacy. In the course of both phylogeny and ontogeny it is often possible to observe that anatomical structures are present even before they are actually utilised. Structure, in other words, antedates function. Consequently, within the animal series it may be expected that both cerebral and peripheral mechanisms will stand ready for use, though not yet productive of mature speech.

Even in the anthropoid there is no valid morphological reason, at a peripheral level, why speech should not occur. At any rate, most authorities would agree with this opinion. The relative coarseness of the tissues would no doubt impart a certain unmusical quality to the articulation, but the phonemic range would probably be not inconsiderable. As Max Müller said, there is no letter of the alphabet which a parrot will not learn to pronounce, and the fact that the parrot is without a language of his own must be explained by a difference between the *mental,* not between the *physical,* faculties of animal and man.

It must be stressed that language is a function which can be looked upon as overlaid, or even parasitic. There are no specific cerebral structures which are peculiar to the faculty of speech. It would be difficult—if not, indeed, impossible—to decide merely from a study of the brain, however meticulous, whether the subject had been a polyglot, an orator, a writer, or even an illiterate or a deaf-mute. Simply by microscopical examination of the cerebral cortex it would not be easy to distinguish gorilla from man. In other words, no essentially human cerebral speech centre can yet be confidently identified as an anatomical entity. Speech likewise makes use of predetermined bucco-laryngeal structures which were primarily destined to serve for acts of feeding and respiration. Certain teleological advantages accrued when the function of communication took over structures which were also being utilised for other purposes. Man did not develop *de novo* some entirely novel means for subserving the novel faculty of language. Linguistic precursors, anatomical, physiological, psychological, and cultural, must obviously have existed in the subhuman animal series. In some creatures like bees, simple communicative acts operate by dint of global movements. In birds and primates, elaborate combinations of cries, intention movements, and pantomimic displays fulfil the role of primitive sign-making or communication. Some birds possess the faculty of mimicking human utterances in a plausible and even startling fashion, but it must be remembered that this is a learned, artificial performance and that their innate instinctive calls are crude, raucous, stereotyped—indeed, anything but human in quality.

We recall Buffon's speculation as to what would happen if the ape had been endowed with the voice of a parrot and its faculty of speech. The talking monkey would, he said, have struck dumb with astonishment the entire human race and would have so confounded the philosopher that he would have been hard put to prove—in the face of all these human attributes—that the monkey was still an animal. It is, therefore, just as well for our understanding that Nature has separated and relegated into two very different categories the mimicry of speech and the mimicry of our gestures.

Koehler has put the question why it is, if there are so many precursors of our own language in the animal kingdom, no known animal speaks like man. It is because no animal possesses all those *initia* of our language at one and the same time. They are distributed very diffusely, this species having one capacity, that species another. We alone possess all of them, and we are the only species using words.

Criteria of Language

Among the prerogatives of *Homo sapiens* the faculty of speech is the most obvious. Other members of the animal kingdom, not excluding the higher primates, are not so endowed, however vocal may be the individuals. By contrast, it can be asserted that no race of mankind is known, however lowly, which does not possess the power of speech. Nay more, the linguistic attainments may be subtle, complex, flexible, and eloquent—even though the cultural level be primitive in the extreme. It is indeed difficult to identify among the races of man anything which can be justly termed a "primitive" tongue.

At the very outset it is important to be clear in what way the cries, utterances, calls, and song of birds and subhuman mammals can so readily be deemed as lying outside the category of language attainment. On enquiry, it is found that no one touchstone of distinction is entailed, but rather a co-ordination of factors, some of which may be present in this or that animal, but which do not come together in integration until the stage of *Homo sapiens* is achieved.

Doubtless the most weighty single criterion of human speech is the use of symbols. Animals betray abrupt fluctuations in their emotional state by making sounds. To this extent they may be said to utilise signs. Whether the sign be perceived and identified as such by other members of the same species is arguable. An alarm-call may act as a signal of danger, and others within earshot may take flight. This effect may be an instance of direct signaling between one bird or mammal and another. Or, possibly, the frightened creature's cry may be interjectional rather than purposeful, and others within call may thereupon be made merely partners in alarm rather than the recipients of a directed message. Be that as it may—and the possibility that both types of concerted action occur in nature cannot be gainsaid—the animal's cry cannot strictly be looked upon either as language or as speech. At most, it is communication. The communicative act may be deliberate, willed, directed encoding, while the comprehending recipients who act upon the signal may be looked upon as decoders. Here, then, is communication in the accepted sense of the term. Or it may be that the communicative act is merely incidental, and no true encoding and decoding can be said to take place.

"Animal communication" is therefore the term which carries with it the fewest drawbacks. In essence it can be said to comprise a series of signs which refer to ideas or feelings within immediate awareness. They do not and cannot apply to circumstances within past or future time. Herein lies an all-important distinction. Man's utterances entail the use of symbols or

signs of signs and consequently possess the superlative advantage of applying to events in time past, present, and future and to objects *in absentia*.
This endowment has been called the "time-binding" property of human
language. It also possesses the merit of beginning the process of storage of
experience, a process which eventually reaches fruition with the subsequent
introduction of writing.

The Evolution of Behaviour

Most of the early arguments concerning the problem of the origin of
speech in man have been either theological or linguistic. In the former case
the doctrine of a divine creation was accepted, but many controversies arose,
including such questions as monogenesis versus polygenesis. The purely
linguistic theories rejected altogether the idea of a special creation of a mature system of language, and while some process of transition between the
communication of animals and the beginnings of speech in *Homo sapiens*
was assumed, there was disagreement as to the *modus operandi*. The sources
of argument included the relative importance of the role of imitation, of
interjectional utterances, of associated motor-vocal phenomena, of gesture
and still other factors, none of which nowadays excites serious comment or
concern.

Attention became focussed more upon the mysterious evolutionary
changes which are believed to have taken place between the behavioural
systems of the highest primates and those of earliest man. The beginnings of
speech, in the strict sense of the term, rank among these changes. However
striking in character and fundamental in importance, speech certainly cannot be looked upon as man's sole perquisite, singling him out from the rest
of the animal kingdom. Several other important developments took place
at more or less the same period of evolution, any one or any combination of
which may actually prove to be supremely significant in the genesis of
speech.

The principal clash of opinion turns around the debate whether the
difference between animal communication and the speech of early man
entail factors which are qualitative or merely quantitative. Expressed somewhat differently, the question has been raised whether the distinction between man and animals is one of kind or merely of degree, as far as the
communicative act is concerned.

Within that stage between the most complex of animal communication
and the speech-efforts of earliest man lies the core of our problem. Obviously, this transition from animal cries to human articulation is but an item
in a much bolder process of evolution. Instinctive responses no longer prove
biologically adequate, and more and more complicated vocal reactions
gradually emerge. Linguistics alone can never afford the whole solution, and
other realms of thought and endeavour will need exploring.

Social Factors Favouring Language

Communal living.

Attempts which have been made to identify these important steps in the evolution of human language fall roughly into two classes. Thus one can distinguish sociological from intellectual hypotheses, the former envisaging some modification in behaviour, the latter implying a change in the mode of thinking as between animals and man. These two attitudes are not mutually irreconcilable, and both types of change may well have operated together.

Many would agree that the ancestry of language lay within the pre-hominid stages, at the same time denying the existence of anything that can be strictly termed "animal language."

Révész spoke of "contact reactions" as being important in the genesis of speech in man. By this expression he understood the basic, innate tendency of social animals to approach one another, establish rapport, co-operate, and communicate. Contact reactions are a necessary precondition of linguistic communication. In a rather unconvincing fashion, Révész seems to have equated the essential differences between human speech and the cries and directed calls of the animal world with an elaboration of this "contact reaction" in the domain of articulate utterance.

Much earlier, Lord Monboddo realised the critical role of communal existence. To convert man into a speaking animal, the factor of society is essential. He posed the question: which is the more important—language for the institution of society, or society for the invention of language. In his view, society came first and had existed perhaps for ages before language developed, for man is by nature a political as well as a speaking animal.

Biologists realise that communal existence is an important factor in survival, which can be traced as a principle throughout the animal kingdom, even in the lowliest species. Indeed, the physiological value of coexistence can perhaps be better demonstrated in the invertebrate phyla. In the higher ranks of Mammalia, there is perhaps a greater co-ordination of group activity, whereby there is a limited degree of sharing of function and a deputing of special tasks increasingly becomes the rule. Allee has shrewdly asked at what stage can an animal group be said to have become truly social: is it at the point when animals behave differently in the presence of others than they would if alone? If this is the case, then we witness in an interesting fashion the first hint of ethical or moral factors in animal behaviour.

One of the principal functions of speech is to co-ordinate the behaviour of the individual members of a group. Grace de Laguna stressed the progressively elaborate communal life which synchronises with the development of speech. Planned hunting forays, the need for securing safety by night, the indoctrination of the young—all these are among the activities of early *Homo sapiens*, and they must have been considerably assisted by the faculty of speech. The power of speech thus confers an important survival value upon its owner.

Tool-using: tool-making.

Allied to this notion is the role of an increasing utilisation of tools, as an immediate precursor of speech. *Homo sapiens* has often been identified not only with *Homo loquens* but also with *Homo faber.* An animal achieves its purposes by modifying its own bodily structure, that is, by making a tool out of some part of itself. Man ventures further by making use of instruments outside his own body. As L. S. Amery said, man also began to employ a "sound-tool"; that is to say, he made use of differentiated sounds as an instrument of precision, in order to indicate not only emotions but also specific objects, qualities, actions, and judgments. Both language and tools are instruments which humans alone employ to achieve definite and concrete actions. "Language, like the tool, and unlike the limb, is something objective to, and independent of, the individual who uses it" (de Laguna) .

We now approach a critical point in the argument. The term *Homo faber* is ambiguous, for it can be interpreted in two very different ways. It can be read as meaning either the "tool-maker" or the "tool-user." This distinction is important and is not to be glossed over. Mere tool-taking or tool-utilising is quite consistent with anthropoid behaviour; tool-making is not. The higher apes are not infrequently to be seen making use of a convenient stick as an implement with which to draw a delicacy within reach. But deliberately to choose and to set it carefully aside, against the contingency of finding at some possible future date an edible morsel just inaccessible, is outside the capacity of the anthropoid. To select an instrument and keep it for future use can be reckoned as analogous to fashioning a tool out of sticks or stones to attain an immediate need or desire.

When the species can do these latter things, it steps over the frontier and qualifies as *Homo sapiens.* Similarly, in the most primitive communal groups of man's ancestors, a piece of sharp stone, a stick, a shell might have been picked up and used straightway as a weapon to fell an object of prey, as a weapon of self-defence, or as a tool for decorticating a tree-trunk or skinning a beast. This sort of activity is consistent with primate behaviour, and speech acquisition is unnecessary. But when the apelike creature breaks a stick in two or pulls it out of a bush or if he puts it aside for another occasion, it is beginning this apprenticeship for qualifying as *Homo sapiens,* and here the first beginnings of speech may be detected.

With the art of knapping of flint core-tools or flake-tools or by shaving down a stake, we have the unmistakable marks of attainment of man's stature, and speech can doubtless be assumed as a concomitant. For here we have the earliest mastery over purely perceptual thinking, the dawn of conceptual thought, and release from the shackles of time-present.

Delegation of labour.

Closely linked with an elaborate communal life and the construction of tools, delegation of labour can also be reckoned as a factor in the ancestry of speech. Greater efficiency in hunting and in the acquisition and preparation of food for the group follows upon the use of speech and leads to the beginnings of a simple form of specialisation. This is an aspect of linguistics which has naturally appealed particularly to Soviet writers. Soviet philosophers of language believe that language began when man—a new species of animal—began to use tools and to co-operate with others in order to produce the means of subsistence. Human labour is a new form of social activity and gives rise to a new phenomenon, articulate speech, and to a new characteristic of the mind, the conscious reflection of objective reality. Stalin —himself a dabbler in linguistics—looked upon language not only as a tool of communication but also as a means of struggle and development of society. Language is connected with man's productive activity and also with every other human activity. Seppe, a Russian neurologist, went further. Work appeared to him as a main factor in the development of higher and abstract thinking of man. Speech functions are created from work. Furthermore, we find Stalin declaring: "In the history of mankind, a spoken language has been one of the forces which helped human beings to emerge from the animal world, unite into communities, develop their faculty of thinking, organise social production, wage a successful struggle against the forces of nature, and attain the stage of progress we have today" (*Pravda, August 2, 1950*).

Such were the progressive elaborations in animal behaviour which immediately antedated and perhaps accelerated the development of speech in man. The alternative group of hypotheses puts the emphasis more upon the elaboration of certain ways of thinking, as bridging the gap between animal communication and human speech.

Intellectual Behaviour

Abstract thinking.

Since Aristotle, many philosophers have stressed man's gift of conceptual thought, whereby he is enabled to deal with general ideas as well as the particular or the concrete. Man's unique power of coping with "abstractions," "universals," "generalisations," has been associated with his endowment of speech. Geiger, a contemporary of Darwin's, was one of the most eloquent advocates of conceptual thought as a human perquisite. In his *Ursprung der Sprache,* he wrote:

> It is easy to see that blood is red and milk is white; but to abstract the redness of blood from the collective impression, to find the same no-

tion again in a red berry and, in spite of its other differences, to include under the same head the red berry and the red blood—or the white milk and the white snow—this is something altogether different. No animal does this, for *this, and this only, is thinking.*

Noiré enquired how man's power of abstraction came about. He attributed it to man's manual dexterity coupled with his ingenuity. More than any other creature, man has the power of selecting objects from his environment and then modifying them to suit his own purposes. Thus he became master of his environment. He learned to create things, and these creations were for him the first "things." Such "things" became endowed with independent existence, and from this point to the endowment of names for the things was quite an easy step.

Terminology readily misleads, however. We now believe that the older, narrow views upon the essentially human nature of conceptual thinking are not warranted by the facts. As Darwin showed, it is not possible to deny that in some animals, as judged by their behaviour, indications of a kind of abstract thinking can at times be traced. Although perhaps an exceptional state of affairs, it occurs often enough to cast doubts upon any notion of a Rubicon separating the brute beasts from man.

Let us recall the very beginnings of philology as a science, which can be said to date from 1772, when J. G. Herder wrote his essay on the *Origin of Language*. Herder rejected the doctrine that language was a divine creation and also the idea that it might be a willed invention on the part of men. Nor did he believe that the difference between man and animals was one of degree. He considered that there had taken place in man as he emerged from the subhuman state a development of all of his powers, in a totally different direction. This abrupt exploration led to the appearance of speech. Language sprang, of necessity, out of man's innermost nature. Herder likened the birth of language to the irresistible strivings of the mature embryo within the egg. In particular, man possessed a keener faculty of "attention" than any other animal, and he was thereby enabled to seize hold of isolated impressions from out of a mass of detail surrounding him. In this way man became able to identify the most arresting feature within his environment. For example, the distinguishing property of a lamb would be its vocalisation; that is, its bleating. Thereafter the lamb would be recollected, and referred to, as a "bleater." So, according to Herder, primitive nouns stemmed from verbs (as indeed we know to be the case in the sign-language of the deaf-and-dumb).

Perception and conception.

Herder's theory, couched in somewhat different terms by Noiré, reappeared a century later. And fifty-five years after that, contemporary animal psychologists state this theory anew. Professor E. S. Russell warned us not to assume that an animal's perceptual world would be like our own: on the contrary, judging from its behaviour, we must conclude that every animal has its own perceptual world, one which is very different from ours. Animals do not ordinarily perceive their environment in the same "articulated" fashion as we do. They perceive things only as ill-distinguished parts of a general complex. Isolated from its habitual context, an object may not be recognised for what it is. Animals respond only to perception-complexes and not to simple and solitary stimuli.

We have already referred to the philologist Max Müller as in many ways an antagonist of Darwin. This would be to do an injustice to both writers, for—as we have stated earlier—in 1861 we find Müller aligning Darwin with Epicurus. The latter believed that primitive man's uncouth instinctive ejaculations were fundamental in the origins of language. In addition, there must have been an important second stage, whereby agreement is made in associating certain words with certain conceptions. For the "agreement" of Epicurus, Müller would offer his doctrine of natural selection, or natural elimination. The phenomenon of the origin of language would then be visualised as follows: Sensuous impressions would produce a mental image or *perception;* a number of perceptions would bring about a general notion or *conception.* A number of sensuous impressions might also occasion a corresponding vocal expression—a cry, an interjection, or an imitation of the sound in question. A number of such vocal expressions might be merged with one general expression and leave behind the root as the sign belonging to a general notion. The gradual formation of roots and of natural cries or onomatopoeia is a product of rational control. Rational selection is natural selection, not only in nature but also in thought and language. "Not every random perception is raised to the dignity of a general notion, but only the constant recurring, the strongest, the most useful." Of the multitudinous general ideas, those and only those which are essential for carrying on the work of life survive and receive definite phonetic expression.

Symbolic Behaviour

Another way of looking upon the development of human speech out of animal vocalisations is to regard speech as the utilisation of symbols. The sounds emitted by animals are in the nature of signs, while man's speech is made up of symbols. Signs *indicate* things, while symbols *represent* them. Signs are announcers of events; symbols are reminders. In other words, symbols are not restricted to the confines of immediate time and place. As "substitute" signs, symbols can refer to things out of sight and outside present experience. When an ape utters a cry of hunger, it can be looked upon as perhaps making a declaration, perhaps an imperative utterance, or even an exclamation of discomfort. No ape, however, has ever uttered the word "banana," for such a word is a concrete symbol, a tool of thought which only man can employ, and he can do so in a variety of ways, irrespective of the barriers of time and space. Man can refer to a banana in past or future tense, as well as the present. Man can talk about a banana *in absentia.* No animal can do these things, the task being far beyond its system of thought and therefore of expression. Likewise no monkey can emit a word meaning "hunger," for this term would constitute, or refer to, an abstract or universal idea.

In Pavlovian modes of thought the use of symbols is regarded as a hallmark of man's cerebral function—although other terminologies are used. Pavlov taught that when the developing animal world reached the human stage, an extremely important addition came about, namely, the functioning of speech. This signified a new principle in cerebral activity. Sensations and ideas from the outer world constitute the first system of signals (concrete signals; signals of reality). Speech, however, constitutes a second set of signals—or "signals of signals." These make possible the formation of generalisations, which, in turn, constitute the higher type of thinking, specific for man.

Man's capacity for dealing with symbols rather than signs or things has been visualised by Korzybski as a specific "time-binding" faculty, peculiar to mankind. Pumphrey has described as many as three considerations which are attached to the human employment of verbal symbols as opposed to the sign-making cries of animals. These properties are (1) *detachment,* whereby man is able to use language to describe events in a wholly dispassionate fashion, if he should so desire; (2) *extensibility,* whereby a proposition can be made and discussed in terms of past, present, or future time; and (3) *economy,* whereby symbols enable man to abbreviate what would otherwise be a long-winded description or declaration.

Many writers view the origins of speech as merely part of a large developing faculty, namely, the beginnings of symbolic behaviour. As Sapir put it, language is primarily a vocal actualisation of the tendency to see reality symbolically, a property which renders it a fitting medium for communication. The problem, therefore, really resolves itself into a search for the earliest indications of symbolic behaviour, as the immediate precursor of speech. S. Langer believed that these beginnings of symbolic thought can be detected when an animal—the highest of the primates, in fact—behaves as if significance were being attached to certain objects or sounds. This attitude may be seen in the anthropoid in captivity, in its attachment toward some inanimate and favoured plaything—a piece of wood, a toy, a rag, or a pebble. Here, then, we are attempting to discern the dawn of symbolic thought; and here, too, we may perhaps descry the remote ancestry of human speech. In other words, the chimpanzee, although devoid of speech, begins to show a rudimentary capacity for speech—an opinion which reminds us of Müller's uneasy feeling that the gorilla is "behind us, close on our heels."

Some of the nineteenth century philosophers who were critical of Darwin, compared the appearance of language in man with the beginnings of religious belief. Certainly, at a very early date in man's emergence we find that there are indications of primitive magical practices, with evidences of ritual or ceremonial. It can safely be concluded that, at such a cultural level, primitive man was surely endowed with the faculty of speech. Noiré believed that the two aptitudes grew up in concert, the rise of mythology being an important and necessary stage in the development of language. This can be looked upon as a period when objects began to mark themselves off from the indefiniteness of the total perceptual processes and to form themselves into independent existence.

Emergence of Speech

The intriguing question naturally arises, at which point in the evolution of primitive man did speech, in the strictest sense of the word, first make its appearance? When did the ululations of the anthropoids give way to the use of verbal symbols, disciplined by phonetic and syntactical rules? Obviously, it is not possible—nor is it ever likely to be possible—to answer this question with confidence. The evidence, such as it is, is meagre, indirect, and oblique. But speculation on this interesting matter is quite permissible.

Anthropological data are of great importance here. They comprise arguments which are of a cultural order and which discriminate clearly between anthropoid and human communities. They also include the weighty evidence which lies within the domain of comparative anatomy. Here are to be found the impressive distinctions between ape and man in respect to the crania and the problems which arise from a study of the fossil skulls of man's immediate ancestors. Here, too, are marshaled the anatomical features in the crania which are to be regarded as specific for *Homo sapiens*. The size of the cranial cavity will naturally indicate brain-volume. This is an important point in that, ordinarily speaking, the human brain differs from anthropoid brain in its greater size, while the cranial capacity of prehistoric man occupies an intermediate position. But the rule is not invariable: one or two prehistoric specimens are characterised by megalencephaly. More valuable than sheer size is the question of the shape and proportions of the cranial cavity. In addition, the endocranial markings may be taken as a likely index of the convolutional pattern of the cerebral hemisphere. In assigning a fossil specimen to its evolutionary rank, the development of such specifically "human" areas of the brain as the frontal lobes and the parietal eminences are all-important. Obviously, clues such as these may be followed when discussing the problem of when in prehistory man developed speech.

L. S. Palmer, a dental surgeon as well as paleontologist, had approached the question of the development of speech in man from a somewhat unusual angle. He distinguished between human speech and animal noises, the for-

mer being regarded as being effected by delicate and voluntary variation in
the size and shape of the oral cavity. The power of articulation (as exemplified in human speech) depends upon a specific morphology of the jaws, and
here man differs in an important manner from the ape. In man the two
rami of the mandibles are splayed apart, whereas in apes they are parallel.
There results a difference in the shape of the posterior ends of the mandibles, together with an increased width between the condyles at the upper
ends of the rami. In man there is consequently ample space for the free
movement of the tongue, in this way facilitating articulate speech.

Another difference between the jaws of apes and men consists in the presence of a bony ledge connecting the anterior ends of the mandibles in apes.
This "simian shelf" serves as an attachment for the genioglossus muscles.
The range of lingual movement is rather restricted. In man, however, the
tongue muscles are attached to a series of small genial tubercles, which,
taking up but little room, permit freer movement of the tongue within a
broader intermandibular space.

Palmer also associated himself with L. A. White (*The Science of Culture*) and believed that there was an important connection in prehistory
between favourable climate factors and cultural acceleration, which naturally includes the origin of the faculty of speech. Palmer set out the chain
of causes as follows:

> A rigorous ameliorating climate → appropriate gene mutation → ex-
> pansion of the skull → development of brain → increased mental abil-
> ity → development of articulate speech and the introduction of written
> words.

Thus we can surmise with no little confidence that Cro-Magnon man
must surely have been endowed with speech, even though no firm evidence
exists that written language was ever in use at that period. The refinement
of the skeletal structure and the large cranial capacity point to a quite
highly evolved type of *Homo sapiens*. But the weightiest arguments are of a
cultural order. The skilful cave-paintings of the Aurignacian, Solutrean,
and Magdalenian periods obviously must have been the work of individuals
endowed with symbolic and conceptual thinking. The frequency with which
hand-prints occur on the cavern walls may also be taken as suggestive of individual personal awareness. Furthermore, the relative preponderance of
left hands over right at El Castillo (4 to 1) must indicate that cerebral
dominance obtained at that period. Perhaps, too, the appearance of obscure
linear markings—red blobs and dots—adjacent to these hand-prints may be
looked upon as the very first modest indications of written communication.
The fashioning of elaborate tools, the use of fire and of clothing, and the
evidence of ceremonial burials as well as religious or magical practices cannot be reconciled with a speechless state. Even the Negroid variant of Cro-

Magnon civilisation, known as the Grimaldi man, as well as the Eskimo-like Chancelate man, is no exception to these arguments. These fragmentary clues take the story of language back to the last Ice Age of late Paleolithic times, that is between 25,000 and 10,000 years B.C.

Can language be assumed in even earlier man? European *Homo neanderthalensis (or mousteriensis)* constitutes a less straightforward problem. Some anatomists were tempted to explain some of the contradictory characteristics of Neanderthal skulls by suggesting that they were out on a side line, away from the main stream of evolution. Thus the anthropoid characters of the supraciliary and occipital ridges, the massive jaw, and the wide orbits and nasal apertures contrast with the large cranial capacity, which actually exceeds that of average modern man. The African Neanderthaloids, including the *Homo rhodesiensis,* and the *Homo soloensis* of Java, present essentially the same problem.

A. Keith believed that the faculty of speech could be traced back as far as Neanderthal man, but no further. His evidence was wholly anatomical, and not very convincing. The left hemisphere was apparently more massive than the right, indicating cerebral dominance. Tilney also believed that Neanderthal man was "possessed of linguistic capabilities not far below the standard of *Homo sapiens.*" His conclusion was based upon the depth of the parietal fossae in the skulls, suggesting a well-developed "auditory area," i.e., the abutment of the parietal lobe upon the outer occipital and upper temporal lobes. This postero-inferior part of the parietal lobe is commonly regarded as a true and specific human perquisite. L. S. Palmer, however, was impressed by the poor temporal lobe development in the brain of Rhodesian man, and he doubted very much whether this specimen of Hominidae ever could speak.

Cultural evidence is more convincing than the morphological. The co-existence of eoliths in the way of sharpened flints and arrow-heads, and signs of the use of fire and the practices of cooking, all point to Neanderthal man's possessing a degree of conceptual and symbolic thinking consistent with the possession of language, just as in the case of Cro-Magnon man. If this argument is admitted, then the story of language can be taken back to about 50,000 years B.C., that is, to the post-Acheulian Paleolithic period, or the last glacial era.

Let us now turn to the early and middle Pleistocene periods. The hominid representatives of this time are exemplified by *Pithecanthropus pekinensis (erectus)* or *sinanthropus,* by *Homo heidelbergensis,* and perhaps also by *ternifine man.* Possibly, too, the Swanscombe and the Steinheim skulls belong here, though admittedly they may represent a transitional or intermediate type between *Pithecanthropus* and *Homo sapiens.* Later specimens within this same period include the skulls associated with Ehringsdorf, Fontéchevade, Florisbad, Krapina, and Mount Carmel.

According to Tilney, the left frontal area of the brain was larger than the

right, a fact which he was tempted to associate with a state of right-handed-
ness. The same author pointed out the development of the inferior frontal
convolutions, a feature which suggested to him that *Pithecanthropus* could
speak. He went on to assert: "Doubtless the linguistic attainments were extremely crude." It is difficult to comprehend exactly what Tilney implied by
this statement, for present-day linguistics has no knowledge of a language
system which can be designated as "extremely crude," even among the most
primitive and uncultured communities.

Upon other grounds, too, there is evidence that speech was an endowment
of *Pithecanthropus*. Implements of quartz have been found in the caves
alongside the human remains, obviously fabricated with some skill. There
is evidence also that *Pithecanthropus* knew how to produce fire and that at
times he produced cooking. Again it is almost useless to conjecture what
manner of speech was employed by *Pithecanthropus*. Oakley was merely
guessing when he surmised that the earliest mode of expression of ideas was
perhaps by gesticulation, mainly of mouth and hands, accompanied by cries
and grunts to attract attention.

By such suggestive paleontological clues, we can refer the faculty of
speech to a period at least as far back as 100,000 years B.C., that is, the middle Pleistocene period. On the evidence of the Javanese and Chinese skulls
(*P. soloensis* and *pekinensis*) the date might even be relegated as far back
as the early Pleistocene era, that is, perhaps 500,000 years B.C.

Few would venture to seek the pioneers of speech at any more remote
period. There arises for serious discussion, however, an interesting series of
fossil skulls found in South Africa, small in size and of an interesting
morphology. These are associated with an extinct series of pygmy man-apes,
originally called the fossil Taung's ape, but more often nowadays as *Australopithecus*. Where these specimens rightly belong is debatable; Le Gros
Clark regarded them as exceedingly primitive representatives of the family
which includes modern and extinct types of man. Leakey called them "near-
men." There is no sure evidence that such creatures fabricated tools; consequently, it is unlikely that the *Australopithecus* can be assigned to the genus
Homo faber vel sapiens and that it was capable of speech. The recent findings of a number of crude stone artifacts in proximity to the bones and the
associated fractured skulls of the fossil bones makes it possible that *Australopithecus* utilised stones as weapons, even though it did not, strictly speaking, manufacture weapons.

L. S. Palmer believed, however, that *Australopithecus* was perhaps endowed with speech. He based his opinion upon the anatomical characteristics of the mandible. The absence of a simian shelf and of diastema (or gap
between the incisor and the canine) and the convergence angle of the teeth
are all features which correspond with a hominoid morphological pattern.
Whether this type of argument is sufficient to militate against such argu-

ments as the small cranium and the lack of sure evidence of tool-making is very doubtful.

Recently it has been suggested that *Australopithecus* had the ability to make fire. If this is really the case, it should be taken as an additional piece of evidence to suggest that speech might have been within its capacity. Obviously, the answer to the question awaits the production of further findings.

The date of *Australopithecus* is remote indeed—probably beyond the earliest Pleistocene era and back into the end of the Pliocene. This means anything from one to fifteen million years B.C.

There is one aspect about the beginnings of speech in man which is only too often completely overlooked. Was speech a consistent endowment in the case of early man? When man first appeared on the earth in the middle and late Pleistocene periods, perhaps only some of the newly evolved *Homo sapiens* were endowed with speech. Speech in those remote times might have constituted an exceptional phenomenon or aptitude, one which was within the competency of only a few highly favoured individuals.

In the case of hand-skills, too, maybe only comparatively few members of *Pithecanthropus* were able to fashion arrow-heads or flints, this expertise being a rare and no doubt highly accorded accomplishment. Then again, skill in handicrafts might perhaps have correlated closely with the faculty of speech. Such especially gifted members of the community probably also had an expectation of life above the average, and therefore speech and the art of tool-making may well have had considerable survival value.

Evolution and the Origin of Language

On rereading these remarks, it appears that perhaps insufficient attention has been paid to the difficulties inherent in a purely Darwinian conception of the origin of language.

It was implicit in this particular hypothesis as to evolution that differences between human and animal structure and function are matters of degree. Were this principle to be firmly established, then it would be difficult to avoid the idea that animal communication leads by insensible gradations to the faculty of speech in man. There are numerous linguistic objections to this view, however. It is important to realise, too, that language does not stand alone in this matter and that there are other weighty considerations which lead to the well-nigh inescapable conclusion that some potent qualitative change occurs at a point somewhere between the anthropoid and *Homo sapiens*.

Animals, at best, may possess a limited store of vocal sounds. These are innate, instinctive, or "natural." Under appropriate circumstances, internal or external, they are emitted. They may happen to possess communicative action in respect to other animals mainly of the same species. It is doubtful, however, whether these cries are always communicative in intent. In ordinary circumstances the adolescent animal does not increase its vocabulary of sounds, except that in one or two strictly delimited circumstances the vocal repertoire may be extended. Thus some animals in states of domestication may amplify their stock of cries and calls. Other animals, particularly certain birds, may elaborate their performance by means of imitation. In this way the innate and instinctive bird song or call is overlaid by learning from other birds, not necessarily of the same species. Finally, certain animals, particularly a small group of birds and a few higher apes in captivity, may be taught to mimic human articulate speech, the specific cries of quadrupeds, or even inanimate noises.

The foregoing recounts the sum-total of achievement in the domain of animal sounds. Between these and human articulate speech lies a very considerable gulf. Even in the case of the most untutored, primitive, and savage human communities the language-system is so far removed in its complexity from the crude and simple utterances of the sagest of the primates as to be scarcely comparable. And nowhere and at no time has there been any hint of an approximation between these two extremes. No "missing link" between animal and human communication has yet been identified.

Can it be, therefore, that a veritable Rubicon does exist between animals and man after all, as Professor Müller insisted when discussing the origins of language? Has a new factor been abruptly introduced into the evolutionary stream at some point between the Hominoidea and the Hominidae, constituting a true "barrier"? Can it be that Darwin was in error when he regarded the differences between man and animals as differences merely in degree?

The lessons gained from comparative linguistics would certainly suggest that there are serious differences "in kind" which interpose themselves at a late stage in evolution. We have been told that the contrasting of differences in kind and in degree is in itself an out-moded attitude. However that may be—and such argument is not easy to follow—it is tempting to doubt whether anything like a smooth gradation has occurred. Outside the domain of language there are other human endowments which are not readily traced in the animal series. As such, they scarcely pertain to our present subject-matter, unless it can be shown that their very existence depends upon the presence of a language system. Here, for example, may be placed the advent in man of what we might loosely term the various "moral faculties." Darwin was not oblivious of this problem, and he believed that a moral sense had been evolved from prehuman ancestors. This aspect of evolution was not mediated by a process of natural selection, however, but it arose from man's newly acquired power of reasoning. So then it is a mechanism of evolution additional to the ordinary natural selection. When early man became endowed with reason and when to that mental accomplishment was added the power of speech, then the way lay open for the operation of conscious purpose or a psychosocial factor. In this way there develops— again indirectly out of the beginnings of language—the beginnings of choice as to conduct. This also implies the power of doing harm as well as the power of doing good. So arise ethical and altruistic considerations. The earlier stages of these aspects of behaviour can be visualised in the animal kingdom in the instinct of maternal solicitude. This instinct is restricted— be it noted—in both time and place. With the achievement of adulthood, the young animal no longer receives maternal solicitude. The instinct, too, is limited to the immediate family group. Altruism extends from beyond the family circle to the clan only with the attainment of human status; and thence, with the growth of social conscience, it expands to embrace the tribe and eventually the nation. This act of stepping outside the strict family circle may doubtless be assisted—if not mediated—by the faculty of language

Reprinted from Critchley, M. (1960) : *Evolution after Darwin*. University of Chicago Press, Chicago.

Lingua Adamica Restituta, or the Future of Language[*]

> *It is unfortunate to find that psychologists have done so little with artificial languages. Language engineers have demonstrated the enormous possibilities that exist and the practical consequences that research can have. As international cooperation becomes more and more of a problem, the need for such information becomes increasingly clear. The reasons why so little has been done are probably the magnitude of the job and the fact that several disciplines must cooperate to carry it off successfully. If cooperative research continues to increase in popularity, perhaps the future will see an increased interest in the business of creating new languages for special purposes.*
>
> G. A. Miller, 1951

The distinction of being a Rickman Godlee Lecturer is one which I appreciate with pride. We are assembled to honour a great surgeon, cultivated and revered. He was born in 1849 at No. 5 Queen Square, a house which I have long coveted, for I have passed and re-passed it day after day for nearly fifty years. In this very house two decades later resided Hughlings Jackson, whose predictive concepts of brain function led directly to that bold gesture of Rickman Godlee when he removed at operation a cerebral tumour. This surgical pioneering took place on November 25, 1884.

Rickman Godlee was a man of parts, and his many talents included a flair for language and an interest in linguistics. I venture to hope that our Patron would have found it not unimportant to project one's imagination and to speculate upon the possible future of our systems of communication.

A century ago the Académie Francaise proscribed all argument about the beginnings of language, but the mandate at no time extended across the Channel. Today, our concern is with the mutability of communicative systems, and we will deal with the dynamic rather than the static properties of language. But while looking forward, we cannot avoid some brief reference to the origins of speech. Are the differences between the communication of the highest primates and that of the lowliest representatives of *homo sapiens* qualitative or quantitative? Currently we favour the former hypothesis. "Species-specific" is the habitual jargon in this connection. Lan-

---

[*] The Rickman Godlee Lecture for 1970.

guage—unlike the calls and cries of the animal kingdom—is a human and sensitive endowment, which is vulnerable to brain pathology. Unfortunately, we are never likely to know at which stage in phylogeny rudimentary language came into being. The evidence is not weighty enough and probably never will be, although we can continue to piece together such tenuous clues as the size of the cranium, the shape of the mandible, artifacts indicating toolmaking as well as tool using, and such skills as kindling fire. Certainly the Aurignacian culture with its wall paintings and hand imprints must have embraced a system of verbal symbols.

It is still in doubt whether the art of language was the perquisite of every adult member of a particular genus. Perhaps in those remote days it was confined to merely a few especially gifted individuals who, by dint of some intellectual or sensorimotor skill, had a better survival rate and a greater fertility.

We need not discuss the various notions of the eighteenth and nineteenth centuries as to the origin of language, however interesting and even amusing this would be. Many speculative ideas were bandied about speech as the elaboration of gesture, speech as the audible concomitant of vigorous physical effort, speech as onomatopoeia emerging from the mimicry of animal cries or of sounds in nature, speech as evolving from the dance, speech as a correlation between delicate linguobuccal motor skills and symbolic thinking, or even speech as a dissociation between sound production and deglutition.

More serious discussion devolved around the question of monogenesis versus polygenesis. Did language begin in one geographical *locus* and in spreading undergo modifications according to accepted rules of linguistic change? Or did pockets of communicative endeavour crop up quite independently here and there throughout the world? The latter idea seems more credible, for anthropologists know well that vast linguistic differences often exist in the speech of undeveloped tribes which dwell in close proximity. The lack of linguistic correspondence may be so extreme as to rule out any simple process of dialectical drift.

In contrast to such materialistic notions there has long existed what we might term the "divine" theory of the origin of language. Theologians taught that after man's creation there was only one language, and this remained in use until the Tower of Babel was shattered. This *lingua adamica* was commonly, though not universally, correlated with Hebrew.

Over the past two centuries a study of contrastive linguistics has shown that there is no such entity as a "primitive" language. However lowly in the socioeconomic scale, however unsophisticated and poorly developed the community, the speech employed is anything but simple. On the contrary, indeed, Sapir well said, "The lowliest South African bushman speaks in the forms of a rich symbolic system that is in essence perfectly comparable to the speech of the cultivated Frenchman." Twenty-one years later Langer said much the same: "People who have not invented textiles, who live under roofs of pleated branches, need no privacy and mind no filth and roast their enemies for dinner, will yet converse over their bestial feasts in a tongue as grammatical as Greek and as fluent as French."

In the grammar, including accidence and syntax, as well as in the semantics of underprivileged peoples, there may be features foreign to the tongues of sophisticates. These represent one extremity of a spectrum of trends. Hallmarks of progress, according to Bonfante, may be enumerated: (1) loss of the dual number in nouns, pronouns, and verbs; (2) creation of the definite and indefinite articles; (3) loss or weakening of the verbal aspects and the introduction of tenses within the verbal system; (4) creation of a passive tense in the verb; (5) elimination of gender, or irregular forms, and of nominal and verbal flexion; (6) transition from a synthetic to an analytic type of grammar; (7) a trend from certain sounds, or systems of sounds, to others; (8) progressive shortening of words, especially through loss of the endings; and (9) increase of abstraction in the lexical sense.

Gabelentz had earlier spoken of a spiral sequence in linguistic change comprising isolation, agglutination, and flexion.

A study of the written and spoken speech of highly developed communities demonstrates how many shortcomings are, unfortunately, attached to verbal symbols. Words are inadequate tools of thought, being anything but precise in meaning, sense, connotation, significance, or reference function. Every term possesses its overtones, so that even the most banal and concrete substantive—"book," for example—implies something slightly different to different persons and, at different times, even to the same person.

At no time is it possible to convey the entire content of one's thought merely by resort to words, for every statement entails an undertext which is not expressed. Some terms are frankly ambiguous, especially when taken out of context. Clarification is aided by recourse to redundancy, pleonasm, or tautology, but, even so, the message remains incompletely encoded. There is always a risk of entropy. The import of words may change over the centuries. On occasions words are expressly used to cloak the content of thought. This device may pass muster in ordinary social intercourse, but actually no experienced psycholinguist is likely to be deceived, for, as Pittenger said, "Within every utterance, however imperfect, there lies a meaning which can be neither disguised nor concealed." Then again, an arrest in speech flow may be used deliberately as a tool in communication, for silence—especially when occurring as a willed contrivance—is only too often meaningful indeed. "Communicative behaviour is continual," as Smith and Trager wrote, "and motionless silence is a special kind of communicative art." Truly within every utterance however sparse, and indeed within every silent pause, there dwells a meaning which can be neither completely disguised nor hidden.

Flaws in verbal communication are often responsible for misunderstanding among ordinary people in everyday usage. This applies even more to the interpretation of the sacrosanct. If we were all sharing completely an identical code, then Holy Writ would cease to be the battleground of warring sects. Attorneys would be halved in number, for those who draft our laws would no longer need to keep a watchful eye on putative loopholers among their own profession. Perhaps even political parties would disappear.

Loose terminology merges into allusive or evocative speech. Sometimes this is a contrived linguistic trick, as when employed by an esoteric clique or cabal. Allusive speech is met with in the "little language" of lovers, as intimate as the bed. J. H. Burns was shrewd when he proclaimed that if everyone in the world were in love there would be as many "little languages" as there are people on the globe, divided by two. Speech of this type also constitutes the bedrock of poetry—the "arresting communication of an arresting perception of beauty." Here the factual content matters less than the ideas it kindles, and through evocative words endowed with qualities of euphony mere reference function is submerged.

Every language holds its complement of "loaded" words which make up the sinister weapons of propaganda. Archbishop Trench spoke of that very solemn and very awful something in the wielding of an instrument like language with such power to wound or to heal, to kill or to make alive. Earlier, Hume had referred to the malefic potency of words in *Weltpolitik*, declaring "Tis not Reason that gains the prize, but eloquence. . . . The victory is not gained by the men at arms who manage the pike and sword; but by the trumpets, drummers, and musicians of the Army."

Drawbacks such as these—vagueness, imprecision, allusiveness—coupled with the arts of deliberate misuse as well as willed silence entail yet another handicap. I refer to the exceeding difficulty, if not impossibility, of rendering a faithful translation from one language to another. To quote the Archbishop again, "language is the amber in which a thousand precious or subtle thoughts have been safely embedded and preserved." How true, but in a linguistic context no two pieces of amber are identical. A given term in one language may possess tenuous or fragile overtones which do not apply to the synonym or homoseme in another language. To transmute a word from one tongue to another is to condone a "compound fracture of an idea," as has been said. A sentence may rate as a polite statement in one language but as a crude, cold, or even coarse assertion in another. What is meant to be humorous may fall completely flat when translated. Every language has its little stock of subtle words which baffle an interpreter.

With etymologically related languages, such divergencies may be few. But in attempts to translate an Indo-European tongue into one which lacks the familiar subject-predicate structure, or vice versa, opportunities for misunderstanding increase. To reduce these sources of potential error, and incidentally to ease the linguistic burden of the parties, trade languages or contact vernaculars accrued. Here is perhaps the first and simplest instance of deliberate linguistic manipulation. Traders and mariners were the pioneer language engineers of history. A contact vernacular represents an amalgam of reduced vocabulary of the visitor's tongue with a simplified grammar of the indigenous language. Thus we have the pidgin English of the seaports of New Guinea and of China; the fanagolo of Zambia; the *petit nègre* of Senegal; *bêche-la-mer;* sandalwood English, Dutch, Portuguese, and French; and the posh-and-posh of Gypsy folk. When in subsequent generations pidgin speech becomes a first language, it constitutes Creole, as in the Jamaican and Haitian vernaculars, Krio, Papiamento, neo-Melanesian, and Macanese.

Still later, Creole slowly changes to a standard or full-sized language. For a time two variants exist side by side to bring about an interesting transition from a transnational language to a purely national one, at first creolised, later conventionalised. Thus, Jamaican Creole merges into the Queen's English, and Sranan into standard Dutch.

Communication of ideas, including those which are scientific, humanistic, and political, clamours increasingly for some medium of expression which all may employ. Eventually the consequences of the destruction of Babel must be replaced by some programme of linguistic rebuilding. A precise yardstick is improbable, but something better than mutual unintelligibility can, and must, be found.

Over the past few centuries various attempts have been made to achieve comprehensibility on an international scale. Chaucer emphasised how a dead language served to keep common folk in ignorance. Latin was demoted by the Royal Society in 1662 as its scientific medium in favour of the language of the artisans, countrymen, and merchants. Thirty years later the Académie des Sciences agreed to employ French. When Latin ceased to be the common communicative system of the educated, various other suggestions were put forward to establish an a posteriori world language. Something was said in support of Yiddish, for at one time it was spoken by eleven million people. It remained essentially the *mame-loshen* or matriarchal tongue, to distinguish it from the *loschen-na-kodesh* or sacred language, and also the Sephardic vernaculars—Ladino, Judesmo, or Judaeo-Spanish. But Yiddish apart, most of these attempts at universal comprehensibility have been Pan-European, or rather Pan-Occidental, if not indeed Pan-Romance, according to Guérard.

The pioneer essay at constructing an a priori world language was in the nature of pasigraphy or an interracial sign talk. The first was devised by a schoolmaster in Guernsey, George Dalgarno, who in 1661 published his *Ars signorum.* He dedicated the book to Charles II ". . . which must have been as great a mystery to the sovereign as to his subjects." Seven years later came the monograph of John Wilkins, Bishop of Chester, entitled, *An Essay Towards a Real Character and a Philosophical Language.* Aubrey described this work as the Bishop's "darling," saying that "nothing troubled him so much when he dyed, as that he had not compleated it." Shortly beforehand there had appeared the *Way of Light,* written by the Moravian scholar Comenius (who had been invited to London by Samuel Hartlib) , as well as the ideas put forward by Cyprian Kinner for a philosophical language.

Best known among the purely verbal systems is Dr. Zamenhof's Esperanto with its numerous offshoots. Earlier, the Volapük of the Abbé Schleyer had come and gone in dramatic style. Other examples include Interlingua, which had a brief heyday in the medical journalism of America. But many others have passed across the scene. In fact, there are 200 systems, some a priori, others a posteriori. Solresol had an interesting claim. Based upon seven fundamentals, it could be transmitted along nonverbal channels— music, song, bells, flags, rockets—and it was available to the blind as well as to deaf-mutes. One of the latest systems is Hogben's Interglossa, a strictly isolating language with a rigid word order, its vocabulary being largely of Greek origin marked by a severe word economy.

As imperialism gave way to the contemporary economic colonialism, English began its strong bid to constitute a world language. The multilinguistic structure of Africa, and the 225 languages of India, have virtually ordained the use of English as a medium of intercommunication, outstripping the whilom claims of Spanish, Dutch, Portuguese, Chinese, Arabic, and Russian. Long ago, Richard Burton foresaw English as the future cosmopolitan language of commerce, stating that it emulates Chinese in being largely an uninflected communicative code which should be made monosyllabic.

English has various merits over many Afro-Asian tongues, for it has dispensed with the grammatical shackles of concord, and it is virtually free from the semantic limitations of a tonal language. Furthermore, English fulfills the four conditions laid down by Guérard. These comprise (1) impersonality—being no one man's invention but rather a discovery stumbled upon by a considerable group; (2) conservatism, which does not rule out progressive improvement; (3) creativity—or "open-endedness" as Chomsky might say—whereby indefinite growth is possible; and (4) an impressive cultural background.

The story of language engineering or language design has been embellished by a number of talented eccentrics within the discipline of linguistics.

One of the best-known was the Polish-American, Count Korzybski (1879–1950) , who, tilting against what he chose to dub Aristotelian habits of thought, founded the pseudoscience of "general semantics." Undeterred by any undue modesty, he described his monograph *Science and Sanity* as the third member of an immortal trilogy, ranking alongside Aristotle's *Organon,* and Bacon's *Novum Organum.* A local manufacturer of lavatory fitments persuaded the University of Chicago to endow an Institute of General Semantics on Korzybski's behalf. Most of his ideas were just provocative, but some were of potential merit. He stressed that a contrast between concretisation and abstraction cannot take place unless one resorts to some process of "indexing," "dating," or "labelling" a substantive. This could be done by attaching to a noun a numeral or a time marker. Thus the differences between an apple on a tree and one at the greengrocers or one in a fruit bowl could be highlighted by some such device as $Apple_1$, $Apple_2$, $Apple_3$, and so on. Or, the overtones which develop with the passage of time could be emphasised by referring to $Mother_{1950}$ as opposed to $Mother_{1960}$ or $Mother_{1970}$.

Unfortunately, Korzybski's useful ideas were overlaid by a superstructure of confused mythoneurology which invoked contrasting roles in articulate speech ascribable to the cortex and the thalamus, with such odd notions as "semantic pauses" and "neuro-semantic relaxation." Korzybski differentiated a state of insanity from one of "unsanity." In the latter, the personal map of reality is out of correspondence with the real world; in the former it is the inner world which is askew. But as Gardner well said, "Where the Count was sound he was unoriginal. And where he was original, there are good reasons for thinking him 'unsane.'"

C. K. Ogden (1889–1957) has been described as "one of those enigmatic figures who pass strangely across the pages of history." A gay, intense, witty, violent oddity of the thirties, he is still remembered as the coauthor of that classic monograph *The Meaning of Meaning*. But that is not all. Anything but. He established a new discipline which he termed "orthology"; founded the *Cambridge Magazine;* and instituted the "Heretics"—a forum of uninhibited debate. As a compulsive smoker he paid the price for his addiction with his life. His career gave the lie to the belief that skill in billiards is evidence of a misspent youth. A "debabelisationalist," as he called himself, he is perhaps most closely associated with his creation "Basic English." Comprising a mere 850 words, it was capable—so he thought—of constituting a second, or auxiliary, world language. So impressed was the wartime Prime Minister that Ogden was afforded a governmental grant of £80,000. Despite this prize, Ogden described himself in *Who's Who* as "1944–1946 . . . bedevilled by officials." One wonders, by the way, whether Churchill— had he known—would have approved the basic rendition of his clarion call as "blood, work, eye-water and face-water." Basic English, far from leading to brevity, proved to be prolix and clumsy. For example, the sentence "He has sprained his wrist" would read in Basic English "He has given a twist to the join of his hand and arm." Its ingrained inability to match the crisp elegance and the concision of standard English led to its death from neglect complicated by derision.

Putting aside these attempts to achieve communication across raciolinguistic frontiers, we may consider the alterations which have taken place and which are presently taking place in our current codes. For obvious reasons we shall confine our remarks to the English language. Students of literature are familiar with the change in connotation of certain terms which has been going on over the centuries. Here we deal with a fixed vocabulary, with deviating reference function. The differences which have grown up between received English and the English of North America and of Australia chiefly entail accretions to the vocabulary. Can one project one's ideas and predict what will be the nature of the English language as spoken and written centuries hence? If we are to look beyond the mere pattern of linguistic drift, this may be difficult, for at some future date the English language may come under the influence of planned language engineering. Natural processes may then become elaborated by the deliberate recommendations of a committee which may seek to mould our vocabulary and our syntax.

Here at least two considerations will arise: tampering with the spoken speech of the community, and changes in the printed modalities. The former may be less malleable to committee work, while the latter, although more susceptible to planned design, has a more precarious vitality.

A forward-looking publisher like Temple Smith has voiced the common anxiety as to where the trend toward audiovisual replacements of printed books will take us. We are already passing through a phase of comic strips, "coffee-table" albums, and closed-circuit instruction. Will literacy ever become an anachronism and will education revert to an electronic form of didactics, with reading material relegated to the museum? Temple Smith is not wholly pessimistic. He believes that 500 years hence libraries will be bigger; that instant bibliographies will be computerised and displayed, but that the books themselves will look remarkably like those we read today. Be that as it may, we are perilously near the time when printed instruction is being overtaken by increasing resort to audiovisual media, a hark-back to pre-Renaissance oral methods of learning. McLuhan contrasts the linear or time-binding approach to reality brought about by current bookish pedagogy with fast approaching, simultaneous, or mosaic form of understanding. Unless some unexpected reversal in teaching trends appears, the time may come when the arts of reading and writing will once again be within the competency of only a specialist minority. This bookish élite of the future will then represent the philosopher-scientist or monastic scholar of the Middle Ages.

In this context we may ask ourselves two questions. What will the situation be not fifty years hence but a millennium? And in that era what kind of printed matter will constitute those so-called books?

Apart from English, we may well witness a shedding of those systems of lettering which do not conform with the conventional "monkish" or Romano-European script, that is, the modern variants of the Latin alphabet. Within the past two generations, we have observed the decline of Gothic lettering in printed and written German, and also the passing of Arabic style in Turkish texts. In China there is a movement to adopt the West

European manner of writing. Arabic, Hindi, Sinhalese, and many other languages are still disadvantageously placed, and so to a lesser extent are the Greek and Cyrillic alphabets. No less a patriot than Lenin once proclaimed to a Pan-Soviet Linguistic Congress that the great evolution of the East would lie in a process of romanisation of Russian typology.

We come next to the question of debabelisation. For the purpose of international communication, will an already existing tongue be adopted and no doubt adapted? Or will some wholly artificial system be devised?

In the latter event certain prerequisites must be met. A Latin vocabulary with a Chinese grammar has been suggested, but this is not nearly enough. An artificial world language will need to dispense altogether with grammar and with tonal encumbrances. It must entail a relatively meagre stock of verbal units. A large audience and a large vocabulary are irreconcilable. To ensure comprehension, messages will depend on redundancy rather than prolixity.

How simple in structure a possible world language can be was shown by Troubetskoy. Fourteen phonemes are enough, instead of the forty-six used in standard English. Words should end in a vowel, or a vowel with a terminal /n/. In this way a vocabulary of over 10,000 mono- or disyllabic words is possible.

The idea of contrived synthetic tongues is, however, not an attractive one. They have been scorned as sickly parasites on other languages. Critics in plenty have protested. Max Beerbohm shrank from any kind of horrible universal lingo begotten on Volapük by a congress of the world's worst pedants. Even Esperanto, the most popular example, though tolerated at various times "from good nature or from weariness" as Jagger said, is largely the endeavour of addlepated amateurs, supported by the adherence of the amiable, uncritical acquiescence of others. Bryden called it mechanical, flavourless, untailored to our personal experience, rather like sex talk.

The alternative is to select from the languages of the world one which is more or less acceptable to the majority. This would be more reasonable. Apart from dialects and patois, there are well over 3,000 languages to choose from. In this connection English has currently the strongest claim as an auxiliary system of communication, not merely because English is the easiest second tongue available to the largest number of persons. Even in its present unmodified form, English has many natural advantages: brevity, conciseness, and comparative freedom from the trammels of grammar.

There is nothing novel about this idea. Gil's *Logonomia Anglica* pleaded for such a state of affairs in 1619. A century later, Swift toyed with the notion. Jacob Grimm, the early nineteenth-century German philologist, agreed. Still later, we find strong advocacy from H. G. Wells, Hugh Harrison, and Hubert Jagger.

But this universal adoption will be the product of no convention or commission. There would be an approved gradualness rather than a revolution in the corridors of communication. These changes will not be ordained; they will just happen, stealing upon us step by step as Guérard said, so that by degrees English will become the Latin of democracy. We can, therefore, envisage a time when nearly everyone will have at his command two media: first, his mother tongue, and then, a simplified and painless form of English which will constitute the auxiliary and universal *lingua adamica restituta*.

If such deliberate bilingualism should ever become the goal of a majority of thinking persons, some revolution will be needed in learning techniques. The drudgery of the unfortunate schoolboy who struggles to achieve Greek and Latin A-levels must disappear. Changes will surely come about in the pedagogic systems whereby bilingualism is acquired. Eventually there will develop a scientific understanding of the modus operandi whereby a very young child picks up his mother-tongue so painlessly and so efficiently. This is the case whether the language concerned is as simple as Farsi or as elaborate as Arabic; whether it be Hawaiian or Hopi, Malayan or Japanese, Italian or Finnish. In the foreseeable future we will possess the key to the riddle so as to apply it to the early and easy acquisition of auxiliary tongues. Only too often we take for granted the veritable miracle whereby a child at a very early age can achieve mastery of one or two tongues in an effortless fashion. How often do we pause to consider—and to utilise—the magnitude of this learning process, especially when contrasted with the laborious attainment of another language in later life through conventional techniques in the classroom? There is nothing novel in this juxtaposition of ideas. Many years ago Jesperson asked, "How does it happen that children in general learn their mother-tongue so well? That this is a problem becomes clear when we contrast a child's first acquisition of its mother-tongue, with the later acquisition of any foreign tongue. The contrast is indeed striking and manifold: *here* we have quite a little child, without experience or prepossessions; *there,* a bigger child, or it may be a grown-up person with all sorts of knowledge and powers: *here,* a haphazard method of procedure; *there,* the whole task laid out in a system (for even in the schoolbooks that do not follow the old grammatical systems, there is a certain definite order of progress from the more elementary to more difficult matter) ; *here* no professional teachers, but chance parents, brothers and sisters, nursery maids and play-mates; *there* teachers trained for many years specially to teach languages; *here* only oral instruction; *there* not only *that,* but reading-books, dictionaries, and other assistance. And yet *this* is the result: *here* complete and exact command of a language as a native speaks it, however stupid the children; *there,* in most cases, even with people otherwise highly gifted, a defective and inexact command of language."

We shall not always be in the dark as to how this marvel comes about, and we shall be able to apply the techniques to adults coping with foreign tongues. Mastery of the international auxiliary language should come early, however. Already Chomsky is thinking that a child possesses inherent knowledge of the universal principles governing the structure of human language. These principles, comparable with the "innate ideas" of Descartes, are in turn activities of the brain and depend upon intactness of cerebral function. Reibel has said that a child acquiring speech operates like a miniature language-learning machine. The child employs artifices like paying heed to what he hears, imitating the sounds, and making up combinations of new words from things already heard and copied. He might have added the ludic activities, whereby a child plays with words like a toy, coining words, reduplicating them, inventing rhymes and jingles. A child is never impeded by fears of making errors in syntax; he is quite unembarrassed. This direct method of language learning could also be studiously adopted by the adult. Language is an important aspect of the total personality, and the adult who has two or more languages is endowed with two or more personalities, and to achieve mastery he must be prepared to adopt as many disguises as Proteus the actor. This is a game which presents no task to a child.

Unless my foreboding as to an ultimate extinction of the printed word is fulfilled, techniques of instruction in reading will need to be severely overhauled and put on a firm scientific basis. The present-day struggle with the problems of dyslexia and reading retardation have fortunately given a great impetus in this direction.

To ensure an acceptable degree of precision, in the structure of this English "cosmoglotta," certain changes must come about. Many would advocate a consistent and logical form of spelling, though there are the many arguments against such a trend. English grammar, simple though it be, must become still easier. Jagger enumerated some of the grammatical forms which might well be shed, for example, the "to" of the infinitive; suffixes which denote comparison in adjectives; the inflective possessive case; all irregular plurals, anomalous verb forms, and many pronomial inconsistencies. In making deliberate syntactical changes such as these, it would be imperative—or so Chomsky asserted—not to violate the transformational grammar made up of the general principles which undertake the sentence construction of all natural languages.

The luxuriant vocabulary of standard English will have to be sacrificed —but only for pragmatic, cosmoglottal, or international usage. Mere condensation along the lines of Orwell's "New Speak" will not suffice. Apart from a deliberate economy, some indulgence in verbal coinage will be needed, partly to correct current ambiguities, partly to assure creative vitality. To dispel equivocacy, novel terms will come into use, some of which might well be borrowed from the tongues of primitive peoples. Without unduly burdening our available vocabulary, we might take cognisance of those unsophisticated races which use distinct words to describe subtle changes of meaning in such ideas as to throw vigorously, to throw feebly, and to throw with a jerk. Enough is enough, however. The verb structure of the Navaho language excels in nicety, elaborateness, and precision, but it would be madness to attempt to emulate it for international use. However, a few expressions in current English are so indefinite as to warrant a change. "Aunt," "uncle," "grandparent," "cousin," and "child" are indeterminate, and require generic clarification. Our pronouns cry out for drastic overhaul. When the sense demands, male and female terms should be combined in a common-sex pronoun. Thus, the possessive "his" in "every man and woman will get his fair share" will have to go. It should be possible to distinguish between inclusive and exclusive forms—"you" (singular) and "you" (plural) ; "you" meaning "both of you," and "you all"; "we" (including you), and "we" (with you excepted). The "and/or" of slipshod commercialese merits a respectable term in its own right. The English use of "thank you" (meaning "yes") should be supplemented by another phrase to indicate "thank you" (meaning "no") as in France.

The demerits of word coinage of this sort will be more than offset by the renunciation of many of the near synonyms peculiar to the opulence of the English language, but the surrender will be only in the context of transworld communication.

In many contemporary languages there are conspicuous differences between the spoken and written varieties. This schism, which is easily demonstrated today even in our own English tongue, is one which is likely to expand with the passage of time. Such a dichotomy will widen all the more with the increasing neglect of the arts of reading and writing which I envisage.

I have already mentioned the probable replacement of alternative forms of printing by the universal use of Romano-European lettering. The change will almost certainly go very much further. Even the common typologies of Western Europe may change, so that no longer will the schoolboy wrestle with a diversity of founts and cases. One day the type of printed books may adhere to a uniform design, and a compromise may be hit upon with cursive. Learning problems will be mitigated for those who seek mastery over printed symbols, even though such students might constitute only a pedantic minority. This standardised typology might well incorporate some of the paralinguistic tricks devised by Korzybski, and by Bell and Wheeler in their challenging "Interscript."

All that I have said applies solely to English in its role as a medium of international communication. I have been describing the English of the technical journal and the symposium, the politician and the trader, the courier and the cosmopolite. This will rank as the common currency of science and of medicine. But beside it, beyond it, and above it there will— let us hope—remain inviolate the richness and the grandeur of our literary heritage; the English of poetry, fine writing, and belles lettres, as elastic, dynamic, allusive, evocative, euphonious, and glorious as ever. In referring to this possible diglossia of the future, Rumdle has contrasted the cold, factual, scientific, and economic vocabulary of the auxiliary tongue with the warm, unreasoning, emotional, self-expressive, cultural language which we will continue to use in literary, homely, and artistic pursuits.

Reprinted from Critchley, M. (1971): *Perspectives in Biology*. University of Chicago Press, Chicago.

The Neurology of Psychotic Speech

Speech has been called a socioeconomic device for saving effort in the attainment of objectives. One of its earliest and most fundamental purposes is to orientate the individual within the community. This socialising effect operates early in childhood, and in a phylogenetic sense it was perhaps one of the greatest factors in the origin of speech in primitive man. As maturity is slowly achieved in the individual as in the genus, the use of language becomes inextricably interwoven within the warp and woof of the organism, as exemplified not only by thinking processes, but also by the complicated structure of personality. The development of speech during the pre-hominoid stage synchronises with the gradual elaboration of communal life; with cries and calls serving as a "sound-tool"; and with the beginnings of delegation of labour. Thus language is primarily a vocal actualisation of the tendency to see reality symbolically. The same is true ontogenetically. As the child gradually acquires speech, the organisation of his thinking slowly changes; it evolves by intricate steps from egocentric to socialised activity; and as he begins more and more to employ pronouns of the second and third person, he also utters fewer "action words". We readily agree with Fillmore Sanford who stated that "there are many indications that language is a vehicle of personality as well as of thought, for when a person speaks, he tells us not only about the world, but also, through both form and content, about himself". The same author quoted Ben Jonson: "Language most showeth a man; speak that I may see thee."

Linguists go deeper and, from a study of man's various preferences, glossaries, and verbal habits, conclude that the choice and use of language is a highly individual accomplishment. This idea underlies Krechel's conception of *Spracherlebnis,* i.e. the personal or specific manner in which we experience and understand words. Each of us possesses his own private idiolect—a specificity which might permit the identification of authorship if only linguistic techniques were adequate. Whether these personal traits reveal themselves better in one's natural spontaneous diction, as stated by Klages or in one's polished, studied, and much corrected fine writing, is a matter of opinion. The link between language and personality may be even more fundamental, for, according to the Whorf-Sapir hypothesis, the structure of a particular language is no accidental morphology, but bears some relationship with the mode of thinking, the prejudices, and beliefs of the racial stock which uses that particular tongue.

Deviations of the inner mental life consequently betray themselves in an unorthodox use of language. Any considerable aberration of thought or of personality will be mirrored in the various levels of articulate speech— phonetic, phonemic, semantic, syntactic, and pragmatic. In written language too, defects may be obvious, and being set out in a medium which is more permanent than the spoken word, lends itself better to linguistic analysis.

The effects of crude lesions of the dominant hemisphere within the area of speech-vulnerability are well known. Here we have the dysphasias, in all their clinical diversity. The subtle, complex, and less consistent deviations of speech which may be met with in many cases of dementia and of schizophrenia, and in some hysterics, also merit attention. The problem, as I have discovered, is an enormous one, and what one might term the neurology of psychotic speech forms a veritable *terra incognita,* a lush and unplotted jungle terrain.

Up to now this difficult topic has been approached from two main directions: the descriptive and the psychopathological. Scarcely any work has been done from the standpoint of linguistics. Aphasiological approaches have also been rare, perhaps because they may have been felt to be unrewarding.

In submitting the various psychotic patterns to aphasiological analysis, we are likely to find striking differences between the phenomena of disturbed language as they show themselves in dements and as they occur in schizophrenes. That is true enough, but there is probably also a certain amount of overlap, at least as far as some of the more superficial features are concerned.

Speech Disorders in Dementia

Let us first direct our attention to the dementias—conditions which imply mental derangement of organic nature. Here the correspondences and analogies with the dysphasias of local brain disease are likely to prove more germane than in most other psychoses.

In dementia, speech impairment essentially entails a poverty of speech due to inaccessibility of those different vocabularies which ordinarily we can utilise and which we may term the speaking vocabulary, the writing vocabulary, and the reading vocabulary. These terms refer respectively to the stock of words which we are in the habit of employing in conversation; to the larger one we draw on in written compositions; and to that even greater depository which also includes terms we recognise but rarely venture to use. With advancing mental inelasticity, bradyphrenia, and memory-loss, the words utilised by the demented patient become severely restricted in conversation and to a somewhat lesser extent in letter writing. But the premorbid reading vocabulary suffers far less. This fact we indeed make use of in our psychometric assessment of intellectual falling-off.

The difficulty in word-finding differs, however, from the anomia of aphasiacs. The demented patient does not necessarily show any hesitancy in putting a name to an object presented to him, even though a faulty use of proper names is common enough. Paraphasic errors in naming do not occur, nor yet neologisms, substitutions, or portmanteau words. Neither does the patient seek to by-pass the elusive term by means of elaborate circumlocutions, as is so common with aphasiacs. But on the other hand the demented patient finds it difficult to retail a series of representatives of a generic class. For example it might be impossible for him to reel off the names of flowers, animals, vegetables, wines, or foodstuffs, unless the specimens lie before him. His halting efforts may at times betray a serious lapse into a bald and concrete attitude, and the names he proffers may turn out to have some special connotation which has facilitated their emission. Thus, asked to give a list of girls' names, a dement may painfully and slowly produce two or three examples, which, on enquiry, turn out to be the names of some who dwell in close association, such as his wife, or daughter, or grand-daughter.

Thus there grows up a taciturn retardation which the patient is reluctant to break through. Prompted by direct enquiry he may reply relevantly enough, but with an economy of diction which is almost telegrammatic. Here indeed is something akin to aphasic poverty of speech. The fragmentary utterances of the dement are capable of linguistic analysis. First of all, the content or semantic values of the speech are altered. Various classifications have been advanced to describe the normal state of affairs. The commonest grouping is into utterances which are (1) declarative; (2) interrogatory; (3) exclamatory; and (4) imperative. It can be demonstrated that the dement—like the aphasiac—rarely embarks upon declarations or propositions, unless to draw attention to some strident bodily need, e.g. hunger, thirst, or a full bladder. Even here the demented patient is in a graver plight than the aphasiac. On the other hand, in their truncated utterances both aphasiacs and dements will resort to exclamations and demands, prompted by egocentric drives. Again, the aphasiac is less handicapped than the dement in this respect.

Another semantic classification of normal utterance speaks of "mands" and "tacts"; or using another terminology, transitive as opposed to intransitive utterances. Mands or transitive speech include requests and questions; tacts, or intransitive speech, comprise comments, statements, and animadversions. Applying this terminology to the dementias, we can say that tacts are rare, for mands constitute the bulk of the meagre pronouncements of the patient.

Another linguist, A. S. Diamond, has divided utterances into (1) requests for action (or commands) ; (2) the statement; and (3) the descriptive-statement. Analysing the content of spontaneous speech in dementia, we can say that only the first of these classes survives.

It is possible to study still closer the fragmentary sayings and writings of demented patients, especially from a statistico-linguistic angle. Thus an estimation of the token/type ratio may prove revealing—and may demonstrate mathematically the poverty of the available vocabulary, and the great tendency towards verbal iterations, perseverations, and contamination. The same techniques are naturally applicable in aphasia, and the results are qualitatively the same, but perhaps more striking in cases of dementia.

Then again there is the verb/adjective ratio which may be found to deviate considerably from the normal pattern, and to show a change as in aphasia. Balken and Masserman reported an upset in this ratio in the speech of neurotics. Again, in the spontaneous writings of dementias such syntactical properties as sentence-length and differential punctuation counts lend themselves to exact analysis.

As Allison described, a patient with early dementia may preserve a façade of normalcy for quite a long time, by resort to a chatter of small talk. As time goes by, his repertoire of things to say becomes more limited and more stereotyped . . . "more laced with clichés and set phrases". Premorbid sequential habits of speech may come to the surface more and more. Later the subject remains taciturn unless directly addressed. This social seclusion —be it noted—does not embarrass or perturb the patient.

There are two other verbal peculiarities which the dement may share with the aphasiac. In the course of conversation he will often resort to the grammatical trick of aposiopesis, whereby a sentence is started but not finished. Again, he often resorts to vague generic terms to avoid a search for the appropriate noun or proper name. Hence there loom prominently such expressions as "things", "what's its name", "thingumybob", "what d'you me call it".

In more artificial and elenctic interviews where the discourse takes the form of question and answer, there may appear deviations from the normal which are far more subtle. Thus the patient may be able to answer well enough ordinary simple questions of a wholly concrete character. But if an enquiry is made which entails notions of a more abstract character, the patient may be at a loss. Typically however he is not distressed thereby. Sometimes the patient interpolates little comments which—though not wholly beside the point—are a trifle unexpected. For example, when shown a watch and asked what it is, the patient may reply to the effect that it is a timepiece—and then go on to say quite unasked for . . . "and a very fine specimen too if I may say so sir". This is the phenomenon of "gratuitous paralogism". Again the patient's replies as to the identity of an object before him may be unorthodox in a different way. What he says cannot be written off as entirely incorrect, but the patient gives a pseudo-description which is inadequate, unlikely, and often prolix. This is the phenomenon of "regressive metonymy", first described by Mrs. Petrie in the case of leucotomised patients. In some ways it reminds one of the *Vorbeireden* met with in the Ganser syndrome. I have reason to believe that this may represent the earliest stage of a sensory- or jargon-aphasia.

Phenomena of a perseveratory character are often met with both in the spoken and in the written speech, and bear witness to the underlying ideational inertia. In the early stages of a dementia this shows itself in the spontaneous letter-writing, whereby a term—perhaps a slightly uncommon one—is introduced into the text quite congruously, but thereafter keeps cropping up in a wholly inappropriate fashion. Aphasiologists speak of this verbal peculiarity as "contamination" for it is familiar enough with local lesions of the brain. Still more striking is the reiteration of common words in the text, some of the errors being detected by the patient and elided, but not all of them. Even more bizarre, and outside the experience in aphasia, is a massive type of echographia which may show itself by a reply to a letter which constitutes an almost word-for-word transcription. Such a phenomenon is unlikely to come to light in ordinary everyday experience, but only in business houses where letters and copies of replies are filed and preserved. An astonishing example is reproduced, taken from the case of a young man with juvenile G.P.I. whose letter to his mother was an almost faithful reproduction of hers to him.

Mother's letter:
   Dear Ern, Just a line in answer to your most kind and welcome letter I received from you and pleased to know you are better than you were and that you will try to steady your nerves for to be home quicker. I am longing to see you as you are to see me Ern but its far better to get well now as you are in the best place for it, but cheer up you won't be long now. Its nice to know you can join in all the sports and get about Ern. Thelma Parry's husband came home this week after four years a prisoner of war. They were all excited in the street. Well, Ern, I had a letter this week from Dave and he told me he had a letter from you. Olive is still home. She did not go to Weston after and Muriel is up at Mervyns home this three weeks. She is coming home next Monday with Mervyn he will be on leave then. I don't know what she intends doing after shes gone back. Well, Ern, Mr. Humphreys and Muriel asks how you are and I told him what the doctor said and he told me to tell you to put your mind and getting well to come home on leave and he also said you promised to write to him when you went back the last time you was home. Well, Ern, I will be sending some more cigs and some bake-scones that is if you would like some later on in the week.

Patient's reply:
   To my dear Mother, Just thank in answer to your most kind and welcome letter I received from you pleased to know you. Pleased I am to

know you are better than you were that will try dry steady your nerves for to be home quicker. I am longing to see you as you are to see Ern, but its far better to get well now as you are in the best place for it. Just cheer up you won't be long now its nice to know you can join now in all the sports get about. Ern Thelma Parry husband came home this week after four years a prisoner of war they were all excited in the street. Well Ern I had a letter this week from Dave he told me he had a letter from me. Olive is still she didn't go to Weston after. Muriel is up at Mervyns home this three ask she is coming home next Monday she will be on leave know what she intends doing after she gone know he gone back. Well Ern Mr. Humphrey tell you to put your mind getting well do come home on leave he also said you promised to write to him when you went back the last time you was home. Well Ern I will be sending some more cigs some bakesdonie that is the week.

Echolalia is a phenomenon common to mental defect, schizophrenia, dementia, and aphasia, in that order of frequency of occurrence. Echolalia or echo-reaction suggests a psychopathological complex which includes a defective recall of verbal symbols, coupled with extreme suggestibility, identification with the interlocutor, lack of insight, an impulse to maintain social contact in the way of speech, and loss of supralinguistic inhibition.

Finally there are the verbal mannerisms in the speech (and less often in the writings) of patients with dementia. They are perhaps more often found in cases of Pick's disease or Alzheimer's disease, than in simple non-specific brain atrophy. Still more are they met with in the late secondary dementia which may follow a life-long mental defect, or a chronic schizophrenia. Such mannerisms are capable of a linguistic division:

(a) *Phonetic.* This type of peculiarity is illustrated in such features as an unduly high pitch of the verbalisation.

(b) *Phonemic.** Several examples might be quoted. A patient in his diction may interpolate an *s* or less often a *t* sound in a frequent but quite unwarranted style. The final silent "e" of the English tongue may be sounded as /ə/ in a somewhat affected manner. Thus "wine" would be rendered as *wajnə*. Such a patient may also break down all diphthongs into their constituent vocalic phonemes. In such patients "soup" would be pronounced as *sow + əp* and not *suwp*.

(c) *Prosodic.* Here the duration of a certain syllable (or word) may be overslow, being extended to an inordinate decree while at the same time a very strong stress is laid upon that particular unit of speech.

(d) *Verbal.* Here certain words or groups of words are emitted in a tic-

---

* One cannot resist drawing attention to the disturbing and idiosyncratic use of the word "phoneme" by some psychiatrists. To students of language "phoneme" is something in the nature of a sacred cow of respected lineage. If not precisely defined, it is at least employed with due consistency. Psychiatrists should really devote themselves to the quest for some other means of indicating *phantasms* of the auditory nerve.

like or compulsive fashion wholly out of context, and not necessarily in response to a bystander.

In this connection we recall the recurrent utterance of some aphasiacs who have available for communicative purposes only one word or phrase—maybe a piece of jibberish. But the functional role, namely that of communication—meagre though it be—distinguishes the recurrent utterance of the aphasiac from the verbigeration of the dement.

On the receptive side of speech, the conversation of others may not be entirely understood, especially if the semantic content is elaborate; or if the diction is unduly fast, or soft in volume; or if the message is masked by "noise", e.g. the rivalry of other people talking nearby. Written and printed texts may not be comprehended to the full, especially if obscure, or elusive or allusive in character. These receptive disorders are no different from what obtains in aphasia, but it can be said that whilst so-called sensory aphasiacs may have a clear or almost clear sensorium, a demented patient with a comparable amount of receptive defect would probably be clouded as to his mentation, disorientated, and severely bradyphrenic.

In the demented, communicative disorders often transcend the use of speech, and may embrace gestural systems. There may be a severe restriction of what has been called the kinesics of an individual, comprising thereby mimicry, mime, gesture, and gesticulation. To such a state of total incommunicado the term "asemasia" was applied many years ago.

"Dysphasia or Dyslogia?"

Another remark is needed as to terminology. We are still seeking a term to indicate disorders of language in cases of global dementia—i.e. in the absence of focal disease of the brain. The term "aphasia" implies to most medical men a state of communicative defect which is by definition, though not explicitly so, the expression of localised disease within the so-called speech centre. In the opinion of many it would not be correct to apply this term to cases of dementia, unless of course the dementia happens to be an epiphenomenon of local disease of the brain. Even the terms "latent aphasia", or "generalised aphasic difficulty" are not beyond criticism. "Non-aphasic speech-impairment" is too clumsy and not self-explanatory. "Pseudo-aphasia" might do; or alternatively "alogia" or "dyslogia", were it not that these last two terms have been sequestrated by Kleist in quite another context.

Attempts have been made to isolate specific linguistic patterns among the demential speech-disorders according to aetiology and pathology. Allison, for example, distinguished sharply between dementia due to global lesions, and dementia due to focal disease (tumour, cerebrovascular accidents). Pichot separated the epileptic and the arteriopathic groups from the senile varieties, and said that subclinical but nevertheless definite language-impairment may be found in the first two types. He applied the term "latent aphasia" here and implicated a particular involvement of the temporal lobes in cases of arteriosclerosis and of epilepsy.

Whether it is of value to form such linguistic subgroups within the phenomena of demential speech impairment is, I submit, dubious. To a neurologist, it is perhaps the mixed clinical pictures which occasion the greatest difficulties in assessment. Two examples may be given. In the first place we may visualise a life-long mental defective who, in his sixties, acquires a lesion of the dominant hemisphere—traumatic perhaps, or ischaemic, or neoplastic. The ensuing picture of dysphasia is likely to be highly unconventional, and difficult to disentangle—particularly if no focal signs of neurological involvement happen to co-exist. The other type of case which is apt to cause diagnostic perplexity concerns patients who have sustained a non-progressive aphasia-producing lesion of the brain (e.g., apoplectic or traumatic) and thereafter begin to develop a superadded steadily advancing brain-atrophy. Or both types of clinical complexity may co-exist. One such case was under my care at the National Hospital, referred from Friern Hospital through the kindness of Dr. Hunter.

A middle-aged institutionalised patient has been known as a life-long eccentric, moody, hypochondriacal, anti-social, a prey to bouts of heavy drinking. At 55 years he suffered a fractured skull from a road accident which produced a right-sided weakness, sensory impairment, and visual field defect, together with a serious and persisting dysphasia. Seen 5 years later the patient was found to have deteriorated intellectually and his speech was larded with an assortment of reiterated phrases of a type and purpose not typical of a simple organic defect. For example his speech was restricted to a small repertoire of recurrent utterances, chief among which were "I ain't got none", "just one", "that's one", "that's one, guv", and—oddly enough—"brown pots run". The patient would wander round the ward, picking up things from other men's bed-tables and lockers, and constantly tidying the coverlets, etc. He seemed to have a compulsive urge towards helping himself to cigarettes. Air-studies revealed gross brain atrophy much more marked in the region of the left temporal lobe. This case might be deemed to represent the picture of a dysphasia combined with a dyslogia.

Speech Disorders in Schizophrenia

If, from an aphasiological point of view, the principal problem of speech impairment in the dementias is one of terminology, the difficulties with schizophrenic speech disorder are far greater.

Very tentatively Rümke and Nijam ventured the query whether the neologisms, confused speech, and disturbed inter-human relationship found in schizophrenics could be reduced to an aphasia. "Might the secret of schizophrenia"—they asked—"lie in a hitherto unknown high-level aphasic disturbance?"

Unlike what obtains in aphasia and in dementia, there is no true inaccessibility of vocabulary. The linguistic *quantum* is probably intact, but the utilisation thereof may be gravely disordered. Resemblances there may be at times between the diction or writings of a schizophrenic and those of an aphasiac, but they must not be overstressed, and analogy must not be promoted to the level of a hypothesis. It is true, of course, that at one time some continental neuro-psychiatrists like Schneider, Fleischacker, Angyal, and Regner were tempted to visualise a linguistic pathophysiology and even a morbid anatomy as an explanation of the aphasia-like states in schizophrenes. Kleist, for example, speculated that there might be cortico-subcortical changes to account for the speech-impairment and he even attributed some of the iterative and perseveratory phenomena to lesions within the basal ganglia. These notions never received credence and rightly so: Kleist in his neurological thinking had always been a deviationist, a heretic, and a materialist. The terms schizophasia and schizographia—though misleading tokens of disordered physiology—may not be wholly unacceptable, for they are convenient descriptive labels, which might be employed even more widely than Kraepelin and Teulié originally suggested.

The briefest description of the diverse schizophrenic speech disorders as a group is to look upon them as a travesty of communication. The message breaks down, and ceases to constitute a conveyer of reference-function. This in turn is the product of the patient's gradual withdrawal from the community. Despite certain superficial likenesses, the situation is basically quite other than what produces speech-impairment in aphasia. The patient with aphasia fails in his communicative intent by virtue of an inaccessibility, if not indeed a loss, of verbal symbols in thought. In schizophrenia the thinking processes themselves are deranged but the verbal symbols are intact and available. The one represents a quantitative and the other a qualitative defect in endophasy, or inner speech. This fundamental pre-linguistic distinction explains why the clinical features vary in the two conditions.

The autism of the schizophrenic may be well shown in the frequency with which pronouns of the first person crop up in his speech and writings. In one letter of 1,241 words a schizophrenic girl used the pronoun "I" 87 times, and this easily ranked as the most frequent term. The runners-up were the articles "the" and "a" which appeared 43 and 33 times respectively. The pronoun "my" also occurred 33 times and "me" 20 times. By contrast we found "you" occurring 11 times, "your" 3, "we" 3, "him" 3, "he" once, and "his" once. This count gave the incidence of "I" as 6.2% (total pronouns of the first person = 11.2%). Fairbank it may be remembered found that "I" constituted 8.4% of the spoken speech of schizophrenics, the figures being 5% in the telephone talk of ordinary people; 3.1% in the diction of college freshmen explaining proverbs; and 1.2% in commonplace written texts. In technical publications the incidence was zero.

This heightened incidence of the first person singular is never encountered in cases of aphasia in speech or in writing.

In aphasia there may be an extreme reduction of spoken and written speech, perhaps to the extent of a single recurring phrase, perhaps to a mere "yes" or "no". Absolute mutism however does not occur, while in the schizophrene there may be a total speechlessness. The schizophrene though often displaying a verbal iteration does not struggle to emit a "yes" and eventually come out with a "no" to his utter distress. Nor will the schizophrene eke out his attenuated vocabulary by a play of gesture. In other words he is not striving to communicate in the face of overwhelming difficulties.

Indeed between the aphasiac and the schizophrenic we observe interesting differences in the total communicative set. The former is an anxious person who may be very aware of his defect (unless he be a jargon-aphasiac) and who strives and strains to achieve mutual comprehension, betraying all the evidences of frustration when he fails. In vain he marshalls every adventitious aid to intelligibility. The schizophrene, by contrast, may be aloof or negativistic. He may display "advertance" by turning away from the one who seeks to converse with him. His voice may be hushed as if secretive, or artificial as in the so-called strangled speech ("Wügstimme").

The similarities between schizophrenia and aphasia are less easy to distinguish when neologisms and jargon speech are concerned. The logor-rhoeic schizophrene may emit a word-salad which apparently carries but little reference-function. Schneider has identified the processes of fusion, derailment, omission, and what he called "drivelling" making up a bizarre combination of telescoped ideas, word-monstrosities, echo-responses, irrelevancies, incoherences, nonsense words, and scattered verbal statements.

The neologisms of an aphasiac however are determined in part by a weakening of supra-linguistic inhibition or vigilance which permits a too free verbal association to exteriorise a medley of synonyms, antonyms, paraphonemic, metaphorical, and metonymous substitutions, and telescoping of words. There is another important factor present which probably does not apply to schizophrenics. The sensory aphasiac has little or no self-criticism for he is largely unaware of the disordered nature of his utterance. Hence the term anosognosic aphasia which is often applied. Moreover he may hotly deny that his speech is disordered and may project the defect of communication on to the stupidity of others. Again there may well be some acoustic perceptual defect like an audiometric scotoma, though this is rejected by some. Luria considered that there is an underlying tendency on the speaker's part to confuse phonemes of somewhat similar sound, e.g. the voiced /z/, /d/, /δ/ with the unvoiced /s/, /t/, /θ/. In other words an essential paraphonemia is hypothesised—a defect peculiar to paraphasia and outside the picture of schizophasia.

This is hardly the place to discuss the asyndetic thinking of schizophrenics in so far as it is responsible for the aberrations in verbal utterance. In any case this would require detailed discussion indeed. Enough has been said to show that the underlying mental mechanisms are quite different in schizophrenics and in aphasiacs, even though the verbal utterances are often similar.

The analogies of disturbed speech in psychotics and in aphasiacs may be carried over into their writings. One striking difference may be made at the outset: aphasiacs are usually very reluctant to write, while schizophrenics often have a veritable *cacoëthes scribendi*. Consequently, genuine spontaneous writings are rare in the case of aphasiacs, though of course they may do their best to perform when directly instructed to do so by the physician.

Another difference between the psychotic and the aphasiac lies in the layout of the text upon the page. The schizophrenic likes to embellish his penmanship with ornate flourishes and elaborate capitals. He often writes vertically in the margins as well as along the lines. The page is barely large enough to contain all that he wishes to impart. Drawings may be inserted within the body of the text, not so much as illustrations, as extensions of what the patient wishes to express.

None of these peculiarities is to be seen in the painful attempts at letter-writing made by the aphasiac. He clearly has a poverty of expression and contents himself with a few lines—either in the centre of the page or huddled along one edge. The verbal disorders of some schizophrenics may be strikingly dissociated as between speech and writing. Either may be severely disturbed, but in complete isolation. This is a phenomenon not met with in aphasia.

Iterations of Verbal and Written Speech

One obvious point of similarity, however, lies in the repetitiousness of the text in both conditions, as opposed to the ordinary verbal diversification of the normal subject. Words, phrases, and word-clusters tend to crop up over and over again, often quite incongruously. The aphasiac sometimes detects his error and makes erasures—but often not. Even when he makes corrections he usually overlooks the bulk of his repetitions.

Those written compositions, whether from aphasiacs or from schizophrenics, are invaluable data for linguistic analysis, being permanent records. They lack, however, the ephemeral paralinguistic overtones which are of such importance in human communication, but which defy transcription.

If, for example, contrasting texts are reproduced—not in their original script, but transcribed into conventional print—some of these linguistically significant features become evident.

The first three letters are written by aphasiacs, and the other two—much longer—are the work of schizophrenic patients.

(1)

21 Westbury Park.

Dear Miss Alice Day,
   My begin with the bing with with with the the old doing into [with] into into [into] with with [with] [with] will [will] with the oldest [older] the oldest the the oldest with the oldest the [the] the oldest.

Yours sincerely,
Maggie Brown.

[N.B. Words in brackets were elided by the patient]

(2)

Thank you ~~very~~ for very ~~yes~~ forget loss lastly forgetful ~~forget~~ to us.
And I should very ~~ve~~ much for your getting to your gratefulness.
I am I singful very grateful rightful and ~~forget~~ forgetful for your gettleftfed, forgetful forgetful and forgetful.

(3)

Dear Doctor
   (Dear) I requirte it the took, I got not why ask when why then, I when you, my shall my you small my, why send sned say, send what why I when (when) I received her (she) she has have a cold, so let recusf the result. I have a resuft takes be to take hate from for from far.
   What change (cal) can (for) for you. What can I for me. All your the for the porter. Tell you your you ponten you will you go.

The foregoing examples differ strikingly in size. The first patient is struggling hard to communicate, but under such difficulties that the message she wishes to impart does not come through. Some but not all of the contaminating words are crossed out—more of them are unnoticed by the patient.

Here are the two instances of letter-writing by schizophrenes:

(4)

. . . . I like Titbits weekly. I like Titbits weekly too. I should like Titbits ordered weekly. I need jam, golden syrup or treacle, sugar. I fancy ham sandwiches and pork pies. Cook me a pork pie and I fancy sausage rools I want ham sandwiches. I want tomatoes and pickles and salt and sandwiches of corn beef and sandwiches of milk loaf and cucumber sandwiches. I want plain biscuits buttered, rusks, and cheese biscuits I want bread and cheese. I want Swiss roll and plain cake, I want pastries, jam tarts. I should like some of your pie you have for second course, some pastry. I want biscuits, fancy biscuits and fancy cakes. I want sweets, bull-seyes or cloves. I want rissols. I want rissols. I fancy fruit, do bring some oranges, apples, bananas, pears. Do brong some fruit, I get dry, oranges. I got tea for all next week from March 10th Sunday, all the week till Sunday March 17th. I shall want more tea Sunday, March 17th, the following week after March 17th Sunday. I want sugar I want jam, golden-syrup or treacle. I like plum jam. I like butter. It would be a treat. We only get margarine. I would like some butter. Bring some butter. I would kile a pot of cream from the dairy and some cherries with the cream. A pot of cream with cherries. Cream with cherries. I like chocolate roll with cream inside. Some nice cake Dundee cake and plain cake. I fancy tomatoes and sause, with bread and butter and salt. I like jam puffs and doe nuts. I like seedy cake, coco nut cake cocoanut cake. I want jam tarts, pastries I fancy pastries, bamberys I want a piece of rubber, a piece of India rubber. I like macaronis. I like macaroni's, macaroni's, pastry, a piece of rubber for my writing letters. Come soon, every week. Send Leslie this Sunday to visit me. Bring another lb. of tea soon, Leslie bring tea and sugar I want sugar and jam. Jam. Soon get me home by Easter I hope. Soon may I come home to you At Easter by my nirthday I hope to be home. I hope to be home soon, very soon. I like chocolate eclairs, I fancy chocolate eclairs. chocolate eclairs. Doe-nuts. I want doenuts. I do want some golden syrup a tin of golden syrup or treacle, jam. I fancy very much some fruit, oranges, apples, bananas. I want fancy cakes, ҡ̶ѻ̶ҫ̶ќ̶ cakes rock cakes, bread pudding jam tarts, doenuts chocolate-eclairs, I would like a pot of honey. I would like some sandwiches of real butter. Ginger bread I like ginger biscuits fancy biscuits ginger breads. I want. I would like sandwiches of milk loaf and real butter Soon get me home from the hospital want you, See the Committee about me coming home for Easter, my twenty fourth birthday. I trust you will have me home, very soon. I hope all is well at home, how is Father getting on. Never mind, there is hope, heaven will come, time heals all wounds, Rise again Glorious Greece and come The Hindoo Heavens, The Indian Heavens The Dear old times will come back. We shall see Heaven and Glory yet, come ever-lasting life and God. I want a new writing pad of note paper. . . .

(5)

. . . . Now to eat if one cannot other one can—and if we cant the girseau Q.C. Washpots prizebloom capacities—turning out—replaced by the head patterns my own capacities—I was not very kind to them. Q.C. Washpots under-patterned against—bred to pattern. Animal se-questration capacities and animal sequestired capacities under leash—and animal secretions. Q.C. Washpots capacities leash back to her—in

the train from Llanfairfechan army barracks wishe us goodbye in Llan-
dudno station and turned in several Q.C. Washpots capacities. . . .

The first of the schizophrenic patients expresses well enough her simple
wants and feelings but the manner in which this is done betrays the underlying thought disorder, mild though it be. The second example—which too
is merely a fragment of a very much longer text—displays not only an
echographia but the incoherencies, apparent irrelevancies, and bizarre
choice of words, which could emanate only from the pen of a schizophrenic.

All these specimens are capable of linguistic analysis (see Tables 1–3).

The samples given are too small, and the scatter of results too wide, for
any conclusions to be drawn. The data are offered merely to show the possi-

TABLE 1. *Type/token ratio in writings by aphasiacs
schizophrenes, Hemingway and Dr. S. Johnson*

Subject		Total number of words "Tokens"	Number of different words "Types"	Type/token ratio "T.T.R."
Aphasiac	(1)	39	11	0.28
	(2)	42	21	0.50
	(3)	89	45	0.50
Schizophrene	(1)	1,241	331	0.26
Schizophrene	(2)	79	52	0.65
Hemingway		167	51	0.30
Dr. S. Johnson	(1)	168	90	0.53
	(2)	127	80	0.65
	(3)	266	170	0.64
	(4)	298	185	0.62

TABLE 2. *Carroll's index of diversification*

Subject		Number of words from one "the" to the next
Aphasiac	(1)	4, 14, 2, 1, 2, 1
	(3)	40, 28, 1, 10+
Schizophrene	(1)	3, 16, 6, 16, 11, 39, 10, 5, 19
	(2)	8, 52+
Hemingway		18, 40, 57, 5, 18+
Dr. S. Johnson (letter no. 846)		6, 43, 26, 40, 2, 9, 7, 26, 20, 4, 53, 37+

Average = 10–15 in normal written speech.

TABLE 3. *Verb/adjective ratio*

Subject		Verb/adjective ratio
Aphasiac	(1)	0.25
	(2)	0.41
	(3)	11.0
Schizophrenic	(1)	3.5
Schizophrenic	(2)	1.0
Hemingway		8.5
Dr. S. Johnson		2.0

bility of linguistic analysis of the writings of aphasic and psychotic patients which, carried out on a bigger scale, might yield interesting results.

Neoteric Literature

Before leaving the subject of schizophrenic writing we can scarcely refrain from referring to something which is, on the face of it at least, analogous. I refer to the unorthodoxies of obscure and reiterative writing as a deliberate art form. Taking first the latter aspect, we readily find in *avant-garde* literature a studied paligraphia which defies traditional syntax. The following example, taken from a well-acclaimed novel, illustrates my point.

This that they were not to have, they were having. They were having now and before and always and now and now and now. Oh now, now, the only now, and above all now, and there is no other now but thou now and now is thy prophet. Now and for ever now. Come now, now, for there is no now but now. Yes, Now. Now, please now, only now, not anything else only this now, and where are you and where am I and where is the other one, and not why, not ever why, only this now; and on and always please then always now, always now, for now always one now; and on and always please then always now, always now, for now always one now, one, going now, rising now, sailing now, leaving now, wheeling now, soaring now, away now, all the way now, all of all the way now; one and one is one, is one, is one, is still one, is still one. . . .

Similar instances are common enough in Joyce and more especially so in Gertrude Stein. Here is an extreme example from post-war French concrete verse, a poem by Louis Aragon.

	Persienne	Persienne	Persienne
	Persienne	Persienne	Persienne
Persienne	Persienne	Persienne	Persienne
Persienne	Persienne	Persienne	Persienne
Persienne	Persienne		
	Persienne	Persienne	Persienne
	Persienne?		

As to obscure writing we need not go further than the existentialist prose of Picasso.

25th March XXXVI
　　Think evening Angelus to see you shattered in the glittering mirror-splintering to the blow of a clog blowpipe to see you nailed upon the quivering pond which stands out and rolls itself up in a pill unfasten the hung naked body of the loved one of the festoon of months remove your hand your hands.

As instances of contemporary verse may I select two poems (by Dylan Thomas) almost at random.

> Sir Morrow at his sponge
> (The wound records)
> The nurse of giants by the cut sea basin
> (Fog by his spring
> Soaks up the sewing tides) .
> Tells you and you, my masters, as his strange
> Man morrow blows through food.

Where does this type of writing belong in the history of literature? Let us quote the interpretation made by David Aivaz, a contemporary professional critic.

> The transition from image to image is by means of the pun, the double meaning, the coined word, the composite word, the noun-verb, the pronoun with a double antecedant. And there is a larger machinery, verbal and syntactical: clauses that read both forward and backward; uneven images that are smoothed by incantatory rhythms, rhymes, word-patterns, verse-forms, by the use of commas in place of full-stop punctuation; cant, slang terms and formal, general abstract wording juxtaposed in image after image, so that the agitation of each becomes the repose of the group.

What does this mean? The words are metalinguistic, but the sense is not. Could the paragraph perhaps be paraphrased using the grammar of psychopathology? Thus a psychiatrist might well be tempted to speak of telescoping of ideas, agrammatism, klang-associations, idiosignificant and obscure allusions. These are perhaps another way of expressing the same opinions. We are even reminded of Schneider's four-fold mechanisms of schizophrenic speech—fusion, derailment, omission, and drivelling. And also of Piro's four fundamentals of psychotic speech, namely: semantic distortion, semantic dispersion, semantic dissolution, and enlargement of the semantic halo whereby meaning is extended like Alice in Wonderland, and language becomes ambiguous, vague, and indeterminate.

Let us examine the other example of Dylan Thomas' verse:

> If my head hurts a hair's foot
> Pack back the downed bone. If the unpricked ball
>   of my breath
> Bump on a spout let the bubbles jump out.

Here let us quote the opinions of two contrasting critics, the one laudatory, the other sceptical. According to William York Tindall writing on this poem . . . "Occasion, theme, and feeling are of less interest than method. We are familiar with the process of conflicting images and with quarrels among words from incompatible areas. But here . . . are advances in rhythm and sound. Excellently sprung . . . the lines unsystematically display all the devices of Welsh sound: alliteration, assonance, dissonance, internal rhyme, and chiming vowels . . . Thomas was learning moreover that sentences need not begin with the beginning of a line or end with its ending. Beginning within the line has rhythmic importance. . . ."

To Henry Treece, however, this same poem seems to be a *verbal compulsion,* almost a psychopathic phenomenon, musical-rhythmic automation, with a possibly unconscious sexual reference thrown in to emphasise the primitive source of the word-group.

The same writer has boldly grasped the nettle by posing—and trying to answer—the question, ". . . is Dylan a fake?" Treece wrote: "I feel that Dylan Thomas is extremely (and unconsciously) ill-balanced; yet, in the unbalance, lies much of his charm. . . . His choking verbalisms, his fixations on certain threadbare or obscure epithets, his inability to resist inorganic alliterations, his wilful obscurity, his deafness to certain obviously poor rhymes, his preponderating rhythmic monotony, his careless use of words, the overstress or understress created by his rhetorical mechanisms, the overemphasized pathos and arrogance, the self-pity, the lack of humour, the poverty of historic background (reflected in his self-sufficiency) , all these are evidence, and to spare, of a lack of maturity. But, unless such unbalance is known to the poet, it is less than just that he should be called a forger, and his works fakes."

Perhaps in conclusion we can indicate two points where schizophrenic writing differs from much of this type of poetry. The one is clinical and compulsive: the other is compulsive too, but it may also at times prove lucrative. One is uninhibited and sincere, while the other may be redeemed by its much contrived euphony. Psychotic writing may or may not have been intended to be read: the other was written not only to be read but also to be declaimed.

This provocative subject could perhaps be clarified by a careful textual study of the works of poets who are well known to have been psychotic, as for example the pre- and post-morbid verse of the Swedish schizophrene Frøding.

Summary

The complicated field of language-disorder in psychotic patients forms an intriguing topic for aphasiological study, especially when linguistic techniques of research are employed.

Demented patients are liable to show a progressive poverty of speech, which may be overlaid by true dysphasic manifestations when the brain-atrophy happens also to involve the mid third of the dominant hemisphere to a significant degree. Terminology offers certain difficulties, and it is suggested that the language impairment in cases of dementia should be spoken of as "dyslogia" rather than dysphasia. Unusual phonemic and other verbal mannerisms may also occur at times in patients whose dementia is associated with a previously existing state of mental defect or schizophrenia.

The diverse and complex disorders of language which may be encountered in schizophrenics may bear a superficial likeness to the dysphasias. The analogies should not be overemphasised, however, for the causation of schizophrenic speech affection lies in an underlying thought-disorder, rather than in a linguistic inaccessibility.

Iterations, both of spoken and of written speech, may be encountered in cases of schizophrenia, and also to a milder extent in dysphasiacs, but for different reasons.

There are interesting problems entailed when the similarities are studied between schizophrenic writings and the non-representational work of certain authors addicted to a cult of obscurity.

Reprinted from Critchley, M. (1967): *British Journal of Psychiatry*, Vol. 113.

The Detection of Minimal Dysphasia

The condition to be discussed entails those subtle impairments in the manipulation of language which constitute the earliest signs of an ingravescent dysphasia. I use the term "manipulation" advisedly, for I wish to embrace the act of verbal communication in all its aspects, receptive and expressive, as well as internal reverbalisation. The conception of a minimal degree of dysphasia can also apply to the latter stages of recovery after a previous episode of loss of speech. Minimal dysphasia may be so mild as to pass unnoticed during the give and take of ordinary social intercourse. Usually the patient himself is unaware of any detriment in his use of language, unless he should happen to be professionally concerned with literature in the widest sense, creative perhaps or merely critical. As might be expected, specially searching tests are required not only to demonstrate the actual existence of a minimal dysphasia but also its extent.

Boller, writing upon this topic, stated: "the preparation of a test highly sensitive to aphasic expressive defects is a task which has not yet been solved, and which deserves to be more thoroughly investigated. The main difficulty with such a test seems to be the risk that, by increasing the verbal difficulty, it will be made more susceptible to non-specific deficits, which frequently accompany cerebral lesions."

But even earlier, certain aphasiologists had devised tests which subjected the patient to relatively stressful situations in order to bring into the open an underlying speech disorder, receptive or expressive. Henry Head's hand-eye-ear test belongs here, and indeed Head was criticised by some of his colleagues for employing a technique which was not strictly linguistic in nature. Even earlier, Pierre Marie had suggested his "three paper test", which is still a useful procedure for uncovering a minimal receptive defect of language. We may also recall the technique devised by Thomas and Roux, as well as the Test of the Absurd Story used by Weisenburg and McBride. These are well worth employment today in demonstrating minimal degrees of dysphasia.

The overall battery of tests for the detection of a minimal dysphasia—or latent aphasia to use the terminology of Pichot—needs to be extended.

Poverty of Speech

An overall reduction in linguistic spontaneity is a common indication of a minimal dysphasia. Although the patient can keep pace with his interlocutor and betray no obvious shrinkage of his vocabulary, he seems reluctant as it were to embark upon the seas of conversation. Inordinately protracted periods of silence are evident when the patient with ingravescent dysphasia is observed in the home, at the conference table, or in the board room. He can and will reply to questions adequately. If sufficiently inspired, he can pose questions on his own initiative. But ordinarily he appears unwilling to break silence with pertinent observations or even with small talk.

This impoverishment of speech is all the more striking when it develops in one who had hitherto been looked upon as constitutionally somewhat garrulous, and anything but squeamish of talking in company. Loquacity is a trait which often increases with ageing and, when the reverse occurs, the possibility of a very early disorder of language should be suspected.

More tangible still is a poverty of written speech. Unless the patient happens to depend for his livelihood upon his writings, he might be expected to express himself on paper far less freely than in spoken speech. With the onset of minimal dysphasia, the reluctance to put pen to paper (or use a typewriter) becomes still more evident. This may show itself in a diminished correspondence on the part of a letter-writer, and in the attenuated output of a diarist.

In contrast to the foregoing remarks, one must not overlook the occasional phenomenon of an *over-reaction* which a minimal dysphasiac may display. An undue talkativeness, or inordinate resort to letter-writing, sometimes represents the very earliest signs of a commencing language-disorder. During the course of conversation, the verbosity of one speaker ordains that he is for the time being the sole master in the use of linguistic tools. The interlocutor's chances of introducing unexpected or difficult material are considerably restricted. This phenomenon of aggressive loquacity does not take place at a conscious level.

Poverty of Speech: Its Linguistic Nature

A verbatim record of the early dysphasiac's spontaneous talk, as well as his written work, may serve as material for linguistic analysis. Various features may be demonstrable:

(a) The discrepancy which ordinarily exists between the two vocabularies may increase; that is to say, the vocabulary which may be regarded as accessible, available, or get-at-able, and the other which is actually in common use.

In normal circumstances the difference between the two vocabularies increases with the intellectual level and educational status, while in the case of the poorly literate there is but little to choose. Nevertheless in minimal dysphasiacs a widening gap becomes evident, the pragmatical vocabulary or the one that is ordinarily utilised being that which becomes attenuated.

(b) This disparity is shown when one estimates the type/token ratio of verbal diversification, or TTR. The latter term refers to the sum-total, while the former indicates the number of *different* words employed. Ordinarily the lower the ratio the smaller the verbal diversity, and this would be likely to characterise the spontaneous writings of a latent dysphasiac.

(c) A reduced sentence-length may be found especially in the written compositions of a patient with very early dysphasia. In spoken speech this may be less evident. Instead one will expect a complicating stylistic or even syntactical imperfection whereby sentences trail off unfinished, or else remain cluttered up with parenthetical clauses, asides, after-thoughts, and qualifications.

(d) Verb-adjective ratio. To establish beyond all question a minimal deterioration in the manipulation of speech, it is necessary to have knowledge of the patient's pre-morbid linguistic competency and habits. When these data are available it may well become obvious that words serving as verbs are reduced in number, while concrete nouns and more particularly adjectival forms show a relative increase. The altered ratio is most striking in the case of the demotic speech of a poorly educated pre-aphasiac. In such, one expects to find a greater incidence of those all-purpose, almost meaningless, fragments of vernacular (such as the Anglo-Australian "bloody") which loom so large in the utterances of the barely literate. Under the stress of growing language-impairment these increase relatively and in actuality.

(e) Enhanced employment of clichés and trite word-clusters. Practiced speakers and writers are less liable to betray in their speech and correspondence a contamination with oft-recurring phrases which are relatively low in reference-function or "meaning". Those who are less well educationally-endowed tend to slip into this habit of usage in a manner which becomes almost idiosyncratic and personally identifiable. Both types of individuals, when under the influence of a minimal dysphasia, are apt to have an increased recourse to platitudinous phraseology, bordering on sheer rigmarole.

Except for the last, the foregoing features are best observed in the written essays of the pre-aphasiac. The last named peculiarity, namely the increased resort to a verbiage which is stale, hackneyed, and threadbare, is particularly evident in the articulate utterance of a patient with minimal dysphasia, being less conspicuous in his attempts to write.

Gratuitous Redundancy

This is a phenomenon that I have described elsewhere, and which may be defined as "the interpolation, by a patient with mild aphasia, of verbiage, comparatively low in reference-function, although not wholly beside the point". This shows itself particularly well in the course of naming tests. In such circumstances, the patient uses too many words, and does not content himself with a simple nomination of the article presented to him. Perhaps he over-reacts against an inability to supply *le mot juste*. The ideal and most satisfying expression on a particular occasion eludes him. Thus, shown an object, the patient may be hesitant in finding the exact term but then, having eventually done so, feels it incumbent to proceed to amplify it unnecessarily. Confronted with a wrist-watch, for instance, the patient may after a pause identify it and then go on to say . . . "My husband has a beauty, but then he's got everything!" My suggestion as to the origins of gratuitous redundancy was that these extrapolated phrases are devoid of any purpose other than a social one, and that the additional words serve merely to oil the wheels of the small-talk of interpersonal relationship. Gratuitous redundancy can be compared with the phatic communion of primitive peoples or the regressive metonymy of leucotomised patients.

Defective Exemplification

This expression refers to an inability to recite a series of instances ex- emplifying some given common property. This ability is sometimes re- ferred to as a process of "word production". For example, the patient may be directed to enumerate as rapidly as possible as many examples of, say, birds, flowers, makes of automobile, fruit, or fish. Slightly more difficult would it be to name articles which are endowed with a common quality or property such as redness, sharpness, and so on. A task of this sort is a higher level abstraction in its nature, and it taxes severely the ability to cull up examples possessing something in the way of a common denominator. Occasionally the patient succeeds by means of carrying out this test but at an utterly concrete level. Thus he may enumerate articles within view, or by resorting to the clues afforded by a clear visual imagery.

There is a marked similarity between the performance of a dementing patient and one who has the earliest (or latent) manifestation of an actual aphasia. In other words, this particular test of minimal dysphasia may re- veal several defects in patients with lesions of either cerebral hemisphere. Two possible explanations arise. Either an impaired word production is a non-specific index of a cerebral lesion—irrespective of its location; or, it is a true and delicate test of minimal dysphasic deficit, which may result from lesions either of the dominant or the non-dominant hemisphere.

Recitation or Revocation

A linguistic test of a searching type is to request the patient to narrate (or to commit to paper) a resumé of some well-known fable, story, allegory, or incident. For example, he might be directed to summarise in a few words the plot of, say, the story of Red Riding Hood or the parable of the Good Samaritan. The victim of minimal dysphasia will demonstrate considerable difficulty in giving a succinct, crisp, and logical account of an incident of this kind, which one would expect to be familiar and accessible.

Somewhat more difficult is the task of directly retailing to the examiner a story or novelette *told to him for the first time.* Many instances can be taken as a model. Because of the pioneer work of Luria it would be appropriate to borrow one or two of his Russian *fabliaux.* For example, there is the "Jackdaw and the Dove" story.

(A jackdaw dyed his feathers and joined a community of doves. As soon as his hoarse cries were heard he was rejected. Disconsolately he returned to his former tree-tops, only to be chased away when the other jackdaws saw his colouring.)

Linguistic tasks presented in succession have proved to be particularly difficult for a patient with minimal dysphasia. One technique for demonstrating the ability to cope with serial tasks, much in favour in the psychological clinics in Moscow, is to relate two short descriptive sentences to the patient who is then required to say them back to the examiner. Two such sentences may be

(a) "On the edge of a forest a hunter killed a wolf";

followed by

(b) "In the garden the apple-trees were in bloom".

The victim of minimal aphasia may hopelessly confuse the two statements, even though he is able to repeat fairly adequately each sentence in isolation. The difficulty can be increased by separating the two test-phrases (a) and (b) first of all by a short interval of time, e.g. 30 seconds; and secondly by a similar interval *which has been deliberately filled by interpolated conversation.* In such circumstances the early dysphasiac may be said frequently to display a "loss of selectivity" of memory-traces, whereby items of the two sentences are combined, and verbal contaminations and perseverations may introduce themselves.

The same type of task may be employed using three sentences instead of two. Each of them may be quite brief, e.g. "The sea is cold. The moon shines brightly. The streets are crowded."

Another way of bringing to the surface an incipient or latent dysphasia, which again introduces the factor of selectivity, is by dint of an *extended naming test.* Shown a succession of common objects, the patient may identify each one correctly, and furthermore when presented with a collection of articles he may pick out to command one item after another. However, if he is shown *two or three articles simultaneously* (e.g. watch, key, collar-stud) he may experience difficulty in correct serial naming. Or being seated in front of a collection of articles, and told to pick out—not one—but three objects, he may be hesitant or even frankly at a loss.

These errors are particularly likely to occur if the articles displayed are not strictly speaking "common" articles, but are objects which are a trifle unexpected, and out of the ordinary.

Other elaborations of these naming and isolating techniques can be employed in order to bring out an underlying inchoate dysphasia.

Thus, the patient, shown a number of objects, may be directed to manipulate them rather than merely identify them. For example, he may be instructed to "pick up the collar-stud and *put it inside* the match-box". This may prove too difficult for the patient, although a moment before he may have correctly identified both articles singly or in combination.

This particular technique recalls the so-called "Token Test" devised by De Renzi and Vignolo. Their test is a valuable one and has been studied with particular care in cases of aphasia, in brain-injured patients with aphasia, and in controls. By this means it has proved possible to uncover mild *receptive* defects in aphasiacs even in those which seemingly were instances of pure motor aphasia. In devising this test, the authors took great pains to ensure that the procedure was short in duration; that no special apparatus or printed material was required; that the instructions were so brief as not to tax the dysphasiac's memory; and that the task should entail the maximum linguistic with the minimum intellectual difficulty. Their "Token Test" materials consist of 20 pieces of paper, in 5 colours, 2 shapes, and 2 sizes. The patient is first instructed to touch one of these papers; and then to touch *two* of them. Finally the instructions become more elaborate, e.g. by introducing a choice (touch the blue circle *or* the red triangle) ; or the factor of position (place the blue circle *on* the red rectangle) ; or of succession (touch the blue circle *after touching* the red rectangle) ; or of condition (touch all the circles *except* the green one) .

The De Renzi–Vignolo test has many merits. Its principal demerit lies in the use of the term "token" in this connection, for in linguistic science "token" has a very special connotation and may be defined as "each particular occurrence of a speech unit" spoken or written. De Renzi and his colleagues would have been on less ambiguous grounds had they spoken of "items" rather than "tokens".

Another useful elaboration of this type of test-situation is to instruct the patient to pick up (or point to) this article or that, *against the competing background of irrelevant noise*. This factor of noise can be brought in by switching on music, or by introducing some distracting element of sound, but best of all by some acoustic handicap of a linguistic character. This last-named can be furnished by an assistant reading aloud a paragraph from a book or newspaper, during the testing procedure.

Linguistic Recall

This faculty may be mildly impaired in circumstances of minimal dysphasia, but may not be obvious until specially penetrating procedures are brought to bear. For example, the examiner may recite to the patient a series of ten substantives of a not unfamiliar sort. The examinee is then immediately instructed to recount these same ten words. Or—to augment the inherent difficulty—to recap the series after a silent gap of thirty seconds; or after a similar interval filled, however, with interpolated talk. Finally the patient may be confronted with a much larger series of words (either verbally or in print) within which he is expected to identify the original ten words which the examiner has recited.

Comprehension and Explanation of Various Trite Linguistic Whimsicalities

This test is similar to, but not identical with, the common clinical test whereby the patient is asked to explain certain well-known proverbs. Here the test is directed more to an examination of verbal manipulation rather than of thinking. In this particular test for minimal dysphasia, the patient is presented with a phrase rather than a proverb which he is asked to paraphrase or elucidate. In the English language suitable test-phrases include such *doubles entendres* as "Players please"; or strained obscure metaphors like "it's in the bag", "the horse's mouth"; or truncated aphorisms like "the hair of the dog"; or untranslatable phrases like "too clever by half". In such circumstances the linguistic abilities of the minimal dysphasiac become severely taxed. It is a debatable point whether the problem lies in a defect in comprehension, or in formulation on the part of the patient, or in both.

Analogies and Multiple Choice Quizzes

Here the patient with minimal dysphasia is presented with three words— audibly or on paper—and is expected to supply the logical fourth term. The following are examples:

winter, snow: autumn ? (rain; fog)
mother, daughter: father ? (son)
lion, teeth: eagle ? (claws)
motor-car, engine: boat ? (sails; oars)
bird, wing: dog ? (paws; legs)

A similar test entails the search for a second word in a common phrase entailing either metonyms or contrasts, e.g.

wet and ?	(windy; dry)
health and ?	(happiness; strength; disease)
fish and ?	(chips)
black and ?	(white)
big and ?	(small)

Rather easier is the linguistic task of word-finding when the testee is assisted by a multiple choice type of presentation, e.g.

water, thirst; food (hunger, meal, mouth)
tree, branch; hand (feet, fingers, glove)
regiment, soldiers; library (readers, books, reading-room)
winter, snow; autumn (falling leaves, harvest, rain)

The patient is required to underline the most appropriate words.

A familiar test-situation which taxes the capacities of a patient with minimal dysphasia can be found in crossword puzzles. In utilising this procedure as a deliberate aphasiological procedure, one should avoid clues which are over-abstruse and which depend almost entirely upon obscure literary allusions. Verbal play, puns, and anagrams are permissible provided they are not too recondite. The following constitute suitable examples:

Clue:	"I'm buried in a small hill. Not a sea." (number of letters 5)
Answer:	Timor
Clue:	"English viewpoint?" (number of letters 5)
Answer:	Angle
Clue:	"If ham's off, you'll have to go hungry." (number of letters 6)
Answer:	Famish
Clue:	"Good folk? Few believe in them nowadays." (number of letters 7)
Answer:	Fairies

This type of linguistic test is unsuitable for general use, but should be reserved where the pre-morbid educational standing is known. A minimal dysphasia might come to light in this way, but only in the case of an individual known to have been a keen contestant in crossword puzzles of the standard set by *The Times, Observer,* or *Daily Telegraph.*

*Comprehension of Instructions Involving Sequential
or Temporal Components*

Here one tests the patient's ability to follow and retain a fairly complicated request. The command may be associated with the notion of interval. Thus, again following Luria, one may say to the patient "I shall count; and when I have got up to 12, and not before, raise your hand . . . one . . . two . . . three . . . four . . ." and so on.

Or the patient can be faced with a series of positive and negative tasks, such as: "When I make a *fist,* lift up your *hand.* When I raise my *forefinger,* you make a *fist*. When I lift up my *hand,* do nothing." This complicated instruction, with the patient attempting to obey the commands, may be repeated a number of times.

Sentence-Building

Here the patient is presented with a series of cards upon each one of which is printed a single word—noun, verb, adjective, adverb, article, preposition, conjunction. The patient is required to arrange these cards so as to form a grammatical and sensible sentence, preferably as lengthy as possible. Thus the normal control subject would have no difficulty in promptly aligning the cards to form some such sentence as the following, "Today the weather is wet, windy, and cold, while yesterday it was quite warm and sunny." Such a performance would be quite beyond the capacity of a minimal dysphasiac, even though he was quite able to read and understand the printed word on each individual card.

Such tests as the foregoing represent a battery of investigations which, in conjunction, endeavour to uncover very mild communicative detriments. Note that all these tests are essentially clinical in nature, and depend upon little more than pencil and paper, together with the efficient utilisation of the examiner's five senses. Elaborate equipment, electrical devices, ancillary aids are dispensed with. But to utilise clinical methods adequately, experience, judgement, patience, and honesty are essential. Every movement on the part of the patient, each gesture, articulate utterance, hesitation, interjection, must be noted, timed, and recorded scrupulously. If the observed data do not entirely conform with the examiner's expectations they must not be glossed over or brushed aside. These "negative cases", these discrepancies, may be all important occurrences, and not just irritating irrelevancies. The history of science shows how often advances have been made simply by focussing attention upon unexpected, exceptional, or nonconforming phenomena. In exploring the garden of language-behaviour, the neurologist must emulate the industry of the bee. To quote Francis Bacon, changing only the last word:

> The men of experiment are like the ant; they only collect and use; the reasoners resemble the spiders, who make cobwebs out of their own substance. But the bee takes a middle course, it gathers its material from the flowers of the garden and of the field, but transforms and digests it by a power of its own. Not unlike this is the true business of aphasiology.

Reprinted from Critchley, M. (1972) : *Scientific Foundations of Neurology,* edited by M. Critchley, J. L. O'Leary, and B. Jennett. Heinemann Medical Books, London.

The Broca-Dax Controversy

The story of the discovery of what is often called "the centre of language" entails the names of five great men. In chronological order these are Auburtin, Broca, Duval, Dax père, and Dax fils.

The scene opens at a meeting of the Anthropological Society of Paris in the rue René-Panhard on 4 April 1864, when Dr. Auburtin (Fig. 1) delivered an address entitled "On the seat of the faculty of language". He pointed out that language is a complex activity mediated by an articulatory organ, a coordinating centre, and a connecting tract between these two. Lesions involving any one of these structures could implicate language.

In opposition to Gratiolet, who regarded the brain as acting as a whole, Auburtin believed that the centre which coordinated the movements underlying language was to be found in the frontal lobe and nowhere else; language alone could be ablated. To support this viewpoint he quoted cases that had been reported by Rostan, Lallemand, Heurteloup, Bernard, Bonnaford, Sedillot, Macquet, and Bouillaud. One which interested him was that of a patient under the care of Cullerier at the Hôpital Saint-Louis; this was a man who had tried to blow out his brains with a revolver-shot but had succeeded merely in destroying the frontal bone so as to expose the underlying lobes. He could still speak, but if the exposed brain was lightly pressed with a spatula, he would temporarily lose his power of speech. This case-report reminds us of the well known story of that beggar in the streets of Paris who would allow passers-by—for a monetary consideration—to press upon his exposed brain, so causing him to pass out. Auburtin stated that the only contradictory case that would be meaningful would need to be one with complete destruction of the two anterior lobes of the brain. "And then if the patient could still speak my theory would be refuted. But I believe that no such case exists."

"As a pupil of Bouillaud (Fig. 2), I have been observing for a long time a patient by the name of Bache who has lost his power of speech. When that man dies I shall jettison my beliefs, if I should fail to discover a lesion of the anterior lobe. As far as I know I have never come across a lesion of the middle or posterior lobes causing a destruction of the faculty of language."

At that particular meeting there was in attendance the Secretary of the Society, namely M. Broca. Two days beforehand he had admitted under his care on the surgical service of the Bicêtre hospital a man named Laborgne, a mental defective who had for long been speechless and hemiplegic and

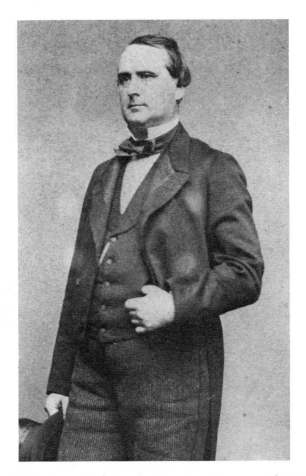

FIG. 1. M. le docteur E. Auburtin (from a contemporary photograph).

who had contracted a cellulitis of the leg. M. Broca (Fig. 3) invited Auburtin to accompany him and see the patient. Some days later Laborgne died. At the postmortem examination there was found a longstanding superficial lesion which had destroyed the lower part of the second and third frontal convolutions on the left side of the brain. When this specimen was demonstrated at the next meeting of the Anthropological Society, namely on 18 April, it aroused little or no interest. But some weeks later a second case was encountered very like that of Laborgne, again with identical autopsy findings. Immediately interest was sparked off not only in anthropological circles, but in medicine throughout the world.

Broca continued to collect cases of hemiplegia with loss of speech or "aphemia" as he preferred to call this latter symptom. Enriched by his imposing series of 22 brains from such cases, he found himself, against his

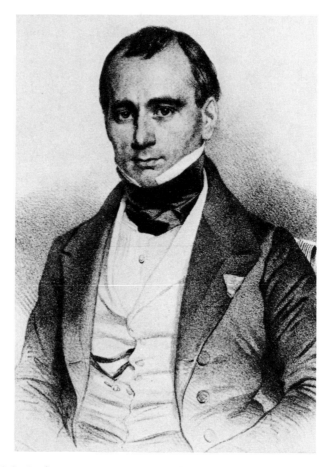

FIG. 2. M. le Professeur Jean Baptiste Bouillaud, b. 1796. Physician and Dean of the Faculté de Médecine, University of Paris.

will, interrupted in his surgical practice to be hailed as a prophet of cerebral localisation, and as the one who had discovered the centre of the linguistic faculty.

The story now takes us four years ahead when on 3 March 1867 at a meeting of the same Society, M. Duval showed two young children afflicted with traumatic aphemia. In both cases it was evident that the lesions were involving the left frontal lobes. During the discussion which followed this paper, Broca said, "I have been struck by the fact that in my original cases of aphemia, the lesion was always localised, not only to the same region of the brain, but always on the same side, namely the left. Since then, and from the evidence of very many autopsies, the lesion has always been on the left side. We have also seen a large number of patients with aphemia, most of them hemiplegic, the paralysis always being on the right

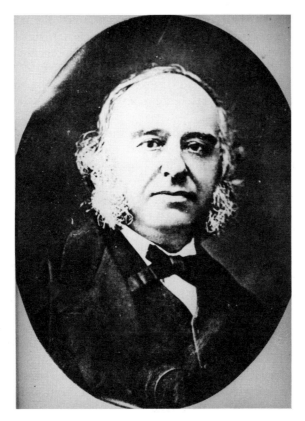

FIG. 3. M. le Professeur Pierre Paul Broca, 1824–1880. Parisian surgeon and anthropologist.

side. What is more, at autopsy, we have met with lesions of F3 on the right side in those patients who were not aphemic. From this evidence, we have come to the conclusion that the faculty of articulate language is represented in the left half of the brain, or at least chiefly so."

At the next meeting of the Society which was held on 21 April, M. Broca demonstrated another specimen with a lesion in the left hemisphere, the patient having lost his speech through a head injury, the vocabulary being reduced to "the head . . . the head" . . . or else "Yes". It was then that M. Broca declared that a certain M. Dax, a little known doctor living at Sommières, in the Languedoc, had complained to the Academy of Medicine that M. Broca had chosen to ignore the work of his late father, who had long been aware that the lesions which destroy the faculty of language are always situated within the left half of the brain. Dax père, it seemed, had written an article on this topic for the Congrès Méridionel of Montpellier.

"I am not fond of debates about priority" said Broca, "but a number of people have suggested that I should have mentioned the name of Dax. I erred through ignorance. The writer of the article was not known to me, nor is he in Montpellier. I have searched through libraries and I have also requested the Librarian of the Faculty of Montpellier to look, but unsuccessfully so. The Meeting had occurred between the 1st and the 10th of July in 1836, but there is no reference to any article by Dax in the Revue de Montpellier."

Thus began the dispute between Broca and Dax which turned out to be still more complicated. Dax had been very much interested in the topic of "alalia" and he wanted to write a thesis on the subject but permission from the University was not forthcoming. Patiently he began to collect cases, and also reports from the literature. He wrote a memorandum for his local colleagues in 1858, and then again in 1860, the title of which was "Observation directed towards proving the association between derangement of speech and a lesion of the left cerebral hemisphere". Later he sent it to the Academy of Medicine where it was received on 24 March 1863.

Dax junior was bitterly wounded by the fact that subsequent authors continued to ignore his work, and furthermore not to accord any recognition to his father. Charles Richet published a paper on aphasia in July 1864 in the *Revue des Deux Mondes*. The contribution of Dax the son and the discovery made by his father were not mentioned. This provoked another protest from Dax that was published in the *Montpellier Médical* in October 1865. On 14 April 1865 another paper on aphasia was published by M. Falret which referred to the work of the father and of the son, but in such terms as to anger seriously Dax fils.

Meanwhile, Dax fils had discovered in a desk-drawer the original manuscript written by his late father, and he published it as it stood in the *Gazette Hebdomadaire de Médecine et de Chirurgerie,* on 26 April 1865. In 1800 Dax père had apparently examined a cavalry officer whose memory for words became impaired by reason of a sabre-wound on the left side of the head. His other patient was the naturalist Brussonet, who had lost his verbal memory and in whom he was able to demonstrate that it was due to a large "ulcer" on the surface of the left hemisphere. Dax had subsequently seen three similar cases, and wrote: "I was impressed with this identical situation in the three sole observations which I had been able to collect over a period of 11 years."

Later he assembled more than 40 such cases, without exception to the rule, and he was able to find similar instances in the literature. From all these data he concluded that . . . "when this (verbal) memory is affected by brain-disease, it is necessary to search for the cause of this symptom in the left hemisphere".

He went on: "I hope that my work will not be without value in the diagnosis and treatment of patients of this kind. When the cerebral lesion is not associated with hemiplegia, or if this latter is delayed in appearance, it is possible to suspect the nature of the illness, or at least the site of the lesion. . . ."

Dax fils added an appendix to his father's article. In his discussion upon speech-disorders it is obvious that he included more than one kind of case, instances of dysarthria as well as dysphasiacs. In this way he repeated the error that for many centuries had deceived physicians and that, in fact, went on to confuse neurologists over very many succeeding years. Like the savants of the Middle Ages, Dax fils tended to ascribe aphasia to a partial paralysis of the tongue. He admitted that at times aphasiacs substituted one word for another, but Dax circumvented this difficulty by claiming that the patient, unable to pronounce a word, groped to find an easier one. Dax was more correct, however, in his belief that the same lesion which could provoke a dyssynergia could sometimes also impede verbal memory, and that in the contemporary state of knowledge, one could not distinguish the two kinds of cases.

Thirteen years later, Dax published a short monograph on aphasia, and his remarks upon the lack of recognition of his father's discovery were bitter indeed.

At that time medical men were too preoccupied with discussions of priority to devote themselves to the more important problems as to the nature of cerebral dominance. Not for many years did physicians begin to debate the explanation of the difference between the right and the left hemispheres.

Lélut commented upon the remarks of Dax fils and threw out the idea how much more mysterious would be that complicated organ, the brain, if it were to be found that the two halves possessed different functions. But Bouillaud interrupted with a penetrating question. "Is it conceivable that we would be left handed, so to say, for certain faculties, like that of language?"

Despite the support accorded by Baillarger in 1865, medicine of that era was slow to recognise the priority of Dax in this problem. Bouillaud, with all his authority as Dean of the Faculty, would obstinately have no truck either with Dax or with the notion of a unilateral speech centre. In his teaching sessions Trousseau continued to support Broca's contention of a left sided centre. This provoked yet another protest from Dax. It is said that Trousseau wrote two letters in reply graciously according priority to the elder Dax, but these two letters cannot be traced. But in the south of France, loyalty towards Dax was consistent. In his 1873 *Thèse de Montpellier,* Trémolet unequivocally recognised the discovery.

Grasset was probably the first in France to accord public recognition to the two doctors of the Midi and in 1873 he was boldly referring to "Dax's law".

Today we ask ourselves in a discreet whisper "where can we find Marc Dax's original manuscript?" "Is it still in existence? Or, has it ever existed at all?" Such accusations are by no means new. Over a century ago the librarian at Montpellier inquired of 20 doctors who had attended the Congrès Méridionel in 1836, but not one had either seen or heard Dr. Dax at that meeting. Some years later, Broca, somewhat appeased perhaps, and, having scrutinized closely the *Gazette Hebdomadaire* for 1865 and noted the difference in style between the two papers, concluded that they had not been written by the same person. But is this opinion justifiable? Nowadays the judgement of a linguist would be needed, and he would be in a position to assert from an analysis of the style whether the text was the work of one author or of two. But this test is not feasible for us. Dr. Joynt was kind enough to bring to my notice an article written in 1879 by Caizergue who proclaimed that he had come across a copy of the original version of Marc Dax's paper which he unearthed when sorting the papers of his grandfather who had been the Dean of the Faculty of Medicine in Montpellier. But that discovery did not establish the date when that paper was written. It would indeed be interesting to know of the present whereabouts of that article.

Dr. Joynt and Dr. Benton have taken up a simple and generous attitude about this business by suggesting that Marc Dax was reluctant of taking the whole responsibility for a discovery of which he was not too confident. From my own personal experience of medical symposia I suggest that Marc Dax's article was never read but was "laid on the table" (in the English— not American—sense), and that he left the meeting without being seen or heard, still less having delivered his communication.

Let us now briefly turn to the biographical details of the five men whose names are associated with this important chapter in aphasiology.

Regarding Dr. Ange Duval, I have unfortunately succeeded in discovering little, except that he was Principal Surgeon to the Navy and a Professor at the School of Naval Medicine at Brest.

Dr. Ernest Auburtin has been far more neglected than Dax by writers upon aphasia. Auburtin was born at Metz in 1825, where his forebears were looking-glass manufacturers. He practised in Paris at 16 rue Saint-Benoît, near Saint Germain des Prés. Previously he had been Chef de Clinique at the Faculty of Medicine. He was the nephew of Professor Lallemand of Montpellier. We do not know what were his principal interests in medicine, but we do know that he was physician to Princess Mathilde Bonaparte who was the cousin of the Emperor Napoleon III. If one can judge from the amusing remark in the *Goncourt Journals,* he was also physician to the comedian Popelin. His chief interest lay in anthropology and he was a founder member of the Paris Society. He was described as a serious thinker with a reflective turn of mind and I like to recall that it was he who really inspired Broca with an interest in alalia. The work of Gall intrigued him in so far as it bore on the question of language. On this topic he was Gall's disciple for he was also a supporter of Bouillaud whose daughter Elisa he married.

Auburtin and his family inherited Bouillaud's estate at Bergerons near Roullet (Charente), between Angoulême and Bordeaux (Fig. 4). There Auburtin died in 1895. Unfortunately there is no longer an Auburtin in medicine, but his grandson is the distinguished Municipal Councillor and the present Mayor of Paris as of 1964.

Auburtin's original contribution was overshadowed by the work of Broca, whose great prestige ensured that he was a man as impossible to overlook as to surpass. Paul Broca belonged to a protestant family and was born in the small town of Sainte Foy la Grande (Gironde) in the Dordogne, just nine years after Gratiolet. Broca's father was an army surgeon who served in the Napoleonic campaigns. Broca was such a brilliant scholar that, when he came to Paris to study medicine, he was already erudite, a polyglot, a talented painter, and an accomplished musician. So hard up was he at that time that he toyed with the idea of emigrating to America. Finally, however, he accepted as a temporary measure the thankless and uncongenial job of a schoolteacher.

In the world of medicine Broca was distinguished as an anatomist and a surgeon. Living at 1 rue des Saints Pères he worked at the Hôtel Dieu, the Bicêtre, and the Salpêtrière, as well as other hospitals. He took part in the

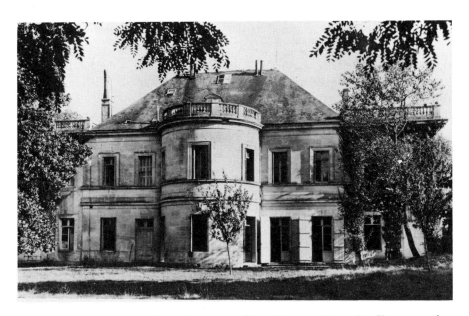

FIG. 4. The Bouillaud–Auburtin estate. "Les Bergerons" at Roullet, near Angoulême, France.

Revolution of 1848, refusing promotion, and also the distinction of the Légion d'Honneur.

Broca's chief interest was in anthropology. He was a founding member and the first secretary of the Société d'Anthropologie. He experienced difficulty in explaining that the new term "anthropology" had no sinister political connotation, and had nothing to do with "the rights of man".

We will not dwell upon Broca's contribution to aphasiology, which was little more than an incident in the course of his remarkable career. Later he established a university department of anthropology where he housed his considerable collection of crania. Again he had to contend with an attitude of suspicion, this time from the Church. During the Franco-Prussian War he was in charge of a military hospital in the Jardin des Plantes. At the time of the Commune he smuggled out of Paris to the government at Versailles gold ingots to the tune of 75 million francs concealed in a hay cart. In 1880 he was elected Senator but lived only a few months to enjoy that distinction.

Finally we come to the two Doctors Dax. Dr. Marc Dax was born in 1770 at Tarascon and qualified at Montpellier. Having coped with an outbreak of cholera at Aigues-Mortes, he set up practice in the small town of Sommières (Gard) on the river Vidourle. Located midway between Nîmes and Montpellier he was outside the main stream of Parisian medicine although he was well thought of as a general practitioner. He worked in the local hospital for 37 years and wrote one or two papers, but showed no interest in neurology beyond his solitary contribution in 1836. He died a year later at the age of 70 and was buried in the hospital cemetery.

His son Gustave Dax was born in Sommières in 1815. Like his father he took his medical degree at Montpellier and practised in his home town. Like his father, too, he worked at the local hospital, but after 23 years service he was invited to tender his resignation. This very unusual step was possibly due to the fact that Marc Dax was a legitimist, a partisan in fact of Henry V. Boisson, who was both the mayor of Sommières and its archivist, did not mention either the father Dax or the son in his official history of the town. Why ever not? Boisson was an Orleanist, his brother was the local pharmacist. Perhaps at some time or other there had been some friction between him and Dax junior, who was from all accounts a rather quarrelsome and obstinate type, fierce in his defence of lost causes.

Dr. Gustave Dax died in 1898. It had been a great disappointment to him that his son did not follow his father's career. Although he had been a medical student he had let the years slip by without sitting his final examinations. He was of a literary bent, being a poet and playwright of some ability. His death was sudden on his honeymoon, probably from *la maladie des amants,* subarachnoid haemorrhage.

Today the contribution of the two Doctors Dax is no longer forgotten in the world of medicine. But even now the peaceful town of Sommières knows little if anything of its two eminent citizens. No plaque adorns the wall of their house in the place du Bourguet; and although there are a number of eponymous streets, visitors will look in vain for any rue des deux docteurs Dax.

Epilogue

This paper was delivered in Paris on 4 June 1964. In the auditorium sat Professor Passouant, the eminent neurologist from Montpellier. Stimulated by these concluding remarks he made contact with the Mayor of Sommières,

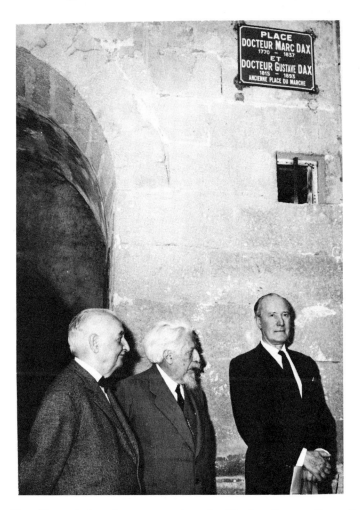

FIG. 5. Unveiling of the plaque renaming the Market Square, Sommières, the "Place Docteur Marc Dax et Docteur Gustave Dax." *Left to right:* Dr. F. R. Ferguson, Professor J. Euzière, and Dr. M. Critchley.

Docteur André, a good friend and colleague of his. Impelled by feelings of justice and the call for reparation, the Municipal Council of Sommières determined to rectify this omission. On 12 June 1966 the town was *en fête* and, amidst celebrations marked by their liberality and their dignity, Professor Alajouanine and Dr. Critchley—accompanied by his friend Dr. Ferguson—unveiled a plaque outside the birthplace of the two doctors, and another plaque renaming the Market Square the Place Docteur Marc Dax et Docteur Gustave Dax (Fig. 5).

With typical gallic wit, Professor Alajouanine referred in his allocution to the embarrassment of the doctors of the Languedoc when they had been made aware that they had been letting one of their treasure-troves drift into a sort of sclerosis and, what was worse, a "sclérose sans plâques".

Reprinted from Critchley, M. (1964): *Revue Neurologique,* Vol. 110.

The Chronic Aphasiac, a Sociological Problem

Language, being a built-in aspect of one's personality, is therefore something specific, idiosyncratic. No two persons possess identical systems of communication. Loss of language when it comes about is never uniform in pattern. The anonymous coterie of uncommunicating inaccessibles holds no two of a kind. Put more simply, no two aphasiacs are absolutely alike.

Such considerations must always be borne in mind when discussing prognosis. Some aphasic subjects fare well, others not. Is it possible to predict those with a favourable outlook? Secondly, can anything be done to influence the rate of recovery, and its degree?

The components involved, some innate, others environmental, are so numerous, that any attempt to establish a "prognostic index" would entail the manipulation of a host of variables, many of them obscure. One hundred and four years ago, Hughlings Jackson had these ideas in mind when he wrote about "the four factors of the insanities". Of course he was not referring to any form of lunacy but to what we would today describe as "highest level brain-dysfunction". He emphasised that the clinical picture depends upon: (1) the depth of the dissolution; (2) the rapidity of the reduction; (3) the influence of external and internal states upon the patient; and (4) the kind of brain affected.

Today we know that these four factors are not enough. Many, many more elements are involved. With a dysphasia from a local lesion of the brain, we have to take count of: its precise location; its size; the rate of onset; its natural course, whether progressive, regressive, or static; the age of the patient; his pre-morbid intelligence; his previous linguistic equipment; his affective stability; the attitude of those around him; and the state of his general health with special reference to his cerebral arteries.

I would like to add yet another imponderable factor, namely the sex of the patient.

Today I want to stress the environmental factor, by-passing all the other important sets of circumstances simply because of the limitations imposed by time.

Let us picture a straightforward case of aphasia. The patient is an intelligent, professional, and well-read man of 65, a lawyer perhaps, or a pastor, who has suddenly sustained a stroke. Consciousness was not completely lost but when examined in his bemused state he is found to be paralysed in his right arm and leg, with a hemihypaesthesia and a hemianopia. His power of speech is shattered, almost completely so. He recognises his family and is apparently understanding the gist of what they say to him, largely from their facial expressions, and their gestures.

He is admitted as an emergency to the nearest university hospital. During the ensuing week his sensorium clears. Some voluntary power returns to the right side of the face and to the right leg. The arm remains immobile. His ability to understand what others are saying to him is obviously improving, and by now he may even be able to articulate a fragment or two of speech, like "yes" or "no"; "goodbye", "please", "thank you". Sometimes it is a profane expletive which is unwittingly emitted.

Days and weeks go by. He has long been encouraged to sit out of bed. With support he can even stand and make a few uncertain steps. Later still he finds he can perform a struggling movement proximally; next, perhaps, a feeble flexion of the thumb. By now he is walking better, but needs assistance. The visual field defect has given way to a one-sided inattention.

His storehouse of available words has now increased and they are better controlled. He watches television but much of what he gazes at moves too fast for him to grasp, and the spoken word, articulated all too often in a diction that is unfamiliar, largely eludes him. Nevertheless he rather enjoys the television, even though he does not hoist in very much of it. His favourite programmes are football, athletics, orchestral music, the newsitems. Comedy is too slick for him; he fails to see the point of the jokes, and he does not quite understand why the audience laughs so often and so loudly.

Physiotherapists come and breezily persuade him to try and do this, or do that. They depart very pleased; he is not sure why. Speech therapists coax him to phonate. This may strike the patient, a High Court Judge perhaps before his apoplexy laid him low, as a little humiliating, and he is glad that his junior colleagues are not there to witness the performance.

A couple of months have now passed. He begins to sense an air of polite boredom on the part of the Professor and his team, as well as the nursing staff. From time to time mention is made of lengthy waiting-lists, quick turnovers. So a spell of convalescence is arranged in a long-stay hospital in the country or at the seaside. New sets of physiotherapists and phoniatricians are involved, and so the months go by. It has become all too obvious that no dramatic cure will eventuate.

The shortcomings of the State medical service now become evident. The patient returns to his home, where the rooms are spacious, the garden agreeable, and where there await him a devoted wife and daughters, possibly even domestic staff.

What then? At first all goes pretty well. He finds he does not miss the physiotherapy all that much. A new speech therapist comes once or twice a week, and the phonetic exercises are resumed. He breakfasts in bed, and when it suits the household, he is washed, shaved, dressed, and helped downstairs to his corner armchair. Meals constitute brief and pleasurable interludes.

Friends and acquaintances call, but their visits become less and less frequent. Sometimes visitors prove tiring, especially when they and his wife and daughters and their friends chat animatedly across the room. What are they talking about? Less and less often is he brought into the conversation, and indeed he is rather glad to opt out. When important guests appear, it is less of an embarrassment if father takes his meal on a tray in the bedroom, and at a convenient moment is undressed early and put to bed.

So day follows day. The scene has been vividly described by Zola in his novel *Thérèse Racquart*, as one of . . . "walled-in intelligence, still alive, yet imprisoned in dead flesh". Despondency follows boredom, and feelings of hopelessness and nostalgia churn up in his mind and lead to utter dejection. This is the picture of grief-reaction coupled with frustration which certain wise aphasiologists have discussed.

Some years ago I described the all too common social scene, in the following words:

> . . . thus we find the unhappy aphasiac, silent and lonely, an alien within a foreign and faintly hostile land. He dwells bewildered amidst a confusion of symbols dimly understood. As often as not he is partially incapacitated and unable to fend for himself. Eager to make communion with others, to share interests, or enlist their aid, he meets a barricade which stands between his ill-formed notions and their expression. Should he succeed in fighting through, maybe he finds his words a gross parody of his will, made up of incoherencies and futile parroting. Thwarted and bemused, he lapses into the security of his silence where he can face the simple things and actualities, leaving unexplored the world of ideas. He lives from hour to hour, with little thought for tomorrow, enmeshed in reverie upon the distant past, the satisfaction of his present needs, while awaiting some immediate simple comfort.

Here comes the crucial question: does regular, skilled speech therapy bring about any benefit over and above the natural process of restoration in an aphasiac? And if it does, how soon should it be started?

Let us admit: it is almost impossible to answer these queries scientifically, mathematically, statistically. To attempt to do so would necessitate research into a series of hundreds of cases matched exactly against a like number of untreated controls. As I have said, the patients must be comparable in both psycho-biological and pathological respects. The latter would comprise the site, size, and nature of the lesion, the state of the general health with special reference to age, and the efficiency of the cerebral circulation. The psycho-biological variables are even more diverse and include the pre-morbid cultural, educational, and intellectual status. I strongly suspect that such exacting demands are not capable of being met.

I submit that the merits of speech-therapy in aphasia are not scientifically established, and probably never will be. However, it is certainly possible to identify various factors which are unpropitious, being harmful to an aphasiac not only to his word-bank, but also to his morale. With the all too common plight which steadily enclosed the patient after he has left hospital, we can witness him sinking into a slough of apathy with depression. Even the most affectionate and best intentioned relatives, finding it hard to establish contact, unwittingly yet increasingly ignore him. Days may slip by without his making a willed effort to utter a word. This state of affairs inevitably leads to mental and linguistic rot.

Here arise for discussion the possible virtues of what has been termed "the Hawthorne effect". Hawthorne found that in mental defectives, and in children with learning disorders, headway begins only when notice is taken of them, even though the intervention may be unskilled, non-specific, and unintentional. Something at least is being done, and the child begins to improve and mature, but only when he has become an object of attention of some sort or other.

Can it be that speech therapy, skilled, sophisticated, and intelligently applied, exercises merely a Hawthorne effect in aphasiacs? This suggestion, shocking though it may sound to some, is rather supported by an important social experiment. At present in Great Britain, at the instigation of Miss Valerie Eaton Griffith, an important experiment is taking place.

A group of chronic, severe aphasiacs was originally chosen—I avoid the term "selected" for they were taken at random from all social classes. Each patient was made the target of intense social stimulation. That is to say, a body of intelligent, pleasant women—quite untrained in any paramedical skills, by the way, volunteered to take part in this project. To each patient, seven of these helpers would be assigned. They were selected from ladies who lived close by, and who if possible shared the patient's pre-morbid interests whether professional or recreational. It was important to ensure that they were *not* friends or even acquaintances of the patient before his illness. From the team of seven, one member in turn would visit the patient daily; sometimes even two visits a day were paid. At these sessions, the visitor would gently chat with the patient, speaking about current news, items of gossip, or of shared interests. To begin with, the interviews were predominantly one-sided; the visitor did most if not all of the talking, but not too quickly and not too loudly, using simple phrases. As time went by, it was found that the dysphasiac began to participate more and more. Usually a warm relationship was engendered and the patient would begin to look forward to each of these visits. In this way the apathy and despondency steadily lifted. This was only the beginning. Later still the speech-impairment, too, began to lessen, and progressively so, and the dysphasiac would talk more and more.

Soon it would become possible for visitor and patient to share in various indoor pastimes, card games, even Scrabble (a word-game). Outdoor trips would be planned, car-rides, outings, film-shows, shopping.

Patients who were by nature gregarious were then encouraged to join clubs where other aphasiacs would meet, share a meal, and indulge in co-operative communication-exercises, like drawing, painting, miming, charades, music, and even talks. As might be expected, some patients are at first reluctant to join such group-activities.

Over the past few years, Miss Griffith's trial-project proved so successful that it has now expanded greatly. At present three geographical areas in England are involved in this scheme, and one in Scotland.

The scheme is by now fairly established being organised with a team made up of the local supervisor, the patient's medical practitioner, and the area community physician. Frequently there is also a warm cooperation with the regional speech-therapists.

One or two interesting points have emerged. Both male and female dysphasiacs prefer to receive female visitors, and of the seven volunteers allotted to each patient, it is usual to choose six female helpers and one male.

The next is a very practical point. The project costs the patient nothing, the family nothing, and the State nothing. The amount of expense entailed is very small and mostly concerns secretarial work. This is met by an *ad hoc* grant from a charity, namely the Chest, Heart, and Stroke Association. The helpers all give their services voluntarily, and each pays his or her travelling expenses.

This particular technique is, of course, pure therapy, but it is treatment of a surreptitious character. The patient is being treated without his realising it, and I believe that for this reason it is often more acceptable, especially to persons with a high pre-morbid intelligence, or those who before their trauma were notoriously successful in business, politics, the stage, or one of the professions. That kind of patient seems to respond better to the informal and indirect approach, rather than being retaught to speak—an approach which he or she may regard as undignified, embarrassing, and childlike. Also, the patient is being bombarded by this surreptitious approach at least once a day, for seven days a week; and the concentration produces better results than less frequent, formal voice-exercises.

To say this I am *not*, let me stress, being critical of traditional speech therapy.

Is it not probable that *social* rehabilitation is the most important single factor in re-establishing an aphasiac's Ego-strength and, out of the benefit which ensues, his shattered language-functions find themselves in a climate most favourable for a *restituto ad integrum*?

Drum-Talk and Whistle-Speech

Students of language are very aware that diverse modalities of communication exist which are of a non-verbal character. Some of these are wholly or partly automatic, such as for instance the involuntary expressive vasomotor phenomena seen in blanching or flushing of the face, lacrimation, dryness of the mouth, and so on. Others are deliberate in character and here belong the sign-languages employed by operatives who work in environments of noise (cotton-mills, steel foundries); or at a distance (railway-shunters, airfield personnel). Sometimes silence is the determining factor, as in the case of electricians working in a broadcasting studio. At other times secrecy is all-important, e.g. the tic-tac or blower system of the race-course bookies, and the surreptitious signals of the croupiers.

On occasions, sensory deprivation necessitates an elaboration of non-articulate systems of communication, as evidenced in the deaf-mute by both finger-spelling and by their international sign-languages. The blind display their very elaborate communicative skill in their Braille symbology.

In addition to the foregoing, other non-articulate communicative systems exist which are not widely comprehended or appreciated, save in the specialised terrain of anthropology. Perhaps the most striking example is to be found in the drum-language or drum-talk common throughout, though not wholly confined to, tropical Africa. For at least a century travellers' tales have hinted at the uncanny speed and accuracy whereby information is coded and decoded over considerable terrains of desert or jungle. Perhaps an element of exaggeration has crept in, but students of comparative linguistics now realise the basis of truth which underlies some of these reports. Furthermore they are now able to comprehend some of the mechanisms with which this form of communication is effected.

The literature is not extensive, and much of it is in the German language. Our knowledge in English is largely due to the writings of Dr. J. F. Carrington, a Baptist missionary who worked in the former Belgian Congo, and also to Stern. Carrington quoted some of the early references, the first of which was made by Francis Moore in 1730. Later, a governmental report of an expedition to the River Niger, published in 1841, described an African who said that his tribesmen could communicate over considerable distances by means of war-drums. These were kept in every village as a means of intimating danger long before the enemy could attack. It was suggested that this method of communication was also employed by the slave-traders to give notice of approaching vessels.

These remarks, as Carrington pointed out, referred to signals on drums, rather than to drum-talk. The latter, however, was specifically reported by H. M. Stanley. Speaking of the baEna tribe on the banks of the Congo at the site of what is now known as the Stanley Falls, he said that the natives possessed a system of communication as effective as electric signals. When struck in various parts, their huge drums could convey language as clear to the initiated as vocal speech.

R. E. Dennett, according to Carrington, described in 1881 the drum-talk of the Loango area . . . "a good operator with his drumsticks can say anything he likes upon it, in his dialect. . . . The drum language . . . is not limited to a few sentences, but, given a good operator, and a good listener, comprehends all a man can say."

As the result of careful field studies, it can now be asserted that communication by way of drums is something more than a matter of a few conventional signals such as Army bugle calls. Based upon the preponderance of the Sudanic and Bantu languages throughout the mid third of the African continent, we are now able to discern the mechanism behind the widespread drum-talk. The all-important factors are those of stress, and tonal patterns. In most of the central African languages, the tone is all-important, in that it conveys meaning, rather than mere emotional nuances. Precisely the same state of affairs obtains in the various tongues spoken in China. In Africa, however, the majority of the languages are strictly bitonal rather than multitonal, and this peculiarity is fundamental and crucial in articulate communication. For example, in the Kele language *lisáká* means a marsh, but *lisaká* is a promise, and *lisáká* a poison. This all-important system of bitonality pervades not only Kele but practically every other dialect and language of central Africa, with the possible exception of Ngwana.

Drum-talk depends essentially upon this significant bitonality. Two principal kinds of drums are used for communicative purposes:

(a) paired tambours, or drums with parchment tops, one high in pitch and the other low; and

(b) all-wooden drums constructed from hollowed tree-trunks; a longitudinal slit is made, with two lips. Percussion of one of these emits a high note, and of the other, a low. Usually the high note is designated "male", and the lower note "female".

In the case of skin tambours reference is made to male drums and female drums. The range of audibility is from five to seven miles.

In conveying a message the drummer, relying on the bitonal properties of his spoken tongue, strikes a male drum to represent a high tone, and a female drum the lower. In this way there is emitted an inanimate or mechanical replica of the spoken message. Thus if a Kele drummer wished to send a message to the effect that "the child has neither father nor mother", he would base his communication upon the sentence which in his spoken speech would run *wána atí la sángó la nyángo*. Consequently he would strike the drums in the following sequence: High-low; low-high; low; high-high; low; low-high (or male-female; female-male; female; male-male; female; female-male).

The risk of ambiguity at once becomes obvious. For example, such a word as *sango* (father) with its simple melodic pattern entails two high tones. Within the Kele tongue there are at least 130 other homotones or disyllabic words with exactly the same tonal pattern. Each one of these 131 words, when transmitted in drum-language, would sound alike. To ensure that the word which is in mind is understood, the signaller resorts to a device whereby he adds various qualifying or explanatory phrases. Exactly the same system is met with, to a minor degree, in that language so rich in homonyms, namely Chinese. Some of these amplifying terms in the Kele language are arresting by reason of their richness in metaphor. Thus "money" is specified in the Kele drum-language by virtue of the tacked-on phrase . . . "the pieces of metal which arrange palavers". A "dead body" in Kele drum-talk is transmitted as "the corpse lying on its back on the clods of earth". While carrying out this method of communication, the drummer can often be observed to hum quietly to himself the actual words.

Sometimes the expressions used to elaborate a message are terms no longer employed in the vernacular. Possibly they are in the nature of archaisms which have long ago dropped out of the spoken tongue, only to be retained in the more conservative drum-talk.

Another device employed to ensure comprehension is that of repetition—a feature which is well-known to contemporary information-engineers who utilise this in current systems of coding.

Hitherto the African drum-language has been a subject of interest only to anthropologists and linguists. To a neurologist, however, the matter offers a suggestive topic of considerable importance. Over a century ago Hughlings Jackson prophesied that by reason of cerebral disease a deaf-mute might well become deprived of his system of sign-language. Years later Grasset and then I proved this to be the case by recording instances of "aphasia" in deaf-mutes. Similarly I suggested over twenty years ago that a blind Braille reader might well lose his acquired tactuo-linguistic skill as the result of brain-damage. Such has since proved to be the case. In the same way it is tempting for an aphasiologist to surmise that an African drum-talker might possibly lose this particular aptitude as the result of a lesion of the brain. No such instance has yet been published, but conversation with physicians in West Africa has led to the strong suspicion that cases of this kind do occur. It would be fascinating to determine whether a unilateral or a bilateral lesion of the brain would be needed to ablate the ability to send or receive drum messages; and to investigate to what degree articulate speech would be correspondingly involved.

This is a research-project for future neurologists of the third world.

Whistle Languages

When serving during the war in West Africa, I first encountered an instance of communication by means of whistles between two Yoruba-speaking nations. Enquiry has subsequently revealed that this type of "language" also exists at times in various other parts of the world, e.g. in Turkish Caucasia, in Mexico, and in the Pyrénées. The most elaborate, and best-known instance of a whistling language is, however, the *Silbo* of the Canary Islands, especially La Gomera.

Neurologists from the Basque district have acquainted me with the capacity and range of this type of communication. Elaborate messages can be transmitted and identified, over a range of about five miles. From those who have studied in detail the nature of *Silbo,* it is clear that the whistling language has many features of resemblance with the drum-talk of Africa. Both depend upon the tonal properties of the underlying vernacular. *Silbo* is little more than whistled Spanish. The *silbador,* as he is called, merely transmutes the spoken language into its melodic components in whistled form. In La Gomera many children pick up and acquire *Silbo* shortly after they attain speech. The comprehension of *Silbo* ordinarily antedates the ability to transmit.

In the Canary Islands *Silbo* virtually constitutes a second language, and the Gomeros are, in a manner of speaking, bilingual. Just as in the case of articulate speech, personal idiosyncracies of *Silbo* gradually develop. A *silbador* learns to identify the *silbo* of his friends, and also to recognise his own whistled speech when he hears it recorded on tape. An experienced *silbador* can play tricks with the language: crack jokes, perpetrate *doubles entendres,* and other *jeux des mots.*

Aphasiologists would not be unduly fanciful, therefore, in expecting that a loss of whistling language, or of the art of perceiving *Silbo,* might well arise as the result of a cerebral lesion, focal or diffuse. A disorder of this faculty might exist alone, or in association with a defect in articulate utterance, expressive or receptive. No such case has yet been recorded in the literature. But as Oscar Wilde proclaimed: "There are two kinds of artist: one brings answers, and the other, questions. We have to know whether one belongs to those who answer or to those who question; for the kind which questions is never that which answers."

Reprinted from Critchley, M. (1968): *Revue de Med. Fonction.,* Vol. 1.

Corporeal Awareness:
Body-Image; Body-Scheme

The modern interest in body-image really began with the writings of the otologist Bonnier (1893–1905) who introduced the term "schematia" to indicate a composite sensory experience embracing the complete anatomical make-up of an individual. With greater precision, Henry Head and Gordon Holmes in 1911–1912 first drew attention—in not very clear language—to the mental idea which a person possesses as to his own body and its physical and aesthetic attributes. In their own words:

> The final product of the tests for the appreciation of posture or passive movement rises into consciousness as a measured postural change. For this combined standard, against which all subsequent changes of posture are measured before they enter consciousness, we propose the word "schema". By means of perpetual alterations in position we are always building up a postural model of ourselves which constantly changes. Every new posture or movement is recorded on this plastic schema. . . .

As practical and authoritative neurologists, Head and Holmes never for a moment realised that they had opened a Pandora's box which let loose a spate of metaphysics, much of it sheer verbiage. The next and very important intervention was made by P. Schilder who, in 1923, brought out his work *Das Körperschema*. Twelve years later it was expanded in his English monograph *The Image and Appearance of the Human Body*. Elsewhere I have described this book as a *chef d'oeuvre manqué*, a work which just falls short of being one of the great monographs of neurology. Like other famous precedents it began well but tailed off feebly.

The immediate post-Schilderian conceptions of the body-image focus around the 1939 monograph of J. Lhermitte. In 1949 Critchley lectured on the topic of "The Body-Image in Neurology" and, wittingly or not, this article when it appeared in print in 1950 triggered off a fresh mass of written material upon this subject at the hands of psychiatrists, neurologists, paediatricians, psychologists, and philosophers, much of which was of dubious value.

Definition and Terminology

The topic began to get out of hand. Terminology blossomed so that terms like "body image", "body schema", "corporeal schema", *"image de soi"* were employed more or less interchangeably. It soon became obvious that thinking was becoming so muddled that the various expressions were made to stand in the literature for wholly different ideas at different times by different writers. At one moment the idea was perceptual; at another it was a conceptual one. Part of the trouble was due to a lack of clear definition, the one put forward by Head and Holmes being more elucidatory than hermeneutic.

Obviously this chaotic state of affairs is untenable. Even though it may require later to be modified, some tentative definition should be advanced, as for instance "The idea which an individual possesses as to the physical properties of his own anatomy, and which he carries over into the imagery of his self".

The notion is a complex one, for it includes such activity as the imagery which one possesses and utilises during states of rumination or brooding, including the predormitum, and also states of dreaming. This is a purely conceptual matter. But in addition it includes actual bodily sensations which may be natural or unnatural in kind, arising from part or perhaps the whole of the anatomy. An obvious example is the phantom limb of an amputee. But the two notions, however cognate, are actually disparate. The former is imaginal, the latter mainly perceptual in nature, and yet both stand within the fabric of the terms "body-image" or "body-schema". Smythies has attempted to correlate body-image with the former and body-schema with the latter aspect of the problem. This, however, was a retrospective attitude and, however commendable the purpose, remains unacceptable. Clearly an all-embracing term is needed; one which combines conceptual with the more tangible perceptual components. The author therefore puts forward a plea for the acceptance of the less definitive term "corporeal awareness" to replace both body-schema and body-image.

It becomes important to determine the physiology of this idea of corporeal awareness and to trace its ontogeny. It is not an inborn entity but is one which grows up slowly as the child becomes older, though always tagging after to some extent. The development proceeds in a step-like rather than uniform fashion, advancing abruptly between the 7th and 8th year of age. Chief among the formative factors are the visual, the tactile, and the labyrinthine components. The visual factors are twofold in character. In the first place they comprise the information which the adolescent subject steadily accumulates from inspection of his own anatomy. This particularly applies to the body-segments, which are ordinarily exposed, e.g. the hands. In some primitive communities within the tropics, the body surface which is ordinarily exposed may be more extensive. The face occupies a special niche. It is an area of the body which is out of the range of sight of the individual. His only clue to his own facial appearance is afforded by inspection by way of reflection in a looking-glass or the surface of a pool. Opportunities for self-inspection are not always available, though there may be exceptional instances as in the case of an actor. Moreover the reflected image is in many ways an artificial simulacrum, for as soon as an individual gazes in a looking-glass, he strikes an attitude. The manifold facial mannerisms and little grimaces cease, and the mirror reflection is often merely a stylised and immobile still-life edition of what every bystander realises as something quite different.

We must remember too that the visual knowledge of one's self is never complete, whether by way of direct gaze or mirror-reflection. Certain areas remain *terrae incognitae,* for they cannot be inspected either directly or by any optical device, e.g. the occiput, the nape of the neck, and the interscapular area.

Ordinarily too the growing individual receives information from the visual observation of other persons. He learns to realise the standard height, the common facial delineaments, the postures, attitudes, and gaits of others, and the abundance of man's gestural world. Even two-dimensional representations in the way of photographs, portraits, and illustrations add their important quota to the visual component of one's own corporeal awareness. By determining a mean he can draw certain conclusions as to his own facial and bodily appearance.

The tactile factors which lead to the development of corporeal awareness consist in the proprioceptive impulses from the joints and muscles, especially in the course of vigorous movement. To these must be added the sum-total of exteroceptive data, e.g. the touch, painful, thermal messages ascending from part or whole of the body-surface. Other sensory components are made up of the complex of visceral sensations, both physiological and pathological.

Labyrinthine factors constitute the third constituent which builds up the body-image. Bonnier was indeed inspired by the considerable upsets in bodily feelings occurring in states of vertigo, and he spoke of the vestibular constituent of the 8th cranial nerve as *le nerf de l'espace.* However, these factors are not as important as the foregoing, which contribute more to the growth of an adult type of body-image.

An individual's body-image is by no means in the nature of a naked mannikin or homunculus. Not only is it ordinarily clad, but, according to the immediate circumstances, it may spread so as to involve inanimate objects which are in contact or in close proximity. The body-image of a motorist, an air-pilot, an equestrian temporarily includes part at least of the automobile, the aircraft, or the horse. A surgeon with his probe, a blind man with his white stick for the time being are endowed with an extension of corporeal awareness. This is the phenomenon sometimes spoken of as the "phantom body" or better still *"le spatialité de situation"*.

The importance of each of these factors can be well realised in those instances of deprivation of special sense-modalities since birth. For example the congenitally blind child year by year develops corporeal awareness in the absence of visual factors. Not only does he have no opportunity of studying his own anatomy or his own mirror-image, but he cannot observe the appearance of others around him. His sole means of acquiring knowledge as to the shape and surface of himself and others is through manual contact.

It is not surprising, therefore, that when a congenitally blind subject makes a drawing or a clay model of a man, odd deformations are displayed. This is particularly the case when the congenitally blind victim is of mediocre intellectual calibre. Those parts of the anatomy which are of special personal significance are apt to loom unduly large and therefore to take a conspicuous part in the drawings and models. For example, the hand with the sensitive fingers constitutes not only a manual tool, but also an organ of perception for making contact with the external world, animate and inanimate. A blind child when asked to draw a man may therefore pay particular attention to the fingers and hands, which may be of inordinate development and size to the detriment of the face and body. In the case of clay models of the head and neck, the mouth may occupy a predominant role, for it is by way of the lips, tongue, and oral cavity that the blind person speaks, feeds, breathes, and even, in certain circumstances, makes tactual exploration. In the models collected by Von Stockert executed by children of rather low intelligence, born blind, practically nothing existed except a sphere for the head and a huge crater with everted lips representing the mouth. Eyes, ears, nose, neck, and so on took little part in the art-form of such children.

Phantom Phenomena

Similarly, in persons deprived of a limb, corporeal awareness continues to operate so as to produce a phantom limb, which represents not the activity of severed peripheral nerves, but rather the body-image which continues to operate as though the individual were intact. One recalls the difficulty with which painful phantom limbs are ablated. Indeed nothing short of a cerebral insult, whether it be the intervention of a cerebro-vascular lesion causing a hemiplegia, or the surgical operation of parietal-cortical topectomy, stands any chance of ridding the patient of the painful phantom. The phantom limb may alter in size, shape, motility, and position in space with the passage of time, but it remains in some form or other a constant manifestation of the will for integrity. Even mental defectives who lose a limb develop a phantom for a while at any rate, indicating that past sensory input is more important than high cognitive levels.

There is a certain difference, however, in the degree of vividness of phantom limbs according to whether the segment has been lost surgically or through the slow intervention of disease. This is well illustrated in the case of patients with leprosy. Here progressive necrosis of the phalanges may lead to miniature stumps representing all that is left of the adult fingers, but in such cases a phantom finger does not follow. However, should the leper lose his arm either as the result of trauma or surgery, then a phantom arm will appear. Moreover, if the gangrenous stumps are amputated surgically, a phantom will follow representing the original intact fingers, and not the mere stumps.

It is of particular interest to enquire whether these phantom phenomena apply only to the extremities as Leriche affirmed. Can it be demonstrated that phantom segments sometimes occur after injury or surgical excision of other parts of the anatomy? Thus after removal of the nose, ear, breast, penis, do phantom organs follow? The question cannot be answered positively because the situation varies from one individual to another, and also depends upon the segment which is involved. Certainly loss of the anus after an abdomino-perineal excision of the rectum may be followed by a phantom orifice, ready for the passage of matter or gas. A phantom nose, a phantom penis, and even possibly a phantom eye have been described in the literature in a plausible fashion. Loss of an ear, however, is less assured and further enquiry along such lines would be rewarding. Riddoch stated that it was a question of prominence or protrusion of segments of the body which determines whether or not a phantom develops after surgery. The question of phantoms following the surgical loss of a breast is more complicated. For example the awareness of the existence of a breast is not ordinarily a conspicuous perceptual experience and it is at first sight not easy to decide what type of enquiry to pursue after mastectomy. However feelings are commonly referred to the breast or nipple in pregnancy, during menstrual periods, and in the course of sexual stimulation. These may well continue to appear after the surgical loss of one mamma. M. L. Simmel studied a series of 77 postmastectomy patients and obtained some evidence of a phantom in about 40%, especially among the younger, more intelligent, and more introspective subjects.

Another point of interest about phantom phenomena concerns the age at which phantom limbs appear; or rather, how often phantom limbs appear in the case of young subjects who have lost a limb through disease in early childhood and infancy. The results of enquiry establish that a body-image may be present at an earlier age than is commonly imagined, so that the loss of an arm or a leg in very early childhood may well be followed by an unequivocal phantom image. In my series a child of $3\frac{1}{2}$ years was endowed with a vivid phantom image of a limb lost two years previously. But in very young amputees the phantoms may be transient and afterwards be forgotten altogether. The situation is probably very different in cases of congenital absence of limbs, as for example in thalidomide babies. Such children as they grow to adulthood might not be expected to possess what might be called a phantom limb, in other words, an engram resulting from years of sensory stimulation. On the other hand it may happen that on the conceptual plane of corporeal awareness, the thalidomide victim of amelia, especially when older in years, during his day-dreaming state, or when planning future activities in which he visualises himself as participating, may possibly regard himself not as a creature apart, devoid of arms and legs, but as one orthodox member of the community, of average height, stature, and endowed with limbs. Thus E. Weinstein and E. A. Sersen, using a special "playing game" technique, have claimed that five out of 30 amelic children possessed phantoms. This observation suggested there might exist in such young persons a sort of built-in frame-work of the body-schema. Perhaps the presence or absence of phantom limbs in congenital amelics depends upon whether cortical and spinal neurons exist corresponding with the musculature of the missing bodily segments. This topic is one which merits further enquiry.

Phantom limbs may also occur, not after surgical intervention, but after paralytic disease, due to lesions at various levels of the nervous system. For example a patient paralysed as the result of a transverse lesion of the spinal cord, whatever the cause, and completely insensitive from the waist downwards, may not feel himself sawn across the middle like a conjuror's partner, but may experience some vague impression of his lower limbs. But the idea which he may entertain as to the length or posture of the limbs may be at complete variance with reality. Thus he may imagine his paralysed legs as being unusually short, or with the middle segments missing, so that the feet seem to be attached to the thighs. Or it may seem to him that the paralysed extremities are flexed at the hip and knees, whereas actually they lie in extension; or it may be the other way round. Phantom limbs can follow lesions of the nervous system not only at the spinal level, but even higher. Perhaps the most likely situation for such a phenomenon to develop is an abrupt vascular lesion deep in one or other parietal lobe. The resulting clinical picture will be that of a contralateral hemiplegia and hemianaesthesia, but the patient in his imagery may conceive of a phantom supernumerary limb, lying in an attitude quite other than is actually the case. The phantom third arm, for example, may seem to be in full extension and abduction at the shoulder, and not folded across the chest as the paralysed limb actually is. Or at times it may appear to move of its own accord, the true paralysed limb being devoid of volitional power. If, however, the paralysed limb be passively placed in the posture occupied by the phantom limb, then the two may merge, and the supernumerary limb disappears for the time being. In one case at least, the patient characteristically personified the phantom third limb, calling it "the intruder" or "that fellow".

That the phantom limb is something more than a mere concept and possesses many perceptual properties is shown by the fact that it can share in sensorial alterations along with the rest of the body. Thus when the patient is cold and shivering, the phantom limb too may seem to be subjected to goose-flesh. In more pathological conditions an amputee who develops peripheral neuritis may experience pains, tingling, and pins and needles in all extremities including the phantom limb. The itching of a generalised irritative dermatitis may also be experienced in the phantom limb. According to Ekbom, the syndrome of restless legs probably does not extend to a missing lower limb, though the stump may be involved in uncomfortable dysaesthesiae.

Some of the foregoing remarks may be exemplified in the following:

(1) A patient with traumatic paraplegia with a level at Th. 8 was given an instillation of intrathecal alcohol. Thereafter, spasticity was replaced by flaccidity, and both legs assumed an attitude of extension and abduction. The legs now felt heavy and very hot, and as if they were tightly touching each other.

(2) A case of traumatic paraplegia with a complete transverse lesion below Th. 7. Though the lower limbs were insensitive, the patient was aware of their existence, but felt as though the legs were perpetually crossed.

(3) An amputee with a phantom foot later became afflicted with a generalised peripheral neuritis of a painful character. These pains were especially marked in the phantom foot.

(4) A German prisoner of war sailor had lost his right arm. Later he contracted diphtheritic polyneuritis following which he experienced constant dysaesthesiae in his extremities including the missing hand.

(5) A Parkinsonian developed tingly discomfort, stiffness, and awkwardness of the right (actual) arm and also in his phantom left limb, which had followed an amputation. The patient began steadily to rely more on the phantom left arm as the right arm became more and more useless.

(6) An elderly man who had lost his two legs in the 1st World War developed phantom feelings of both feet, sometimes with pain. After a right-sided hemiparesis due to a stroke the patient completely lost the phantom sensation on *both* sides.

The Body-Concept

Turning for the moment to the more conceptual aspect of corporeal awareness, and dealing with one's own notion of self in certain situations past and future, we find considerations of striking interest. A striking lack of correspondence may be met with in the discrepancy between the true appearance of the anatomy as obvious to everyone around, and the notion which the individual himself entertains. The two may be entirely different. Although on an intellectual plane the patient probably realises and is able to express graphically the fact that he is bald-headed and gray haired, wrinkled, cadaverous, bowed in stance, and altogether changed, nevertheless he rarely for a moment regards himself in that way when he is thinking about his recent activities or what he was doing in the remote past, nor when he comes to project his thoughts into future plans. When he visualises himself on an intended holiday or business-trip, the body-image that he nurses in such circumstances is that of an individual considerably younger than the actual one. In other words, the body-image does not keep pace with the increasing alterations in the features and build so obvious to others, but lags behind. The degree of difference varies: first of all according to age, the gap becoming wider and wider as the years go by, and secondly according to the state of the individual's well-being. If he should happen to feel well and vigorous, healthy and refreshed, then his body-image becomes that of his far younger self. However, if the contrary is the case, and the ageing individual feels tired, depressed, or in pain, it is more likely that his corporeal awareness will conform closely with that of his actual appearance. A discrepancy between image and reality is often strikingly brought home to the person concerned when he inspects snapshots which were taken of him by other members of the family, and with which he expresses rather shocked dissatisfaction, protesting perhaps that the photograph is a bad one and is nothing like him.* Some inkling as to the nature of the body-image in the crippled may be discovered through the medium of a "draw-a-man" test. A child with cerebral palsy is liable to omit one or more limbs. One of my patients who had been afflicted with alopecia drew an elaborate figure of a man, but omitted the usual scribble depicting hair. It is also apt to show itself at a reunion of alumni, where his class mates at college who qualified together, and then parted, meet at some function 20 or 30 years later. Each individual probably looks at the others and thinks to himself how old his contemporaries are looking, never for a minute realising that he too appears to them at least as changed.

Another interesting discrepancy probably occurs between persons who are markedly unconventional in body-build, height, or appearance. Such crippled or deformed persons may in an intellectual fashion be able to describe precisely their configuration, but not for a moment do they visualise them-

---

* D'Annunzio wrote in his old age, "I have just received the photograph which was taken yesterday. It is ruthless, for it shows me as I am, and my face just as it is. Nevertheless, whilst riding today, I experienced inexplicably youthful sensations." (Quoted by J. Todd and K. Dewhurst.)

selves as such in their browsing or day-dreaming moments. The stunted achondroplasiac, the man who is unduly tall or grossly overweight; the individual who has been disabled from old poliomyelitis and is left with a withered limb; the albino; the man with a grotesque rhinophyma; and the old pottique stunted from extreme scoliosis, may not for a moment imagine himself as being different from anyone else although, in his sober moments of cold reflection, he knows full well the extent of his anomaly. This particularly applies to those who are well below the average height—the midget, the achondroplastic dwarf, and the victim who has lost both legs at the hip-joints. If we accept for a moment the notion put forward by Claparède that the focus of most vivid imagery lies at a point somewhere between the two eyes, and that one looks out onto the world from such a height, then the midget must be someone quite different. In his ordinary waking moments, instead of inspecting his entourage from a height of five to six feet, he is always peering upwards. But what about his times of loneliness, as for example when dropping off to sleep at night? Does he, in thinking forward or reminiscing backward, still gaze up at a world of pseudo-giants; or does he imagine himself an equal? It is probable that at such times he does and that the discrepancy for the moment does not exist.

Another consideration regarding the body-concept concerns its location in outer space with reference to the actual body. A difference probably occurs according to whether one thinks forward or thinks backward. Perhaps it can be said that when an individual indulges in a reverie and broods upon some past event in which he has participated, then the imagery becomes concentrated on himself, and he stands entirely within his own self and looks around. In other words his own body-image occupies the central or nodal point whereby he looks upon himself as an actor and not an on-looker. However, when the individual switches from the past and looks into the future, in order to plan some activity—a voyage, a piece of work, a social occasion—then he probably sees himself as a participant, looking upon himself not from afar, but as an *alter ego* standing close by, perhaps to one side of the imagined actor in the future scene.

These statements may hold for conditions which are more or less normal. If, however, one considers the situation when the subject is not in vigorous health, but very unwell, then the situation might be different indeed. Even with the normal person, subjected temporarily to a state of ecstacy, as for example when passively or actively participating in music, there may occur an intense depersonalisation leading to a wide dislocation between the actor and the onlooker. The singer who is carried away by his song may visualise himself as seated at the back of the theatre. The same applies to an orchestral conductor who, as the music sweeps him on, seems to drift further and further into the distance, looking on at a miniature performer. Something comparable may occur in orgasmic experiences. The relevant literature contains one piece of fine writing on the part of a female observer . . .

Gradually there is a very acute awareness of every individual component of my body as if each part had a separate longing of its own. All these longings gather together, drawn towards my innermost being, and then fall away from my insignificant matter. A state of fluidness seems to supervene and I discover to my great delight that my body does dissolve and that *I* can, and have escaped. For a brief moment I know myself without a body—only thus can this experience be described—and, on one or two occasions, from my exalted position, which is always to the left diagonally from and facing the body, I have been able to look down upon my shell. Surely the reality must be that complete self which has flown so swiftly out of the body, for it is *that* self which gazes so confidently upon what had seemed to be such a disordered array of meaningless parts each with its own sensation striving to assert itself, and which now lies immobile, inanimate, and totally unaware of the immense change that has overtaken it. It is only the material tool of my true reality.

On reflection, when the excitation has receded, I often wonder, provided consciousness could be retained, if dying would produce a similar experience. Fainting, a bodily lapse I have experienced a few times, has nothing in common and is certainly very dull and unpleasant when compared with the exhilaration of a being set free.

To a minor degree, I have felt a similar exhilaration, like a "walking on air" feeling, when listening to music, i.e. the fifth symphony by Sibellius, Beethoven's Pastoral, piano music of Chopin, and a Bach organ fugue. Wagnerian compositions and similar music give me a very real feeling of evil as if in giving myself to it completely I would awake to find I had sold my soul to the devil.

Heautoscopy

There is a phenomenon which approaches closely to this physiological phenomenon, namely the rare and very interesting instances of specular hallucination or heautoscopy, whereby an individual experiences not a vivid image, but a veritable visual hallucination of himself. This is a theme which was originally mentioned by Aristotle when writing of Antipheron and has since become dear to the writers of romantic literature even more than to neurologists and psychiatrists. The circumstances in which a veritable heautoscopy can occur—as apart from fictional notions—are states of ecstacy, of confusion, as well as during epileptic or migrainous equivalents. The first reference in pathology is perhaps that of the Swedish naturalist Linnaeus who from time to time had a very vivid image of himself, situated in natural circumstances and behaving in a natural fashion. Once he entered his study to find the image of himself seated in a chair writing or reading. Or as he would wander through his garden studying a plant or picking a blossom here and there, he might see some little distance away his *alter ego* performing the same actions, stopping to gaze at a flower and pluck it.

Corporeal Awareness in Various States of Disease

The notion of body-image is very much influenced by intercurrent physical disease, not necessarily neurological. Thus in almost any condition of localised pain the segment involved may obtrude itself unduly into the patient's awareness, and may be inescapable from the imagery. For example the pain of a fractured wrist may cause the affected arm to appear too big, too heavy, or too long. The same applies to regions of the body other than the limbs. Again during states of diarrhoea the focus of attention may be somewhere perineal. In dyspepsia, or even in the physiological circumstances of hunger, thirst, undue coldness, uncomfortable heat, sexual arousal, the body-image may undergo a more or less local enhancement. This would correspond with what Bonnier termed "hyperschematia" (or "macrosomatognosia"). Something similar is also met with in patients afflicted with states of partial paralysis. A limb which can be moved only with difficulty may appear unduly awkward, cumbersome, too long, too broad, and excessively heavy. Phenomena of this order are commonly experienced by patients with disseminated sclerosis. On the other hand, there may be a contrary state of affairs whereby a segment of the anatomy may seem to shrink, and even drop out of awareness. This is particularly so when a limb is completely paralysed and insensitive. Thus a patient with a total paralysis due to a brachial plexus injury may feel that the affected limb is shrunken and excessively light. He may or may not have a phantom limb as well. In some cases of hemiplegia, especially when the lesion lies in the non-dominant hemisphere, the affected limb may seem to the patient to be withered, and either too light and yet at other times too heavy. These phenomena correspond with a "hyposchematia" or "microsomatognosia". Something like this may be vividly experienced during states of vertigo. The famous surgeon John Hunter, who was liable to Menière-like attacks, described in arresting language how he would seem to shrink at such times and recede into the distance. In those rare conditions where the victim suffers generalised pain as opposed to localised pain, something similar may occur. The trauma of severe electric shock represents one of the few circumstances where pain is universally experienced, and there are vivid descriptions on record of how the electrocuted individual seems to shrivel up and almost attain the dimensions of a doll or puppet. In other pathological circumstances there may occur not so much an enhancement nor yet a decrement of the body-image, as a distortion which cannot strictly speaking be described in terms of plus or minus. Some of the most telling descriptions of this dysschematia, as we may call it, or deformation of the body-image, are to be met with in the delirious states due to certain drug intoxications. Here mescalin and L.S.D. are particularly potent, and the literature on this subject is rich in incisive descriptions of the personal feelings of distortion.

A few clinical instances may be quoted in illustration:

(1) During the acute symptoms of his cardiac infarction a patient felt as though he had become elongated and was 12 feet high. This feeling lasted two hours.

(2) In each attack of migraine, one hand would seem to be a very long way off.

(3) A woman of 41 with a left hemiparesis due to a fractured skull sustained when she was 5 also developed post-traumatic epilepsy. For the past two years she had had epileptic equivalents in which she would feel as if she were in two halves which would not connect. If she were to try and clap her hands they would miss each other. "I have to keep moving my left arm and leg to make sure that these limbs are part of me."

(4) A woman of 57 sustained temporal lobe attacks . . . "My head does not seem to be on my body any more, and the right side of the head is not there. The feeling is as if I were in the air, seeing my body lying on the bed, and I say to myself . . . 'get back there'."

(5) Following childbirth a woman of 28 sustained a sudden dysphasia and right-sided mild hemiparesis with severe right hemihypaesthesia. Lying relaxed in bed she would feel as though there was nothing there on the right side—even when she proceeded to move the paretic limbs.

(6) A patient with a left parietal meningioma had life-long attacks of migraine. In each of these the right side would feel bigger and swollen, as if there were a sharp line down the middle. The left side however would remain "calm, cool, and collected, while the right side would be tense, anxious, agitated, and highly-strung".

(7) D. D. Williams has described a case of traumatic temporal epilepsy. On the occasion of his first attack he was, as an engineer, engrossed in a problem entailing $\frac{1}{16}$th of an inch. Suddenly he experienced the feeling that if the $\frac{1}{16}$th were to leave the unit one (i.e. himself), he would lose consciousness. This indeed happened, and he sustained a convulsive seizure.

Corporeal Awareness: Hyperschematia and Narcissism

The body-image experience is, of course, a perfectly natural and normal one, but ordinarily it is by no means obtrusive, and is more likely to loom large only in states of solitude when the lonely individual is cogitating about his actions past or his future activities. It is a notion which possibly may elude the descriptive powers of one who is not of high intelligence or whose vocabulary is limited. Therefore it is more likely to be comprehended by those of high intelligence, particularly introspective and intelligent psychopaths, where we find perhaps the most flamboyant descriptions of all. In one particular psychiatric anomaly, body-image is all-important; I refer of course to states of narcissism. Here the subject takes an inordinate and un-conscionable interest in his bodily appearance and his subjective sensations and he may constantly alter his activity so as to check up his appearance, or to embellish it or to commit it to posterity. Mirrors and portraits may occupy an unduly important role. He or she may adorn the visage with cosmetics to an inordinate degree. The male may indulge in elaborate and unconventional hair-styles and grow whiskers, beards, and other facial adornments as if obeying some urge to express his odd personality. Elabo-rate headgear may be an instance of narcissism and play an important and deliberate role in the scheme of things. During the German occupation of France some women were able to express their personalities only by wearing the most outrageous headgear which became more and more complicated and extraordinary as the restrictions of the invader increased. Narcissism may be exemplified in primitive persons by deliberate deformation of the anatomy. For example scarifying the body, tattooing the face, inserting discs of wood into the lips or into the lobes of the ears, or transfixing the nose with skewers. A pathological state of the body-image can also be pointed to in the well-known case of the ageing beauty which might be called the "Miss Havisham Phenomenon".

Disorders of Corporeal Awareness and Parietal Disorders

The story of the manifold anomalies of corporeal awareness which may follow brain-disease has often been told and is now familiar to neurologists and psychiatrists. For this reason the various disorders may merely be enumerated. At one end of the scale of defect is simple passive neglect of one limb during what should have been a bimanual activity. More patho-logical is the syndrome of active unilateral neglect whereby the patient fails to wash, dry, make-up, or clothe one side of the anatomy. When hemiparesis is a conspicuous feature the patient may display various degrees of aware-ness. There is anosognosia which, though strictly speaking indicates lack of knowledge of the defect, is often extended to the more grave condition of denial of paralysis. Intermediate reactions include illusory projection of the defect on to some unimportant peripheral disorder (e.g. a sprain, rheuma-tism, etc.). Another is met with in an unexpected lack of concern over the fact of paralysis (anosodiaphoria). Patients who display deeper levels of disintegration may go so far as to deny the ownership of the paralysed limb, and indulge in fantastic confabulation. Quite different is the case where awareness of hemiplegia exists but with a morbid and almost illusory reac-tion towards the paralysed limb. This misoplegia or hatred of paralysis may be associated with the idea that the palsied arm is shrivelled, ugly, claw-like. Much commoner is the attitude of the chronic hemiplegic who may come to look upon his affected limb as if it were a puppet or play-thing, in a sort of playful semi-detachment. This so-called personification of the paralysed limb is illustrated by the patient's facetious or semi-serious habit of endowing it with a nick-name.

It is conventional to regard these organic anomalies of corporeal awareness as the expression of disease of the non-dominant parietal lobe. Although the volume of clinical supporting evidence is impressive, there are other attitudes which merit serious consideration. Briefly, the current hypotheses comprise the following:

(1) That corporeal awareness is a faculty localised within the non-dominant parietal lobe;

(2) That it is a parietal faculty in essence, but that lesions of the dominant hemisphere preclude the demonstration of defects, owing to concomitant aphasia;

(3) That the various types of unawareness are not necessarily parietal symptoms, but may occur with lesions of the brain in any situation. This is the "denial syndrome" of Weinstein and Kahn;

(4) That the reaction of a patient towards his hemiplegia is the resultant of his previous personality;

(5) That the demonstration of these various types of unawareness is largely as iatrogenic clinical artefact, the product of the peculiar interpersonal relationship as between doctor and patient.

Space will not permit full discussion of these points. Suffice it to say that these foregoing hypotheses are not mutually exclusive.

Reprinted from Critchley, M. (1955): *Encephale (Paris)*, Vol. 6.

Man's Attitude to His Nose

In many respects the human nose is a vestigial organ. Aside from its function as a respiratory passage with its perpetual vulnerability to infection, its olfactory activity has waned. Instead of the macrosomatic brains of certain mammalia, man becomes endowed with a pallium. In the ontogenetic development of many of the lower mammals the well-developed smell-brain is associated with a specialisation of the cranium. The fore-part elongates so as to constitute a conspicuous muzzle or snout-formation. At the tip we observe a highly sensitive cap of mucous membrane which is kept continuously moist. This delicate organ is receptive not only to a rich variety of olfactory stimuli—most of which are too subtle for human perception—but also to purely tactile impressions. Behind and alongside are *vibrissae* or feelers which enable the creature to "nose its way around". This combined olfacto-tactual sensitivity is what Edinger spoke of as the "oral sense". With a change from a terrestrial to an arboreal mode of life, the smell-brain becomes down-graded, for the tree-dwelling mammal no longer requires for its survival a supersensitive olfactory sense, but instead a combination of keen sight, binocular vision, and prehensile fore-limbs.

G. K. Chesterton well expressed in verse this inferior function of man's nasal organ:

> They haven't got no noses
> The fallen sons of Eve;
>
> They haven't got no noses,
> They haven't got no noses,
> And goodness only knowses
> The noselessness of Man.

In man, therefore, olfaction is of subordinate importance. Its presence, however, is dramatically brought to the surface in certain disease-states, particularly in the temporal epilepsies, where the most bizarre and complex hallucinatory experiences can develop out of olfaction bringing into its ambit diverse, almost ineffable, synaesthetic phenomena. So complicated are these hallucinatory aurae that they often defy verbal description. This explains the patient with temporal lobe seizures reported years ago by Sir David Ferrier, who said that each of her attacks was preceded by a smell which reminded her of "green thunder".

My object is not to discuss the chemical and psychological aspects of the world of smell—much as I would like to do so. I only wish I had the time to discuss the olfactory accomplishments of the dog, with its abilities to perceive and discriminate odours, to attach meaning to them, and thereby derive curious pleasures which we can but dimly comprehend. The rival theories of chemical reception are intriguing, but we must pass on. . . .

What concerns us more is not the sense of smell, but its anatomical receptor, the nose. More particularly I would like to discuss man's attitude towards his own nasal organ.

Of course this problem is merely part of a larger topic, namely that of the body-image. This is a term which is applied to the notion which a person entertains as to his own body—its size, shape, appearance, and so on. It is essentially an "image", being partly perceptual, partly conceptual, partly an intellectualism. The body-image is not present at birth but is something which slowly develops as the result of an interaction of various factors, visual, tactile, proprioceptive, and experiential.

Corporeal awareness—a term which is preferable to the more common expression body-image—is by no means a simulacrum which reflects the actual configuration of the body like a statue or portrait. The focus of awareness may shift from one segment to another according to a complex of circumstances, exogenous and endogenous, physiological as well as pathological.

For many reasons, the finger-tips, the hands, and the face occupy a particularly important role. One obvious explanation is that of visual availability, for these structures are ordinarily uncovered and readily scrutinised either directly or in a mirror.

A very special category within the total complex or corporeal awareness is occupied by the nose—"that bone and gristle penthouse", as it has been termed. Though sensitive both to superficial and deep modalities of stimulation, the nose is largely devoid of proprioception. It possesses only a very limited range of motility. Perhaps it was for this reason that Coleridge said that the basic reason for the existence of a nose was to take snuff. It cannot be directly viewed by the subject, though in a mirror-reflection it is perhaps the most conspicuous landmark, and one which immediately comes into view. For this reason Ambrose Bierce called it "the extreme outpost of the face". Although invisible to the owner, it is open to the gaze of all and sundry, particularly as it is almost always stark and unconcealed. At a peculiar disadvantage, the nose stands exposed with all its physical attributes, of which the subject is the sole person whose knowledge is obtained at second-hand. Although Shakespeare spoke of the nose as being "inscrutable, invisible—like a weathercock on a steeple", it is so only to the owner: to everyone else it is a beacon, cynosure, or a spectacle.

Edward De Bono explored the developing body-image of the child by getting a number of youngsters to draw pictures of possible elaborations of the human anatomy which might come about in some ideal technological age of the future. One little boy made a drawing with the nose away from the face, relegating it to some situation on a lower limb near the ground. The young artist explained this by writing "I whant my nose on my legs, so that I can smell if any bad man have come my way, and I would like my nose a very strong smelling nose and a very long nose so I can smell a long way like a cat. It will work when you press a buton evrething hapens. . . ."

With these inherent shortcomings, the individual—who has only the recollection of a mirror-reflection to guide him—is very liable to harbour an incorrect notion as to its physical properties, or to be unduly sensitive as to its blemishes. Everyone suffers a potential organ-inferiority when it comes to one's nose. According to a Scottish proverb, "he that has a muckle nose thinks everybody is speaking of it". Anomalies in size, or shape, or colouring are liable to be magnified in a way which rarely applies to other body-parts, e.g. eyes, mouth, hands, legs. Those with a dermatological problem show a particularly severe reaction when the eruption invades the skin of the nose. That grotesque deformity which is known as rhinophyma often evokes a serious consequential depression. Pierpont Morgan was a victim of this deformity. Perhaps this explains his perpetual misery and his twin obsessions, the predatory collection of art treasures and the acquisition of other people's gold. A red nose is a source of shame, all the more so because of its common correlation with alcoholic tippling. This was emphasised by Shakespeare when he referred to Bardolph's nose as ". . . all bubukles and whelks and knobs and flames of fire". The Restoration playwright, Beaumont, rightly indicated that dyspepsia rather than strong drink was the immediate factor:

> Nose, nose, jolly red nose,
> And who gave thee that jolly red nose?
> Nutmeg and ginger, cinnamon and cloves,
> And They gave me this jolly red nose.

This verse illustrates the ridicule commonly attached to an inflamed nose, particularly when of blatantly large size. Immediately we think of the circus clown, and, of even greater antiquity, the *Punchinello* of the *Commedia dell'Arte*. George Speaight has recently afforded us a scholarly history of the origins of this particular puppet show. *Punchinello* was already in 1625 depicted as having a prominent hooked nose, which over the subsequent years became more and more exaggerated so as eventually to extend to his wife Judy—originally Columbine. Swift wrote in the 17th century:

> If Punch, to stir their fancy, shows
> In at the door his monstrous nose,
> Then sudden draws it back again;
> O what a pleasure mixed with pain!

On the continent the conspicuous feature of the principal marionette player is illustrated in "The Nose" of the Antwerp cellar theatres, and "Long Nose" of the puppet shows of Lille. Occasionally the victim makes deliberate capital out of his imperfection by a process of over-compensation, as with the American comedian "Schnozzle" Durante. We have only to throw our memories back a few years to recall Barbra Streisand of *Funny Girl*. Critics were unanimous in praising her great talents despite her nose which was likened now to a sign-post, now to a snow-plough. A classic case is that of Cyrano de Bergerac who, according to Rostand, boasted "My nose is huge! Vile snub-nose, flat-nosed ass, flat-head, let me inform you that I am proud of such an appendage, since a big nose is the proper sign of a friendly, good, courteous, witty, liberal, and brave man, such as I am."

Then he went on to enumerate these attributes in the following way: *Aggressive:* "I sir, if that nose were mine, I'd have it amputated—on the spot!" Friendly: "How do you drink with such a nose? You ought to have a cup made specially." *Descriptive:* "'Tis a rock—a crag—a cape—A cape? say rather, a peninsula!" *Inquisitive:* "What is that receptacle—a razor-case or a portfolio?" *Kindly:* "Ah, do you love the little birds so much that when they come and sing to you, you give them this to perch on?"

These various remarks recall the sexual connotation of the nose and the implication of size with masculinity. In a woman a nose which is too long, or too fleshy, is often aligned with a lack of apposite feminancy, and bears ugly hints of sexual inversion. Nevertheless, a too-small nose in a woman is rarely attractive, and Pascal stressed *"Le nez de Cléopatre si'il eut eté plus court, toute la face de la terre aurait changée."* Incidentally, the independent and current evidence is all to the effect that Cleopatra was none too glamourous in profile and that her nose was disappointingly fleshy.

In Spain, the word *chata* means literally a small, flat nose, and it is often applied to a woman as a term of endearment. But to speak of a man as *chato* is to cast aspersions upon his virility.

Patrick Miller has graphically expressed some of these ideas:

. . . the nature of the feminine nose cannot be fully appreciated, in its delicacy as a central feature, unless compared with the masculine feature; and that such comparison emphasises the invulnerability of masculine beauty. A man's nose . . . need have no bones about it. It is clearly an organ which smells, and which is used for sniffing both up and down. It is none the worse for being weather-beaten. Nor is its attractiveness necessarily spoilt by a slightly swollen or reddened appearance. Even a nose which has a slight tendency to drip does not matter so long as the man, its owner, is large-boned, dark in colour, and preferably a Scot. It is understood, of course that such a man should carry his handkerchief in his sleeve. But a woman's nose, like a camouflaged aerodrome, must not betray its function. It must only say, "I am a central beauty." A woman shows her disappointment, pleasure, or disdain with her nose, by means of hardly perceptible tilts, tiny dilatations. Some men—stockbrokers, merchants, house agents, and antique dealers —betray their calculations by movements of the nose; but they betray themselves, while women explain themselves. We . . . will only refer to one common superstition about noses. It is said that women prefer to put them in most things, and can seldom follow straight behind them to any given point. [*Women in Detail,* 1947]

In the male, a large nose, even thought unsightly, is often popularly endowed with certain advantages, particularly virility. Napoleon always selected a man with a long nose when he wanted good handwork done. In Italy a big nose correlates with intelligence. According to Guadagnoli . . . *"[che] indizio e un naso maestroso e bello, di gran . . . e di gran che? Di gran cervello [i.e. uccello]"*.

Correlation of a large aquiline or beak-like nose with the qualities of determination and martial skill is shown in our imagery of de Gaulle and more particularly the Iron Duke.

Other titbits of facial folk-lore have identified the aesthetic nose of Tennyson, the melancholy nose of Charles Kean, the busybody nose of Colette, and the executive nose of John Ruskin.

Other historical personages have been noted for their large noses, like Numa Pompilius (6 inches long), Plutarch, Lycergus, and Solon. But the accolade belongs to Thomas Wadhouse of Yorkshire, a mental defective who lived in the 18th century and whose nose measured $7\frac{1}{2}$ inches. Contrariwise, an undersized nose was observable in the Duc de Guise, the Dauphin d'Auvergne, and William of Orange.

Perhaps this question of size was the idea behind Proust's statement " . . . if the eyes are sometimes the organ through which our intelligence is revealed . . . the nose is generally the organ in which stupidity is most readily displayed".

If only plastic surgeons were as skilled in psychological thinking as in technique they would doubtless have much to impart of significance. Perhaps this was in Proust's mind when he wrote, "Thus a particular woman . . . who had now acquired an unforeseeable bridge on her nose, occasioned the same surprise, often an agreeable one, as a sensitive and thoughtful remark, a fine and high-minded act which one would never have expected of her. Unhoped for horizons opened around that new nose."

Since the time of Taliacotius in the 16th century, the nose has perhaps been the object of more cosmetic surgery than any other organ or body-part. Big noses have been chiselled; retroussé noses have been built up; deflected or fractured noses have been straightened in clinics all over the world by reason of feelings ranging from bleak inferiority to sheer vanity.

A surgeon who tinkers with the contours of an unsightly nose lays himself open to risks greater than he may envisage. I know at least one rhinologist who perished at the hands of a particular patient dissatisfied with cosmetic surgery to his nose which he had endured.

The actor Derek Nimmo has explained how the shape of his nose influenced his career: how when he first went into show business his director advised him to specialise in baby-faced villains. He was born with a straight nose but in the wolf-cubs he tripped and fell on to his face. His nose became squashed, and it was then that he was cast for sinister roles in the theatre. Eventually his mother advised him to submit to a plastic operation. When the surgeon took off the bandages he realised something had gone wrong, and offered to take a bone-graft from his hip and give him a beautiful straight nose. Derek Nimmo did not take advantage of this offer, but is keeping it up his sleeve in case his comedy parts dry up.

Racial implications must not be overlooked, and we are mindful of the ethnic aspects of the nasal structure of Jews and Amerindians. Throughout the centuries a comparison has been drawn between that which rates high in the scale of beauty and desirability—the Grecian nose, the Roman nose, the aquiline nose—with the converse, where the bulbous and the fleshy proboscis and the ridiculous snub-nose are relegated.

The modest, if unusual, rank of the nose within the hierarchy of corporeal awareness raises one or two questions for consideration. Why do young children display so strange an interest, if not in the nose itself, in the nostrils—a preoccupation which they perhaps extend to other bodily openings and orifices? Their folk-lore is eloquent on the subject. They associate nasal configuration with personality-traits, and align a turned-up nose with "cockiness" or disdain; a long nose with "nosiness" or inquisitiveness; and a Roman or "beaky" nose with courage. Young children have a rich store of descriptive adjectival terms like ferret nose, jelly nose, pig nose, cucumber nose, Peggy parrot nose, cheese-cutter. A red nose is known as Rudolph (the red-nosed reindeer). Rude little boys have an unpleasant habit of digital exploration or nose-picking. Indeed this manoeuvre constitutes one of the shoddier functions of the human thumb, the adductivity of which is man's proudest prerogative. Little girls, and boys too for that matter, not infrequently insert various foreign bodies for obscure reasons forgotten by most adults. Sometimes they cannot be retrieved, and every casualty surgeon acquires skill in dislodging such intruders as dried peas, beads, coffee beans, cherrystones, and (fifty years ago) shoe-buttons. Occasionally the child is reluctant to confess, and years later rhinoliths have been discovered which turn out to be concretions surrounding forgotten steel-rings, thimbles, and many other unlikely objects. But quite apart from the sly and secretive invasion of the air-passages, the nostrils are not infrequently the bolt-hole of inquisitive living creatures. The offbeat literature of surgery contains records of flies, worms, leeches, centipedes, and maggots, living and breeding here in security often to the serious detriment of the host. There is an account of a small lizard which crawled up the nose of an unwary Indian.

The creature's pungent urine caused local blistering and ulceration, which terminated in death.

The nose as a promontory rather than an air-passage is often incorporated within the gestural language of children. Almost international is that mark of derision, the cock-snook. Its origins are mysterious, and students of sign-language remain uncertain as to why a thumb to nose with full digital abduction should be used in order to infuriate the onlooker.

Gordon H. Wright made an interesting anatomo-linguistic study of the popular nomenclature of body-parts. He listed from the general literature the names of 65 organs which occur most often, from which he was able to construct a "linguistic body-image". According to Eaton's 1940 "Semantic Frequency List" with scores which ranged from 1.0–10.0 the nose rated comparatively high, namely 1.7 (being exceeded by such conspicuous regions as the arm, body, eye, face, foot). Wright then proceeded to make the bold step of invoking the mythical *homunculus* of Penfield, believed to be represented upon the sensori-motor cortex of the brain. Of the 43.8 mm which was the speculated extent of cortex devoted to the "representation" of the head and neck, 1.7 mm was allocated to the nose.

The impact of linguistics upon the neurology of the nose reminds us of the rich vocabulary of synonyms which are attached to this organ. Thus in the English language we find snout, snoot, nozzle, muzzle, proboscis, beak, bill, pecker, nib, neb, smeller, hooter, beezer, bugle, snot-box, snorer, schnozzle (Yiddish), conk, snitch, boko. The same language is endowed with a wealth of metaphorical terms associated more or less intimately with the nasal organ (e.g. nose in the air = disdainful; to turn up one's nose = to look down upon; putting one's nose out of joint = to offend; under one's nose = immediacy; to nose around or nose into = to inquire over-zealously; to nose out = to uncover; nosiness = undue curiosity). Not surprisingly Dickens referred to Conkey Chick in Oliver Twist as "Nosey".

Still on the topic of linguistics, it can be mentioned how often the phonemic cluster /sn/ at the beginning of a word seems to imply words of a pejorative kind, arising out of the audible expiration of air through the nostrils, and standing for ideas which are something more or less concerned with olfaction, or with something which is disagreeable, something which "stinks". Thus in the English language we have such terms as snout, snot, sniff, snort, snarl, snooty, snitch, sneer, snide, snail, snatch, snuffle, snag, snivel. For some obscure reason the German language illustrates this type of phonemic-semantic linkage in the case of the initial /sm/ as well as /sn/. Thus to quote Guy Endore, we find: "Why have we so many words beginning with SCHM all of which refer to something dirty? There is the word itself *schmutz. Schmeissfliege, Schmutziges Geschmeiss, schmatzend im Schmadder. Und warum beginnen schnappen, Schnabel, schnalzen, schnauben, schnauze, schneuzen, schnufflen, schnupfen, schnurren alle mit 'schn'?"*

Strangely enough this sort of onomatopoeia does not apply to Latin, French, Italian, or Spanish.

Lastly, we turn to the question of the phantom nose. Although it was at one time stated that phantom sensations follow the loss of the extremities only, this we now know not to be the case. Riddoch believed that the surgical ablation of any protuberant part of the body could be followed by a phantom. This certainly applies to the nose, and a particularly vivid instance has been recorded in 1955 by J. Hoffman.

A 14th century surgical treatise dealt with the question of prosthesis. "Are there any authenticated cases" it was asked, "where caoutchouc, or any other substance, has been used to make a false nose when a real one has been removed by a sword-thrust or by some accident?" Even gold has been used as in the case of the Danish astronomer Tycho Brahe. But an early monograph is that written in 1816 by J. C. Carpue, Surgeon to the York Hospital, Chelsea. According to the *Oracle* 1883, ". . . every surgeon of any practice has made false noses. The materials are various. From caoutchouc, or similar substances, they are usually but a very imperfect makeshift. A better plan is to make a real living nose from the skin of the arm or forehead. The operation is a good one; usually quick, successful, and with the additional advantage that one can have the choice (not accorded to ordinary mortals, whose noses are born with them) of a Grecian nose, or a Roman nose, or a nose 'tip-tilted, like the petal of a flower'. Any good surgeon would undertake the case."

May we in conclusion backtrack from the nose as an anatomical excrescence, to its principal function as the organ of smell. Though vestigial in many ways in man, olfaction is capable of refinement in circumstances of increasing maturity or civilisation. Contrast the crude gustatory pleasures of primitive peoples with the delicacy of the *bon vivant*. What a gulf separates the table habits of the Naga, who relishes the flesh of decomposing dogs, with the *gourmet,* who can assign a vintage to a Chateau Mouton Rothschild and can experience to the full the fragrant bouquet of a Pouilly fumé. Thus we find a renaissance of the essential function of the nasal organ, and in the truly cultured and sophisticated gastronome we witness a resurrection of the smell-brain. In this connection we may quote Brillat-Savarin, the greatest authority on food and cooking, who proclaimed that "for unknown foods, the nose acts always as a sentinel and cries 'who goes there?' "

No one has expressed these ideas better than Poulain and Jacquelin, authors of *Vins et Vignes de France*. "Now watch this gourmet. His face becomes vacant. His eyelids close and his gaze becomes lost in some far off mist. The nose alone remains alive. And what a nose! A nose with nostrils spread, diabolically voluptuous and mobile. A nose full of curiosity delicate as amber. A nose dainty with aromas, a great virtuoso of their gamut of a thousand scents. A lucid cultured nose which evaluates, classifies and compares. A wise, translucent nose. A nose which knows! In fact, a nose!" (*"Maintenant, observons ce gourmet. Son visage s'éteint. Ses paupières se ferment ou son regard se perd dans on ne sait quelle lointaine brume. Seul, le nez manifeste l'existence. Et quel nez! Un nez aux ailes éployées, voluptueux et mobile en diable. Un nez plein de curiosité, fin comme l'ambre. Un nez friand de bouquets, grand virtuose de leur gamme aux mille et une senteurs. Un nez lucide, cultivé, qui évalue, compare et classe. Un nez sagace, transcendant. Un nez qui sait! Enfin, un Nez!"*)

Reprinted from Critchley, M. (1970): *Transactions of Hunterian Society of Lonodon*, Vol. 29.

Misoplegia, or Hatred of Hemiplegia

Misoplegia is a term applied to the phenomenon whereby a hemiplegic patient develops a morbid dislike directed towards the offending immobile limbs. It is not a hostile or paranoid reaction towards the actual fact of his being crippled or paralysed. Misoplegia is not a common state of affairs. Perhaps it is more often met with in patients with a left hemiplegia than with a right, assuming, of course, that they were right-handed before they sustained their brain lesions.

Since Babinski's original description in 1914, we have been familiar with the conception of an anosognosia whereby a left hemiplegic after an abrupt paralysis is obviously temporarily unaware of the fact that his limbs are paralysed. This, of course, is a commonplace reaction, but only when the cerebral lesion is of an acute or fulminating character. If the patient's sensorium is cloudy, he may go further, and proceed to deny the fact that he is paralysed when directly questioned. As yet neurological nomenclature holds no single term to stand for this *denial* of hemiplegia. Superimposed upon this phenomenon, and from searching cross-examination at the bedside, it may be found that the patient is developing various degrees of confabulation. That is to say, when directed to move his affected limb, he may proclaim he has done so, when indeed he has done nothing of the sort. Or he may move the opposite limb and attempt to persuade the examiner that he has satisfactorily flexed or extended the paralysed limb. Or, in a most bizarre fashion, he may deny the actual ownership of the limb. As the interrogation continues, and he is asked to whom the paralysed limb belong, he may resort to a confabulatory projection and proclaim that the paralyzed arm and leg are the limbs of someone else, close by or remote, real or imaginary.

This anosognosia—so well described and elaborated by the studies of the Mount Sinai School of Neurology—tends to fade in the ensuing days or weeks after the acute onset of the illness. This change in attitude is, in part, due to the intervention of nurses in attendance, visiting relatives, and the doctor in charge of the case. In other words, the patient eventually becomes aware not only that he has a left arm and leg but that they are actually helpless and out of control.

Here again, we may view at the bedside a number of diverse types of confabulation, associated with various anomalies of corporeal awareness or body-image. Thus, the patient may perhaps admit grudgingly that he is well and truly disabled. However, he may seek to explain away the disability as being due to some peripheral disorder, fancied or factual, but in the latter case quite insignificant and irrelevant. Thus the patient may attribute his paresis to an arthritis, sprain, old fracture, etc. This again is a transient state of affairs. Later he may come to accept the paralysis for what it is, a hemiparesis of cerebral origin. However, he displays not so much a euphoric attitude, as a light-hearted acceptance of the disablement, shutting his eyes and ears to the probable repercussions of his stroke regarding his future employability and wage-earning capacity. In other words he treats his illness in a peculiarly carefree, almost jaunty fashion, and may even joke about the curious heaviness or awkwardness of the affected arm and leg. Again, this phenomenon was also described by Babinski under the term "anosodiaphoria", which literally means "lack of concern over the existence of a disability". This frame of mind may persist and may prove detrimental to the success of his treatment in that the patient may fallaciously regard re-education and rehabilitation as quite unnecessary.

As even commoner, and very intriguing experience is that which I have described under the term "personification of the paralysed limbs". Developing sometime after an initial anosognosia, it can in some ways be regarded as a diametrically opposite attitude, perhaps a pattern of over-compensation. A patient so affected has now come to accept the paralysis as a fact, but he appears to be almost detached about it, somewhat of an onlooker. The paralysed arm and leg now come to be regarded almost as things apart from the rest of the anatomy, as if they were foreign bodies. The useless limbs are referred to as though they were invested with a personality or identity of their own, but in a semi-facetious and proprietary fashion, as one might perhaps show towards a plaything or pet. The patient perhaps speaks of his arm and leg in a sort of baby-talk. A hemiparetic male may refer to the paralysed arm as "she" or "it", while a female patient more often speaks in terms of "he" or "him". More often still nicknames are attached to the affected limbs in a childish fashion. I have personal knowledge of patients who have called their paralysed arm "George", "Toby", "silly Billy", "lucky Joe", "Baby", "Gammy", "Hermione", "the immovable one", "the curse", "lazybones", "the nuisance", "old useless", "silly Jimmy", "floppy Joe", "Fanny Ann", "Dolly Gray". A patient recorded by Gilliat and Pratt referred to her paralysed arms as a "poor little withered hand" and would often pick it up and kiss it. An Australian designated his limb as "the bugger"—a term of affection in the Antipodes. Another patient dubbed his paralysed arm as "the communist" by which he meant the limb that refused to work. To another patient the paretic left arm was "James", and the leg "lefty".

I suspect that this phenomenon of personification is far commoner than we neurologists realise, and family doctors, physiotherapists, and the relatives are perhaps better informed. It is odd that until my original description in 1955 it had not been referred to in the literature of neurology.

Personification of this kind often coexists with some degree of anosodiaphoria or abnormal cheerfulness over the existence of a hemiplegia. This is shown by the nature of some of the foregoing nicknames. I think it likely that in every case unawareness of the hemiplegia comes first, perhaps even a temporary denial of the paralysis. As in the case of anosognosia, personification is commoner in left hemiplegics than in right hemiplegics. Nonetheless, I have encountered at least one such case in a right-handed man who had developed a mild dysphasia and a right-sided paresis, the lesion presumably being in the dominant cerebral hemisphere.

Sometimes the personification becomes part of a frank delusion. A man with a right temporo-parietal meningioma, speaking of his weak left upper limb, said "He gets tired sometimes; he doesn't keep time with you; he gets out of step. He gets very lazy; he sits and hangs about and when he does get hold of you he doesn't want to leave you. He's been doing this for a week." Asked to open his fist, he held it up before him, still clenched, and then began to cuddle and caress it, patting it and rubbing it, talking to it and encouraging it, e.g. "Come on, you little monkey, don't let us down. Come on, 'Monkey'. I used to call him 'lucky'. We're doing nicely now, so we'll call him 'lucky'. Come on, 'lucky'." After nursing and cajolling the left hand and arm for about three minutes, the fingers began to extend. Asked what was wrong with the left hand, the patient explained, "he doesn't know what the other one's doing; he's so slow, sitting idle". The nursing staff observed that at meal-times he would "feed" the "little monkey" with a spoon, saying, "come on, have a bit".

Apart from hemiplegia, patients with non-neurological disease rarely adopt this curiously detached attitude towards painful or crippled extremities. I can recall one or two exceptions, however. Thus, when the librettist W. S. Gilbert was unwell, he was in the habit of addressing his gouty limbs as "Labouchere" and "Clement Scott", who were the respective editors of *Truth* and *The Theatre*.

Amputees very occasionally personify their phantom limbs. Perhaps the most bizarre, non-neurological example which came my way was a patient who spoke of his colostomy as "George".

In receiving the diverse instances of personification shown by hemiplegics when they are thinking or talking about their affected arms, it is obvious that many patients adopt anything but an affectionate or even wholly detached attitude. Some patients assume a frame of mind towards their paralysed segments which is critical, disapproving, or hostile. This is mirrored in such terms as "the delinquent". One hemiplegic patient designated with bitterness her affected arm as "the dummy", and she characterised herself as "a broken doll". A doctor patient of mine was a keen musician with strong likes and dislikes. When he developed a left hemiplegia, he specified his paralysed left arm as "Schumann"—explaining that he was "not much good", whereas the normal right arm was "Chopin", for whom he had a profound admiration. When, as a visiting professor to Melbourne, I was examining a hemiplegic female patient, she suddenly proclaimed in the words of St. Paul, "Oh! Wretched woman that I am! Who will deliver me from the body of this death?"

These critical attitudes are the minor manifestations of what I have called a *misoplegia*.

From this mildly paranoid reaction, frankly psychotic types of thinking and behaviour may insidiously develop. In a patient whose left hemiparesis was mild, but was complicated by a gross loss of postural sensibility and a hemianopia, the affected arm would spontaneously wander around in space often without the victim's knowledge. The patient was heard to address his affected limb in the following terms: "You bloody bastard! It's a lost soul, this bloody thing. It keeps following me around. It gets in my way when I read. I find my hand up by my face, waving about."

A female patient who sometimes denied the ownership of her paralysed arm, while at other times reluctantly admitting that it was hers, would often thrust it violently away from her, out of her sight.

Still more hostile was the persecutory type of personification shown by a patient whose paretic left arm was frequently the seat of focal involuntary jerking movements. The patient confided to the doctor, "The old swine! The stinker! Don't talk about it, it might hear you and start twitching again."

Not infrequently the patient develops illusions as to the size and appearance of the affected limb, often describing it in extravagant language. "Like a bird's claw"; "Like a heavy iron bar"; "A piece of dead meat"; "Wooden . . . it won't cooperate"; "Shrivelled and shrunken, like the hand of a mummy". Sometimes the patient will endeavour to conceal the limb under the shawl, or inside the suit jacket, or the bed-clothes. At times, he will avert his gaze by turning his eyes, head, and neck towards the opposite direction. Not infrequently the patient may be observed to strike violently the affected hand, over and over again, screaming abuse at it.

This is misoplegia in the highest degree.

What underlies these variable attitudes on the part of the patient towards his disablement, which may run through the gamut of unawareness, denial, unconcern, disownment of the limb, somatoparaphrenia, insouciant acceptance, affectionate personification, paranoid hatred, and delusional ideas as to the physical properties of the limb? No dogmatic answer can be made but many considerations arise which need study in depth.

In discussing this problem, one might well refer first of all to the more serious question of the varying modes of reaction of a patient rendered completely blind from an abrupt cerebral lesion. Reaction to the disability, we find by experience, varies from simple unawareness of the visual defect, to blatant denial of the blindness, confabulation, reluctant admission that the sight has perhaps deteriorated to a minor degree, projection of the disability to the environment such as inadequate illumination. We also see in the sphere of defective sight from cerebral insult something which we might call "visual anosodiaphoria".

These reactions follow the same pattern as the hemiplegic, but these unexpected reactions are the more striking in the blind than in the crippled.

Four principal hypotheses have been put forward in an attempt to explain some of these various attitudes towards the disability of blindness or paralysis.

In the first place there is the notion that anosognosia, whether for blindness or hemiplegia, is a *specific manifestation of involvement of the parietal lobe,* particularly on the non-dominant half of the brain. In other words that it is quintessentially a focal manifestation.

On the other hand, we have the shrewd observations of Weinstein and Kahn that these diverse aberrations in awareness may represent something more fundamental and not focal, and that they are all various examples of an organic repression, or a far-reaching *denial syndrome* which is inherent in every victim of brain damage. There is some reason too for thinking that the greater the disability the greater the degree of mental adjustment. This hypothesis is supported by the experience of patients with anosognosia, disavowal, and so on following cerebral lesions far removed from the parietal lobes.

Thirdly, there is an interesting suggestion that lack or presence of insight into the effects of a cerebral lesion depend almost entirely upon *the nature of the premorbid personality.* There is a phrase within the Koran which bears this implication, "Your illness is within yourself, but you don't see it." A century ago, Hughlings Jackson repeatedly referred to this possibility. Speaking of the "four factors of the insanities", Jackson had in mind the clinical consequences of a localised lesion of the brain, and not necessarily a psychotic state. According to his teaching, the effects depended upon (1) the site of the lesion; (2) the size of the lesion; (3) the degree of abruptness of the onset of the lesion; and (4) the kind of brain which was in existence prior to the appearance of the lesion. It is this fourth factor which may be argued as being all-important in determining the nature of the clinical picture.

Lastly, there is the hypothesis submitted by Jaffé and Slote to explain patients with unawareness of cerebral blindness. They have suggested that the principal explanation is one of iatrogenicity. In other words, the interpersonal relationship between doctor and patient is all-important. The patient is suggestible, and reacts with exquisite sensitivity to the attitude of the doctor in charge of the case. As the authors put it, "anosognosia represents a symbolic adapted mechanism to be observed under the conditions of communicative interreaction".

In the case of misoplegia, which is under consideration here, we may find the third hypothesis the most acceptable one, though the other explanations are not necessarily wholly excluded. Morbid dislike of the paralysed extremities may prove to be evidence of a hypochondriacal notion bordering on the delusional, which in turn is the operation of an acquired cerebral lesion upon a susceptible premorbid personality. Such an individual has perhaps always been an obsessional and a candidate for hypochondriacal trends by reason of an innate preoccupation with bodily efficiency and physical fitness. Perhaps the patient was once a man of exceptional muscular prowess and of athletic proclivity. We know that by easy stages this may in later life lead on to a certain faddiness, eccentricity, or crankiness. The sudden development of a hemiplegia in such a subject will then constitute much more of an affront to the *amour propre,* one which would scarcely occur in the case of the "cracked pitcher"; the weakling of indifferent physique. The novelist, Christopher Morley, was shrewdly correct in the statement which he put into the lips of Kitty Foyle: "When anything goes wrong with a man, he sure lets you hear about it. If they'd been athletes, I guess they just think of bodies as something to have fun with until the works begin to gum up. They don't realise the way women have to, that it's a damn complicated piece of doings."

Reprinted from Critchley, M. (1974) : *Mount Sinai Journal of Medicine, New York.*

Ecce Homo: Observations upon Self-Portraiture

In the Uffizzi gallery repose over 700 self-portraits. Rembrandt was responsible for almost 100 such paintings. Wandering through the art museums of the world and pondering upon the history of portraiture, one might well wonder what could be the reason why so many artists have depicted themselves upon canvas.

An obvious answer suggests itself at once. A penurious artist can thereby dispense with the assistance of a paid model, expensive perhaps and not always available. But this hypothesis does not really account for all the facts. Cezanne, for example, was anything but hard up. Artists varied in their *penchant* for painting themselves. To some this was an occasional happening, while others—like Rembrandt, Munch, Cezanne, van Gogh, Liebermann, Corinth, and Beckmann—painted themselves year after year throughout their professional careers. Why?

Ingres, Tintoretto, and Monet have each left on record but two self-portraits, separated in time by many decades.

A purely technical point of interest concerns the question of spatial orientation as between right and left. The artist with brush in hand, holding his palette and malstock in his left, stands before the mirror. The blemishes of the right half of the face now appear in the right side of the portrait, which is actually the painter's left side. Van Gogh cut off his left ear: in his self-portrait the lesion seems to be on his right. But when the artist's gaze drops below the level of the upper trunk he often makes a rapid adjustment and paints in a plausible fashion the left hand holding the palette. In other words, the face is reversed but the hands are not. The artist depicts himself as a sinistral. This was the common practice; but there were exceptions.

Other questions pose themselves. Can one recognise that a painting is a self-portrait? If so, what are the clues? Most connoisseurs would hit upon a certain penetrating or disconcerting stare whereby the eyes seem to follow the observer all around the gallery. Gowing was close to the current psychological conception of the body-image when he wrote, "What is this shape . . . that a man grows like a shell around him? Investigating it, the painter separates himself from it, like a creature that sheds its carapace. He identifies it coldly as himself—and yet not himself, unless at two points, the pupils of the eyes, the two fixed and transfixing points of a self-portrait which fasten that which is seen to we know not what, and fasten as remorselessly to the riddle."

If then a self-portrait is no faithful photographic simulacrum, what of that allied phenomenon, known technically as an *Assistenzbild,* whereby the painter interpolates himself somewhere on the canvas, but not necessarily in the forefront? He may introduce himself backstage as one of a crowd, like many Italian painters in the Middle Ages. The Dutch-Flemish school of artists would often relegate their auto-portraits to a homely indoor scene. Later, this technique was elaborated in an extreme fashion, as by Velasquez and by Courbet. Annigoni has a trick of putting himself *in petto* as a little mannikin tucked away in the background of some formal portrait. In the Middle Ages this practise at times assumed grotesque or even macabre properties. Caravaggio's own features were depicted in the severed head of Goliath. In his "Last Judgment" Michaelangelo's face is shown in his painting of St. Bartholomew carrying his own flayed skin. Dürer identified himself in his painting of Christ. Brouwer portrayed himself with grim realism as a scowling debauché in a tavern. In modern times Buffet painted himself as a strained victim of some inner mental anguish. Dürer once painted himself naked (Fig. 1).

What is the nature of the tie-up which surely must exist between self-portraiture and aberration of the body-image (corporeal awareness)?

According to Oscar Wilde, "only in mirrors should one look, for mirrors do but show us masks." A mirror-reflection—which is, of course, the starting point of an auto-portrait—is in many ways a mask. When deliberately gazing in a looking-glass, one does not behold the tic-like grimacing and all the ugliness of uninhibited mimic movement, but an almost flattering visage which stares back at the beholder. But these are not what others discern. Marcel Proust referred to the discrepancy between portraits according to whether they were drawn by oneself or by another, and he spoke of those "grinned frightful faces" invisible to the owners. As Gasser said, "self-portraits rarely attain the degree of honesty we are accustomed to look for in autobiographies. With few exceptions, indeed, painters clearly sought to present a handsome, attractive or imposing exterior to later generations —one that the facts can hardly have justified with quite such a high degree of regularity." Friedlander's interesting comments deserve quotation ". . . Man does not take up a neutral or objective attitude towards his own appearance; his participation is coloured more by his 'will' than by his 'idea.' Self-portraits do not confirm the view that we know ourselves better than others. They are not in a particularly high degree 'good likenesses.' Observation is interfered with by vanity, by ambition. The painter wants to cut a figure; he takes himself over-seriously, portrays himself in a definite situation, namely, as gazing, with open eyes, in tension and action. The ordinary sitter on the other hand—the person whose portrait is being

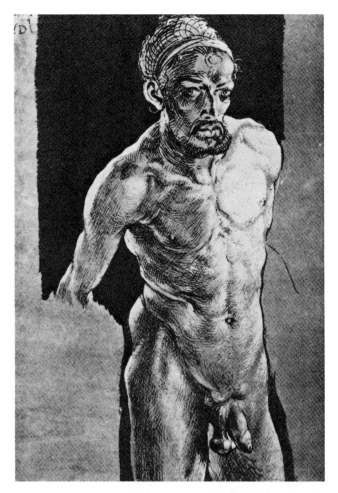

FIG. 1. Dürer's self-portrait naked, 1503, one of the illustrations in *High Renaissance*.

painted, gets tired and bored. For this reason self-portraits are aggressive and dramatic, and not infrequently theatrical. They convey to us less what the painter looked like than what he wanted to look like. One may speak of a rhetoric of the self-portrait."

The same idea crops up in the lines written by Robert Graves:

> "You ask the person you see reflected in
>   your shaving mirror why
> He still stands ready, with a boy's
>   presumption
> To court the queen in her high silk pavilion"

Vanity, of course, comes in. The urge for graphic self-perpetuation must have been a potent influence during the centuries before the advent of photography. This is evidenced by the work of some painters who, though notorious for other kinds of painting, nevertheless occasionally succumbed to the temptation to depict themselves. Why, for instance, did Picasso paint himself 40 times, but cease to do so after the age of 26? On occasions Klee and Léger departed from their usual techniques, as did Toulouse-Lautrec whose autopictorial sketches were little more than uncanny doodles—almost caricatures. Arnold Schoenberg gave us a back view, so that the artist glossed over his grotesque ugliness and his myopic peer.

The so-called "intimate" self-portrait did not really appear until the last

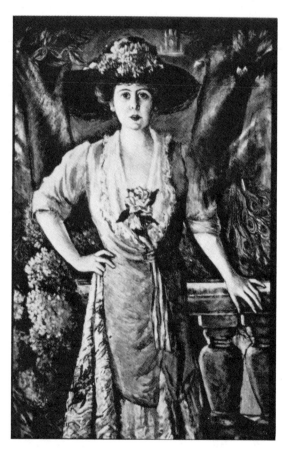

FIG. 2. Beatrice Turner: At 58 she still painted herself to look like a woman years younger. To the end she wore dresses fashionable in her youth. (From *Life Magazine,* July 10, 1950.)

century. Here we meet Dérain, Chagall, Kirchner, Schiele, Soutine, Miró, Jawlensky.

What of those artists who indulged freely in self-portraiture and whose paintings did not with honesty represent actuality? Edvard Munch comes to mind. In the picture "Between clock and bed," painted when he was 78 years of age, he is shown as a far younger man. This is clearly shown when one compares this picture with the one painted a year before and entitled "The wanderer in the night," which certainly does not flatter. The work of the Czech painter Škréta also showed a comparable Peter Pan phenomenon. Perhaps the most astounding instance of a youthful arrest of the body-image is to be met with in the numerous self-portraits of Beatrice Turner. Kept immured at home by her wealthy but puritanical parents, she indulged her natural talents. In her secluded state she painted herself again and again, but always appearing decades younger. Hair, features, figure, and dress were all those of an attractive adolescent (Figs. 2 and 3). The syndrome represents an amalgam of Dorian Gray and Miss Havisham. Lonely and eccentric, she frenziedly continued to paint, but she meanwhile neglected herself and died from malnutrition. When the executors took possession they were amazed to find a collection of over a thousand self-portraits, those painted in her last days displaying herself as a seductive nude.

But the reverse phenomenon can also be discerned when we study Val-

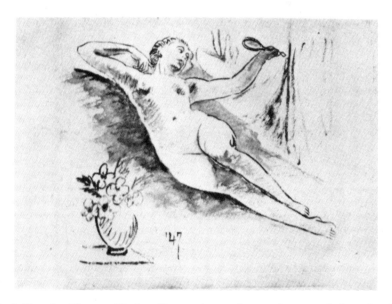

FIG. 3. Beatrice Turner: Nude self-portrait was done only a year before she died. Her figure looks ample though in her last years she grew thin from inadequate diet. (From *Life Magazine,* July 10, 1950.)

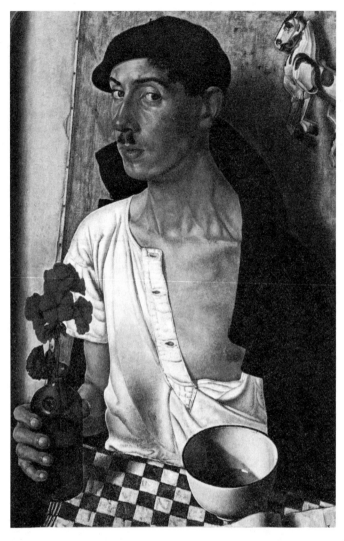

FIG. 4. Self-portrait with red geranium by Dick Ket, 1932. The artist died in 1940 from heart-failure, still a young man. His realisation of his ill-health is shown by his half-bared chest, the cyanosis of his lips and clubbed fingers, the medicine-bottle, and the open book with its one word FIN (the end).

lottoni's self-portrait. Though the artist was but 17 years of age the picture represents a man very much older. Chagall's self-portrait showing him with two right hands and seven fingers reminds us uncomfortably of schizophrenic art. Rembrandt's final self-portrait, painted when he was 63, indicates ill-health and premature aging coupled with sadness. In Dick Ket's self-portrait, we also observe symptoms of his declining health (Fig. 4).

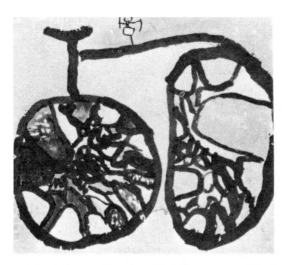

FIG. 5. Self-portrait by 3½-year-old girl entitled "Me and my bike."

Van Gogh wrote, "to know oneself is difficult—but painting oneself is not easier." His 22 self-portraits are of psychological interest, for the close observer can detect traces of the waxing and waning of his psychosis. Though a great deal of nonsense has been written on this theme, van Gogh's last effort cannot be dismissed as anything but the picture of a crazy individual, disturbed, even paranoid.

Still on the topic of body-image as revealed in self-portraits, we may turn to *l'art naïf* of young children. It is well-known that corporeal awareness is a fluid conception which may extend into extra-personal space and embrace material prolongations like clothes, walking-sticks, tools. A most striking instance is seen in the vivid painting by a girl aged 3½ years which she entitled "Me and my bike" (Fig. 5). Her picture is dominated by a highly coloured machine, but perched upon the saddle of which is a miniscule figure—"me" in fact. The relative difference in the scheme of things as between self and non-self is unmistakeable.

Finally there is that extension of the narcissistic trends in portraiture—the phenomenon of self-sculpture, a somewhat uncommon feature in the history of art. Phidias left a graven record of his own appearance, but this was in a product of that tweenie technique—bas-relief. An example can be seen in St. Stefan's Cathedral in Vienna, where the architect Meister Pilgram engraved himself as peering through a window to admire his work (Fig. 6). Mĕstrović certainly constructed many personal busts, a task which entails prolonged and deliberate creative activity. A self-portrait can be sketched in a matter of minutes. To paint oneself in oils may entail hours or even days. But to perfect a three dimensional replica must surely neces-

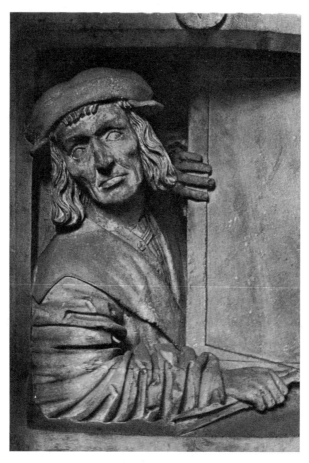

FIG. 6. Self-portrait of Meister Pilgram engraved in St. Stefan's Cathedral in Vienna.

sitate a process of introspection, appraisal, and representational craftsmanship extending over days or weeks. Mirrors constitute but feeble props.

Perhaps the apogee of narcissistic self-sculpture is to be found in the life-sized effigy constructed in wood by Ito Hamashi. Painstakingly over a period of ten years he assembled piece by piece so that he eventually constructed a completely faithful model made up of 2,000 chips dove-tailed and glued. Every item of surface anatomy was portrayed—musculo-tendinous or venous. The sculptor had even depilated himself little by little and, after boring minute holes, had inserted every single hair into its appropriate facio-cranial, axillary, or pudendal situation (Fig. 7).

Neurologists and psychiatrists may well agree that the story of self-portraiture and auto-sculpture is one that merits their professional scrutiny.

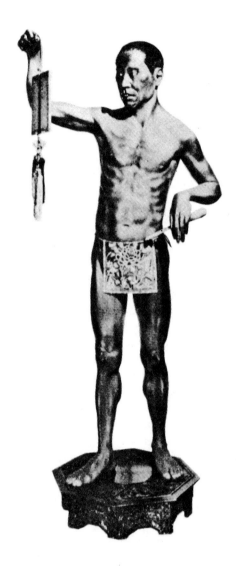

FIG. 7. Life-sized self-sculpture by Ito Hamashi.

Certainly it is a topic that fascinates the closer one observes. It offers the traveller zest to his sight-seeing expeditions. There are interesting links with a critical aperçu of psychotic art and the paintings of young children, especially the handicapped. The definitive work upon the subject still awaits authorship.

Reprinted from Critchley, M. *History of Medicine, Ltd.* Ridgeway Mill Hill, London.

The Mask in the Mirror

This chapter is about the human face, and its rank in the behavioural sciences. The title is taken from Oscar Wilde's dictum that "only in mirrors should one look, for mirrors do but show us masks".

In many respects the face stands aloof. It is not only the organ of articulate speech, but by its play of mimetic movements it is itself communicative in a silent fashion. It also stands supreme in the hierarchy of the body-image, even though every single individual is at a unique disadvantage in being the only one who has no direct knowledge of its physical attributes. What imperfect information we have is based upon the indirect and inadequate evidence of the mirror, the camera, the portrait. Except in strict Muslim communities the face is always exposed, and is, therefore, blatantly obvious to others with all its beauty and all its blemishes. There is also something unique about the face, namely its individuality. No two faces are absolutely identical even though the resemblance may be very close in young homozygous twins. Theoretically it should be possible to match the face with the individual, but this is a skill which is attained by relatively few, like forensic professionals. Even here identification is assisted by such factors as body-build, gait, voice, and gesticulation. Such an expertise is slowly acquired, and we find its extension to sheep-farmers who can pick out individual lambs and ewes in their flocks, or to the farmer's wife who can confidently distinguish one stupid-looking chicken from another.

Many believe that the face is an index of character and personality. A face may be deemed aesthetic, austere, lugubrious, stern, severe, dour, sulky, arrogant, cruel, tight-lipped; contrariwise, jovial, jolly, sensual, kindly, sympathetic, gentle. In the United States we sometimes hear of a "smile belt" which runs roughly parallel with the Mason-Dixon Line. To the south the inhabitants have warm and friendly countenances, while the Yankees in the north are cold and hard-faced. All this is very interesting but as a matter of fact attempts at physiognomy are only approximate and dangerous.

As across the orchestra of a Greek theatre, a play of emotional movements may add a meaningful vitality. Some of these are essentially deliberate; others are automatic, being outside of awareness and yet controllable; others again are wholly involuntary. Within the first group are such actions as scowling and smiling. Laughter and tears belong within group 2, while the third is made up of such manifestations as pallor or flushing, watering of the eyes, and horripilation.

All these panorama are highly communicative, more eloquent perhaps than articulate speech. Words may mislead, but facial mimicry, unless the product of play-acting, is more honest, for it gives a sincere indication of the speaker's actual thinking.

These revealing items of facial mimicry deserve closer attention.

A smile is usually a social grimace which serves to establish a climate of warmth. But at times a smile may be wholly insincere. Then there are quizzical or enigmatic smiles, as in the Egyptian Sphinx, in the Mona Lisa, or in the statue of Voltaire. A neurotic trick well-known to psychiatrists is that of the inappropriate and obtrusive smiling of the nervous and insecure. Then there is the secret smile of the schizophrenic and also the broad yet mirthless grin so characteristic of victims of Wilson's disease. We must not forget, too, the Japanese smile, that is simply a mask of politeness or of diffidence, yet to a European it often seems wholly inappropriate.

Laughter is a far more complex subject, and has fascinated philosophers for centuries. In the context of hilarity it is closely linked with gregariousness. A man may smile to himself. That is acceptable, but if he begins to laugh aloud in solitude, it is time for his family to worry. As a sign of pleasure, laughter is singularly ugly and cacophonous to others outside the circle. It becomes louder and more raucous under the influence of alcohol, as any cocktail-party hostess knows, or any restaurant-goer. But when the food comes in, relative silence ensues, and the peace and comfort of other diners are restored. Uncontrolled laughter may involve the entire body musculature. The face flushes, eyes water, limbs and trunk contort, and one observes such contact-gestures as elbow-digging. Later the muscles lose tone so that the subject sags limply at the knees or in his chair. "Laugh, I should have died" is a cliché which happens to be scientifically correct.

A neurologist can find plenty to interest him in the topic of laughter. He is familiar with laughter as a factor that provokes the cataplexy of narcoleptics, so that the victim falls helplessly to the ground. Then there is gelastic epilepsy, where ribald laughter culminates in a fit. The neurologist is also aware of the pathological hilarity of the arteriopath with pseudobulbar palsy, where a trivial pleasantry may trigger off peals of uncontrollable laughter, merging insensibly into crying.

The topic of laughter leads us to discuss tears. These are commoner in infants than in adults. Though weeping is ordinarily a witness of mental or physical discomfort, it is uncommon when depression is deep, and likewise in patients with chronic pain even of great intensity. We also recall the story of crocodile tears, and of fabulous bloody tears. In the warfare of the sexes ready evocation of tears is one of woman's most deadly weapons—the "hydraulic force through which masculine willpower is defeated by feminine waterpower".

Earlier we spoke of the specificity of the human countenance and the ability to recognise a person even across a room, the face perhaps of some notoriety one has never seen save in a photograph. The picture may have been in profile, the actual situation being face to face, yet though the spatial dimension is different, recognition is prompt. Some persons are far better at this game than others. We have already spoken of the experts at this rare but striking talent. Others are not so clever.

There is a curious state of affairs whereby, as the result of a brain-lesion, a patient loses—not his visual acuity—but merely his ability to recognise faces, even those of near relatives and friends. This is the phenomenon of *prosopagnosia*. The voice, the footfall perhaps, affords the appropriate clue, but the face alone is a meaningless blur. Cases have been known where the victim of prosopagnosia has sustained a broken engagement because he failed to recognise his fiancée.

Enthusiasts have been led away into regions of speculation. They have said that a prosopagnosia may be partial and spare the area around the eyes. On the analogy of central or macular vision they have hypothesised an "ocula" or eye-region which they regard as the kernel or most significant segment of the face, asserting too that an infant begins to recognise its mother or its nannie first by learning to identify the ocula. Such notions are far-fetched and unimpressive, to say the least of it.

Prosopagnosic patients also have difficulty in recognising photographs or pictures of well-known personalities. This is by no means rare in many victims of brain-damage. Failure of identification may even extend to a nonrecognition of portraits or pictures of themselves. Indeed a patient may fail to recognise his own reflection in a looking-glass. An extreme example of this is the "phenomenon of the mirror", when a patient gazing at himself sees in the looking-glass nothing at all. Such a phantasy was admirably described by Guy de Maupassant in his novella "The Horla".

Many medical articles or addresses have dealt with art and its medical aspects. Unfortunately the authors do not touch upon the topic of self-portraiture. When we recall the important role of the face in the body-image, it is not surprising to find how common has been the practise of auto-portraiture throughout the ages, as discussed in a previous paper.

Returning to the theme of this talk, namely the human face, we may try and explain why a mirror-image reflects but a mask and not the real thing. Charlotte Bronte touched upon this topic when she wrote in *Jane Eyre*:

> Returning, I had to cross before the looking-glass; my fascinated glance involuntarily explored the depth it revealed. All looked cooler and darker in that visionary hollow than in reality: and the strange little figure there gazing at me, with white face and arms specking the gloom, and glittering eyes of fear moving where all else was still, had the effect of a real spirit. I thought it like one of the tiny phantoms,

half fairy, half imp, Bessie's evening stories represented as coming out of love, ferny dells in moors, and appearing before the eyes of belated travellers.

However often, however closely, we study our features in a mirror—single or even triple—we never see the same features that everyone else beholds. As soon as we look at ourselves, we strike an attitude, a pose. The manifold tic-like mannerisms, the oral dyskinesias, so typical and yet so inelegant, do not appear in the reflection, and we go on wearing our dream-mask oblivious of its artificiality. The ravages of age slowly proliferate and yet we do not detect them even though we constantly shave, wash, and titivate our faces in the mirror. Of course, others note them, but not the individual, and that is why he is shocked when he unexpectedly meets a contemporary after a lapse of years, or when he is shown the holiday snapshots taken by his grandchildren.

Sometimes this relationship between anatomical actuality and the conceptual body-image attains abnormal standing. There is the grotesque phenomenon of the faded beauty who continues to apply more and more cosmetics and to dress in the peak of fashion of thirty years ago. This is the Miss Havisham syndrome.

If the face is so important in the body-image, why is it that the nose should occupy the supreme role? Men and women are hypersensitive about its size, shape, and colouring. Any true or imagined deviation from the norm is a source of undue distress to the owner as every dermatologist, every beautician, can testify. A nose is not a very useful or attractive contrivance. As a piece of anatomical engineering built to house a vestigal organ of smell, it could be improved upon. Perhaps the principal function of the nose is to meet the supertax of cosmetic surgeons.

Leaving the nose, let us explore some other areas of the face with all their oddities and quirks. Take for example the eyes. These have been accorded a position in the scheme of things which I regard as being too lofty. From poets to peasants, we all tend to write and to talk as though eyes constitute the principal apparatus for betraying thoughts and feelings, even more sincerely than speech. This exalted rank is, I submit, an exaggeration.

To explain what I mean: piercing eyes cannot possibly pierce anything. Eyes cannot flash. They cannot melt or soften or harden or blaze. They say that Irish eyes are smiling, but that is inconceivable: the most that can happen is a narrowing of the palpebral fissures and a crinkling at the corners. A look of horror is no more than a rigid retraction of the lids.

In other words the attributes which are popularly applied to the eyes all depend on mimic movements of the upper part of the face.

Let us admit that the eyeballs are little more than blobs of jelly. True, they can be moved about at will; sometimes they are seen to squint; some-

times they oscillate involuntarily; but at no time do they function as ve-
hicles of communication. These globes are fully occupied by their important and specific role as visual receptors, where messages are handed in to
be transmitted to higher cerebral centres for interpretation.

But what of the mouth? Here, I submit, is that segment of the face which
is more revealing than any other feature. Lips may be contorted deliberately
to demonstrate the feeling-tones which lie behind pouting, sneering, smiling. When the mouth takes part in articulate speech it adds overtones of
sympathy or displeasure, roguery or scorn, liking or dislike. Do you wish to
judge a man as he speaks? Watch his face, but not his eyes; certainly not
that pinnacle, the nose, or those ridiculous flap-like appendages, the ears.
No; you must study the mouth. You need not be a lip-reader, but subtle
movements of that colligation of tiny peribuccal muscles of expression will
tell you much—even perhaps the race, the social rank, the breeding, the
education of the speaker, over and above the content of what he is saying,
and its emotional undertext. The totally deaf know all this better than you
and I. How ironic it is that in the aged, loss of teeth combine with unwilled
dyskinesias, chomping, chewing, and popping out of the tongue, and anal-
like wrinkling of the lips to make a caricature of man's most expressive
feature.

But even greater fundamentals lie behind this topic. The face is more
than a mask, more than a mirror. Very many questions crop up for discussion: why is it that for thousands of years man has considered it ex-
pedient or necessary to embellish, adorn, decorate, or distort the visage?
Why do the Maoris, Amerindians, Mesoamericans, and Bedouin women feel
an urge to uglify or disfigure their features with elaborate tattooage? Or at
times, as in the Soudanese, with facial scarifications? What compels African
savages to insert wooden platters into their lips or their external ears, or
to transfix their nostrils with bodkins made of metal, bone, or wood? Why
are elaborate masks so all-important among primitive communities, in ritual
dances, or in their efforts to avert disease or ill-omen?

It is perhaps easier to understand the practise of earrings and facial orna-
ture by women with unguents, powder, paint, and pigments, while among
Aboriginals ritual dancers employ an elaborate painting of the whole body
as well as the face with light-coloured clay. Why? On a more homespun or
artless level there is the question of eye-glasses or spectacles. Nowadays,
over 50% of adults resort—or should resort—to the provision of convex or
concave devices in order to visualise the environment with adequate definition. And yet the history of art shows how late it was before these particular
contrivances became acceptable. It was not until the 18th century that
Chardin made the first self-portrait of an artist wearing spectacles. Not until
recent years were glasses deemed not only to be admissible but even at
times a trifle erotic, as I am assured by my junior colleagues who study
girlie magazines. Why do men's fashions in facio-cranial hairiness fluctuate

so much from one generation to another, so that the keen cut and clear features of the Aztecs, Mayans, Amerindians, Egyptians, and Romans gave way to the shaggy tangle of the Assyrians, the Greeks, and the Jews. Later the vogue was again for hairlessness as in the 18th century, while early in the 19th century whiskers again became respectable, only to be frowned upon for some decades and then to go to the modern extremes of grotesque hirsutism. In Catholic circles, clean cut features denoted high rank in the Roman Church while in the Russo-Graecian Orthodox circles, bushy beards were obligatory. What does it all mean?

It would take volumes to do justice to this topic of ostentatious facial adornment as an aspect of psychology and anthropology. We can but give it but a passing mention here.

Let us have done with the face as a mask, to hark back to the human body-image. This elusive concept is largely the product of visual experiences as learned from oneself (though this does not apply to the face), from portraits, from reflections, coupled with the evidence gained by looking at other people. What then of the person who is born blind, and who grows up never having seen anyone's face—either in reality or in a looking-glass or in a picture? Surely the body-image of such a one must be in some way different.

One final thought, fanciful perhaps, but not without interest. I refer to the origin of speech in primitive man. Verbalisation was certainly preceded by pantomimic movements, and for a time both played a partnership in communication, as in the apes. *Homo sapiens* differed from the anthropoids not only in the acquisition of language, but also in the lesser distribution of hirsutism and in particular the facial hairgrowth. This relative baring of the features permitted visibility to the facial mimicry. But the sexes differ here. Could it be that the remote beginnings of speech in the hominoid species were the product of the female rather than the bearded male? And why not indeed, for common experience supports the evidence of linguistics that greater prowess is displayed by women rather than men in the manipulation of words.

The Miss Havisham Syndrome

Both as a stylist, and as recorder of the *comédie humaine,* Charles Dickens is still insufficiently acclaimed. His shrewd observation, or maybe his inspired thinking, has enriched our culture by way of at least a score of oddities. *Great Expectations*—perhaps his finest novel—depicts one of the most unusual of these types, one which merits the attention of the literary psychologist. Miss Havisham, an attractive young woman, spoilt child of a wealthy brewer, was cruelly jilted by her fiancé on what was to have been their wedding day. Following the shock of this rebuff, Miss Havisham continued to live on as a recluse, clothed perpetually in the fading satin of her bridal dress. Years went by. She had stopped the clocks at 20 minutes to 9, the moment of her calamity. Not once did she put foot outside her gloomy house. Never did she allow sunlight to filter through the shutters on to the dust and cobwebs around her. When, 25 years later, young Pip comes to the scene, he found the strangest lady he had ever met. Bridal flowers were in her hair, but her hair was white, and the flowers withered. Jewels sparkled on her neck and hands. Half-packed trunks were scattered around. Everything was white, but lack-lustre, faded, and yellowing. Pip was reminded of a ghastly waxwork in a fair representing some fantastic lying-in-state, or an exhumed skeleton with a rich garment crumbling around it.

Thus Dickens described the prototype of what I like to call the "Miss Havisham syndrome". Though a fictional figure, this imaginary eccentric anticipates other comparable cases in reality.*

Consider, for example, the story of that Florentine beauty, Virginia the Comtesse de Castiglione (Fig. 1). Born in 1835, married at 15 and widowed five months later, she grew to be a sulky young woman of extraordinary loveliness, and of calculated frailty. At the age of 18 she was deliberately introduced by the King of Piedmont into the court of Napoleon III, with the express purpose of subtly influencing him in favour of the policy of Italian unity. Her success surpassed every hope, and for a while the Comtesse held the role of supreme favourite within the Imperial seraglio. "If only I had said 'no' I could have been Empress." But in due course she was discarded. There followed an unsatisfactory procession of liaisons with one

---

* According to J. R. Tyrrall, Dickens based the Miss Havisham legend upon what had been told to him about the daughter of Judge Donnithorne of Sydney, Australia, who died in 1886 at an advanced age in such a state of living mummification.

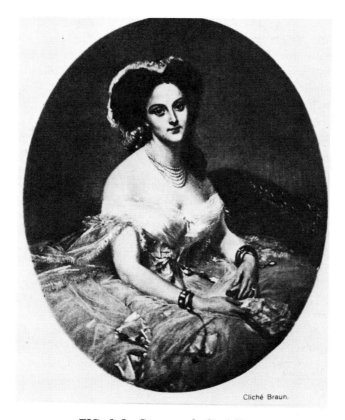

Cliché Braun.

FIG. 1. La Comtesse de Castiglione.

man after another. This did not suffice. Disappointment over the Imperial snub caused her to cut herself off from Parisian society. The last 20 years of her life were spent as a recluse in receipt of a pension from the Italian government. The daylight was perpetually shut out from her apartment in the Place Vendôme by heavy curtains drawn across shuttered windows. Only after dark did she venture out of doors, and then heavily veiled. Indoors, the mirrors were draped so that she never glimpsed her reflection. She continued to wear the heavy and out-of-date crinolines, her appearance becoming more and more grotesque. By the age of 45, her beauty was declining. Her dull complexion was accentuated by heavily blackened eyebrows; her dyed hair set in elaborate kiss-curls. She had put on weight; her limbs had thickened; her ankles, formerly so slim, were now hideously swollen. A favourite garment was a dressing-gown of black velvet and white quilting over her naked body, but when she went out of doors she protected herself against the cold with a pair of leggings of the same material lined with ermine, which came to the top of the stockings.

The rooms were dark, ornately furnished, and befouled with the excrement of her two podgy and nondescript dogs. Some nights she wandered through the streets for hours, halting now and then to talk to herself. There were times when only the police could persuade her to return.

"I see her", wrote Frederic Loliée "in one of these fantastic flights and peregrinations through her usual haunts—putting off, as long as her infirmities will allow, her return home to the place she abominates yet refuses to leave. Sometimes she counts her steps, or now lowers her gaze to the pavement as she wanders along . . . unconsciously stopping in front of the refuse boxes, starting desperate conversations with the reconnoitering scavengers."

Eventually she had to leave her apartment for a dingy pair of rooms nearby at 14 rue Cambon overlooking the courtyard well. Much of her time was spent in scribbling pencilled and angry scrawls, barely decipherable, to various notables. Strange persecutory notions disturbed her. Her health began to fail, and she took to her bed. In her correspondence she referred to her "thirteen chronic ailments, all serious, and two of them mortal". She drew up an extraordinary will with detailed instructions proscribing all the orthodox funeral rites, and specifying that in her coffin her two dogs, now stuffed, should lie at her feet like cushions. She was to be buried in the nightdress she wore in 1857 at Compiègne when she first lay in Napoleon's arms . . . "*batiste dentelles, et peignoir long raye, velours noir, peluche blanche; au cou, le collier de perles petite fille, neuf rangs, six rangs blanches et trois noires, collier habituel que j'ais toujours porte. . . .*"

She died during the night of 28 November (1885), paralysed down the left side, possibly from a cerebral metastasis.

Let us now take a third example, namely Jane Francesca Elgee, mother of Oscar Wilde. A dazzling, intelligent, and striking figure in political Ireland, she was a poetess who wrote inflammatory verse under the pen-name of Speranza. In due course, successive troubles assailed her. Her dissolute husband, the scandal of a Dublin prosecution, her ne'er-do-well elder son, and finally Oscar's disgrace accumulated so as to constitute an insupportable series of mental traumata. More and more eccentric in dress and manner, she retired to Chelsea where for a time she strove to maintain a bohemian salon. W. B. Yeats has told us that Lady Wilde received her friends with blinds drawn and shutters closed that none might see her withered face. Recklessly she resorted to powder, rouge, and the posticheur's skill. Her callers dwindling, she turned to occultism. Horace Wyndham wrote "In the darkened room where she sat brooding hour after hour and day after day, all she had left with which to occupy herself were memories, the memories of 70 years." According to an obituary notice in *The Athenaeum* ". . . bereaved of husband, and assailed by misfortunes for which the only sympathy was silence, she finally hid herself in the greatest of all hiding-places, London; and fled the light of day, bearing her heavy cross in silence and stoical patience under the cover of darkness and the cloak of oblivion."

Yet another example can be quoted in the case of the writer Marie Corelli. For 30 years she had been the best selling novelist in the world and her *Sorrows of Satan* sold more copies than any other English novel had achieved. An infatuated and jealous admirer of Shakespeare, she retired to Stratford-on-Avon so as to reside as close as she could to his birthplace. In her hatred of literary critics she would not allow her publishers to issue review-copies. Photographers, amateur and professional, incurred her deepest displeasure and the mere peep of a camera caused her to cover her face. Sharing a menage with a much trusted woman-friend, she shunned society. In appearance she was short and stoutish. Anyone who happened to glimpse her in the street described a dwarfish figure with huge hat of a kind which had long been out-of-date. Her pretty dress was a concoction of frills and floral flounces, baby-blue or shocking-pink, with a fresh nosegay at her bodice. According to her biographer, Brian Masters, it was the kind of attire which might have suited a demure sixteen-year-old in the mid-Victorian era, but the lady wearing it was, in 1905, fifty years old.

The Miss Havisham syndrome is not always irreversible. This is well shown in the case of Queen Victoria, widowed in 1861. From his private sources of information, Lytton Strachey described the suite of rooms within Windsor Castle perpetually excluded from the gaze of all except the most privileged. There everything remained as it had been at the time of her beloved husband's death. On the Queen's command Prince Albert's clothing was laid pressed and ready on the bed each evening, with basins filled with fresh water as though he were still living. Such was the fantastic ritual which was carried out with scrupulous regularity for nearly 40 years. Meanwhile the Widow of Windsor immured herself within her palaces, shut off from public gaze, but immersed in even the trivialia of routine office work. Years later, however, the Queen emerged from her semi-retirement, bowing to the pressure of mounting public protest.

Doubtless many other examples of the Miss Havisham syndrome could be brought to light. Certain fundamental conditions seem to emerge. The syndrome appears to be confined to the female sex. The usual setting is that of a young woman of exceptional beauty, domineering and intelligent, of aristocratic or well-to-do parentage. Then, at a climactic point in the personal history, comes some catastrophic disappointment: a bereavement, or a callous rebuff. From this moment the victim chooses to opt out of life. Time stands still, and this is reflected both in her material entourage and in the realm of her body-image. No longer does she keep pace with her contemporaries; self-exclusion is a means of avoiding social intercourse, either gradually or abruptly. No longer does she attempt to keep up with the changes ordained by fashion and social custom. Frequently she obstructs the daylight from her sanctuary, and surrounds herself with the mementoes of her past, heedless of the inroads of time. Dust accumulates. Dressed in the old garments belonging to her prime, over-jewelled, the fading beauty goes to extremes in her maquillage. Her yellow skin is increasingly encrusted with paint and powder; her lips are heavily carmined, and eyebrows and eyelids darkened to excess. Her hair is crudely dyed and curled in girlish manner. To some extent this extravagant use of cosmetics may be put down to failing eyesight and poor lighting, but such an explanation is certainly not the whole or even the most important factor.

To this scene is often added the phenomenon whereby a study or bedroom is preserved intact. Particularly is this so when adjustment to a bereavement proves impossible. The personal belongings of the loved one may be left *in situ:* the bed unmade.

It may be argued that minor degrees or incomplete variants of the Miss Havisham syndrome are not uncommon. This may well be so, if one includes those instances where ageing Aphrodites go to great extremes in their attempts at beautification and personal adornment. But such eccentric figures do not necessarily shun society; indeed they may strive in an inordinate fashion to keep up with their younglings. If seclusion with its arrest of time is to be looked upon as the *sine qua non* of the Miss Havisham syndrome, then strictly speaking these latter specimens of the faded belle do not belong here.

The same applies to the over-dressed old men who cling tenaciously to the fashion of their youth to a ridiculous degree. Unlike the derelict beauty, these old peacocks have not tried to halt the passage of time by retreat. On the contrary, they are sweeping along too fast in the contemporary scene, like desperate anachronisms.

The Miss Havisham syndrome, and even more so the phenomenon of the ageing beaux and belles, can be analysed along the lines of the body-image, or—to use that more appropriate term—corporeal awareness. It is perfectly natural that with advancing years the body-image should lag behind the actual morphology that is so obvious to everyone else. Despite the evidence of the looking-glass, the elderly usually do not in their imagery or when in a brown study regard themselves as wrinkled, bowed, or grey. Candid snapshots come somewhat as a shock. But the normal subject accepts the situation, and unlike the victim of the Miss Havisham syndrome, does not reject actuality. Still on the topic of the body-image, one can also recall the rejection of the loss of a limb by way of a continuing phantom feeling. This is normal enough. But in the realm of neuro-psychopathology, the anosognosic phenomena of unawareness of hemiplegia; or of denial of palsy or blindness; or of repudiation of the ownership of a useless limb; and the extraordinary instances of confabulation can be equated on a different plane with the syndrome of Miss Havisham.

Reprinted from Critchley, M. (1969) : *History of Medicine,* Vol. 1.

Tattooed Ladies, Tattooed Men

Small adv. Personal.
Tattooed lady—wishes to meet gentleman with similar views.

T. E. Dunville, 1910

Years ago in a receiving ward I saw an acutely demented and agitated male patient who until a week before had been an inoffensive God-fearing bachelor. He lived with his sister and journeyed each day from Tooting to the City of London and then home again. Nothing had disturbed this humdrum routine until the dramatic development of a crazy and uncontrollable excitement. Taken to a psychiatric acute hospital he was undressed and for the first time his sister discovered that, over his torso back and front and all four limbs to wrist and ankles, her brother was tattooed to such an extensity that it was impossible to place a coin upon an unmarked area of skin. It transpired that this bank clerk had daily slunk into a tattooist's shop on his way home, and subjected himself to the ministrations of the artist, who was the sole co-partner in the secret.

The clinical diagnosis of the mental break-down turned out to be an acute dementia paralytica.

A reflective student of human nature may well ponder over the motives which compel the man in the street to submit the virgin territory of his dermis to permanent assaults of such a graphic or pictorial nature. Not only *why* should this be, the onlooker may muse, but what decides the choice of a particular *motif*. Who are they, those who elect to be marked—if not marred—in perpetuity? Do they belong to any recognisable psychological type, or social bracket, or professional class? Or even sex? Are there such beings as tattooed women? Or are men alone the self-appointed victims of this peculiar type of attention?

The ethnologist may intervene at this point to demonstrate here an age-old propensity towards skin-markings with their magical, cultural, tribal, even medico-prophylactic implications.

These interesting facts do not necessarily throw light upon the problem of tattooing as found currently in our Caucasian civilisation. It seems improbable that the tattoo marks observed in our fellow men have been placed there to indicate rank or social status; or to ward off disease, local or generalised. With certain rare exceptions, the purpose of modern tattooing is decorative.

Permanent ornamentation of this sort obviously does not possess a universal appeal. By and large it is more commonly seen in service personnel than in civilians; and in the lower orders rather than the upper classes. Even now it possesses a vogue among the criminal population. The painless electric techniques of today have eliminated the earlier circumstances, whereby to submit to tattooing was to afford a visible and permanent proof of stoicism, virility, or hardihood.

Ornamentation of the skin suggests not so much an aggressive masculinity

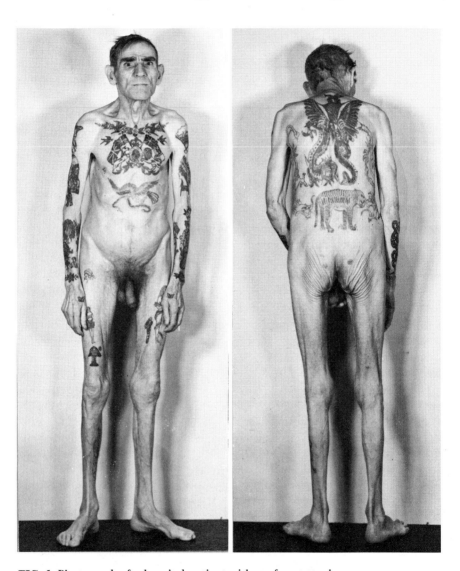

FIG. 1. Photograph of a hospital patient with profuse tattooing.

as a mark of simplicity, naivete, or immaturity. The tattooed subject is, on the receiving end, the counterpart of the *graffito* who expresses his turgid uncomplicated feelings by way of wall-writings, executed in anonymity but designed to attain the widest possible publicity. Indeed it would not be difficult to visualise a spectrum of communicative effort ranging from the cave-paintings of primitive man, through the scratchings on the catacombs of esoteric religious sects, the wall-newspapers of the Pompeiian Romans, the scurrilous art, obscenities, and political *olla podrida* in the world of graffiti; blotting-paper and note-book doodles; skin markings whether pigmented or not; the coloured transfers favoured by pre-war schoolboys; and even the accepted and highly sophisticated techniques of the cosmetic art. We see here the same urge for self-expression, if not for communication, an endeavour which characterises *Homo sapiens,* irrespective of the frontiers of time, place, language, and culture. Self-decoration, whether it takes the form of tattooing, cosmetics, clothing, or auto-mutilation, is merely one aspect of a wider and more fundamental narcissistic trend.

It is not surprising that the early Christian Church forbad tattooing, for the Emperor Constantine asserted that man's body, being made in God's own image, should not be disfigured.

Within living memory tattooing was also forbidden in Nazi Germany, for reasons not dissimilar. The *corps d'élite,* however, received special dispensation. Thus the S.S. were compelled to have their blood-group tattooed in the axilla to assist priority in surgical contingencies. Among the Allied Forces the Russians alone were shrewd enough to realise this and they forced their German prisoners to strip and hold up their arms. Those with this tattooed identification were shot. When it became clear how the war was going, some of the S.S. anticipated that eventuality by demanding plastic surgery. In turn this merely led to the Russians taking violent action when an axillary scar was discovered, without further enquiry.

In considering contemporary tattooage, it seems necessary to discuss separately this practice as applied to males and to females. This very fact is, in itself, important and significant.

Modern white men elect to get themselves tattooed for a variety of excuses, but behind them all is the urge for self-adornment. Of greater interest is the question of choice of pattern. Provided that the victim is sober enough at the time, he has a diversity of opportunities. Briefly the decorative themes can be divided into:

(1) Religious and sentimental (crucifixes, mother-motifs) ;
(2) Patriotic (ships, flags, regimental crests) . The army has its own means of displaying battle-honours. Men of the 2nd battalion of the Royal Welch Fusiliers (the "White Ghurkhas") often have their thumbs tattooed with a mosquito, to commemorate an onerous march across India during the second World War.

Surgeon Captain Scott is the authority upon tattooing in Royal Naval personnel. Out of every 100 ratings, almost 50 are tattooed, four-fifths of them within the first two years of their service. There is a correlation between tattooage and intelligence: artificers and writers are less often so adorned and those who are advanced from the lower deck to officer rank have but few adornments. Feathered birds are the sailor's favourite. A bluebird represents 5,000 miles sea-service, a heart a further 5,000. Capt. Scott said that 70 per cent of tattooed sailors regret their adornment by the time they marry, and even more when they leave the service. One of Capt. Scott's favourite stories is of an American sailor in the Orient who had staggered from one bar to another proclaiming how he despised "those Goddam Limeys". The Royal Naval contingent quickly drank him under the table and then bundled the unconscious mariner into a taxi. The sailor woke next morning to find tattooed across his chest "Rule Britannia, Britannia rules the waves";

(3) Amorous-erotic (ranging from a girl's name to nudes of all grades of pictorial obscenity). Allied is the Rabelaisian theme of which the classic example is the tally-ho picture. Here the back is tattooed with an elaborate hunting-scene with mounted horsemen and hounds chasing a fox who has gone to earth into such a hidey-hole that only its bushy tail is visible;

(4) Aggressive-horrific (dragons, tigers, daggers);

(5) Mainly decorative (butterflies, bracelets, etc.)

Obviously a certain amount of overlap may occur, as between (1) and (3), while (4) may prove to be mainly ornamental, the more particular choice of pictorial violence depending upon the nationality of the tattoo-artist.

According to Delarue and Giraud (as quoted by Ebensten) tattooing often constituted a sort of sign-language among French criminals. Thus the mark of a pimp was a woman carried aloft by an eagle, and the insignia of a burglar was a butterfly. But the criminal is ordinarily less selective. A common mark among French prisoners is MAV, meaning *morte aux vaches* (i.e. the cops). Yet another piece of cynical art is a bracelet-like mark around the throat, beneath which is written *Fatalité*, or perhaps even *Promis à Deibler* (reserved for the executioner).

Anyone who has inspected with admiration the widely tattooed torso of a sailor will be able to identify, at a single viewing, patterns which belong to each and every one of the 5 foregoing classifications. This in itself suggests that most tattooing, if not all, is more self-expressive than communicative, although these two functions are related and not conflicting. There are exceptions, of course, and it is these which ordinarily apply to the factors underlying the phenomenon of tattooing in the female.

Tattooed prisoners of a rather different type are nowadays appearing, namely among the political detainees in Siberia. It is unlikely that the complete extent of this practice or the diversity of *motifs* will ever become general knowledge. We secure a glimpse of the situation from the rare accounts afforded us by ex-prisoners. According to Marchenko, for example, it is not unusual to observe that the cheeks or foreheads may be the site of such writings as "communists—butchers", "communists drink the blood of

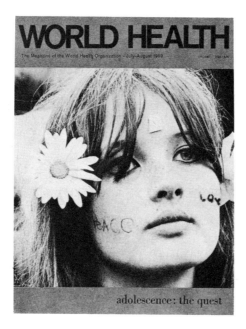

FIG. 2. Cover of World Health Magazine, July–August 1969.

the people", "Khruskev's slave" or "Slave of the C.P.S.U." (Communist Party of the Soviet Union). One man, in a special regime camp, was as tattooed as a Maori. On one cheek could be read "Lenin was a butcher" while on the other was "millions suffer because of him." Beneath his eyes appeared "Khrushchev, Brezhnev, Voroshilov are butchers". A hand clutching the throat was tattooed on the neck, with the letters C.P.S.U. decorating the fingers, while on the thumb gripping the Adam's apple appeared "KGB".

Up to the time of the Second World War, medical students were taught that tattooing in a woman was tantamount to a positive Wassermann reaction. The implication was that she had been a low-class prostitute consorting with seamen of all nationalities. Thus one sometimes observed an arrow on the inner thigh, directed upwards, and labelled "Excelsior". According to Moraglio (quoted by Zucker) a German prostitute's thigh was tattooed with a phallus, inscribed *Immer Linnen* (always inside). Incidentally a tattooed beauty spot on the right side of the upper lip was sometimes a lesbian trade-mark. The sociological pattern has since changed. Today a forearm tattooed with a set of numerals may indicate that the unfortunate woman (or man for that matter) had been an inmate of a concentration camp during the Nazi regime. The cynic observes darkly the antinomy between the self-preservatory tattooing of the Nazi high officials, and the contemptuous cattle-like branding of their victims. In female remand homes and gaols, it is a not uncommon practice for the prisoners to

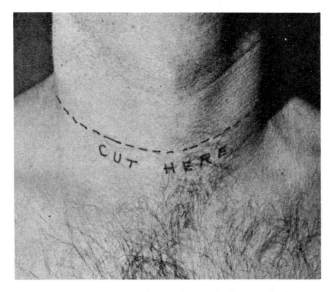

FIG. 3. Tattoo marks on the neck of a criminal.

scratch their skins indelibly with a pin, to record the names of pop singers and boy friends. This more strictly falls into the category of scarification, as practised by the Sudanese for other reasons. Here we embark upon the topic of tribal marks, a subject which merits a monograph to itself. But actual tattooing is also carried out in some female reformatories, certainly in Hungary. A girl of 16 years whom I saw in Budapest displayed many marks over both forearms, including a palm tree, a skull and crossbones, various boys' names, and one or two slogans such as "beat me" and "life is a crime". Over the first phalanx of each finger was a letter, and the ten put together formed the sentence "I am a vagrant". This girl had been found abandoned in a field as a baby; was raised by cruel and drunken foster-parents; she was rescued and put into a childrens' home, from which she repeatedly absconded. Later, because of truancy and promiscuity she received rough handling by the police, and was sent first to a gaol and later to a mental institution as an incorrigible psychopath and dullard.

A New Zealand study investigated the tattooing habits of the inmates of a female Borstal institution. A sample of 61 girls showed 27 with seven or more tattoo-marks, 14 with a few, and 20 with none. Of those who were heavily tattooed many were active homosexuals, most of whom bore the names of their "darls" or female partners. There was a direct correlation between the profusion of tattooage and the masculinity of their behaviour and sexual orientation. Many girls bore on their faces the letters **BOG** meaning Borstal old girls.

However, tattooing in women may be practised for quite different rea-

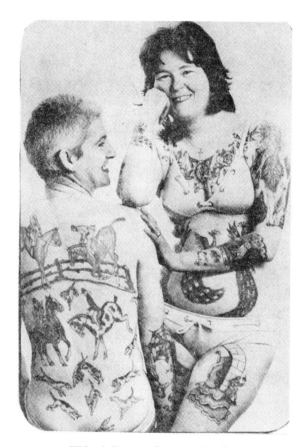

FIG. 4. Tattooed man and wife.

sons. Thus Armenian women in the Levant may submit to tattooing to indicate that they have made a pilgrimage to Jerusalem.

In a group apart belong the tattooed women of the show-ground and circus. The female, rather than the male, is more prominent in this role.

Within show business the prestige of the tattooed woman is not high. She is regarded not as an exponent of a difficult or dangerous technique like the rider or acrobat, but as an individual on display, inferior even to the contortionist or stripper. It is not surprising that tattooed ladies have rightly or wrongly been identified with certain unpleasing personality traits, such as conceit, aloofness, and inaccessibility.

Let us, in conclusion, give due credit to one of the earliest writers upon this subject, Dr. James Bulwer. In 1653 he published his monograph upon this topic upder the startling title:

Anthropometamorphosis: Man Transform'd: or The Artificial Changling Historically presented, In the mad cruell Gallantry, foolish Bravery, ridiculous Beauty, filthy Finenesse, and loathsome Loveliness of most Nations, fashioning and altering their Bodies from the mould intended by Nature; with Figures of those Transfigurations. To which artificiall and affected Deformations are added, all the Native and Nationall Monstrosities that have appeared to disfigure the Humane Fabrick. With a Vindication of the Regular Beauty and Honesty of Nature. And an Appendix of the Pedigree of the English Gallant.

The subject of tattooing constitutes an interesting off-beat aspect of contemporary social anthropology. Doctors occupy a particularly advantageous role in this matter, and they could, with care and tact, contribute an interesting chapter to this topic, although the tattooist is becoming more and more a rarity. In fact he may slowly disappear from the contemporary scene leaving, as the sole perpetrator of decorative anonymity, the faceless individual who writes on walls.

Reprinted from Critchley, M. (1969) : *History of Medicine*, Vol. 1.

Perseveration in the Domain of Vision

Whenever I pass the Hotel, which I do constantly, I see the same man. Scientists call that phenomenon an "obsession of the visual nerve." You and I know better.

Unpublished letter from Oscar Wilde to Robert Ross

Chronogenic aspects of disordered perception, although alluded to many years back, are perhaps not yet sufficiently borne in mind. One example—namely, visual perseveration—has even now scarcely passed into the *corpus* of neuro-ophthalmology, although cases constantly crop up in clinical practise.

Briefly the term *visual perseveration* can be made to cover more than one unusual subjective experience:

1. A visual stimulus may be sensed in the ordinary way but, after its removal, there may occur a hallucinatory and recurring reappearance of the object. This may be termed *palinopsia.*

2. A disappearing visual stimulus may not fade from the patient's gaze, for he may continue to imagine he can discern the object for some time—usually a matter of seconds or minutes—when it is actually out of sight. This is *visual perseveration* in the strictest sense of the word, and unlike what happens in the case of palinopsia, the "phantom" does not keep recurring.

3. A visual stimulus may be sensed, but over an unduly extensive area of environmental space. This usually happens when the targets are exceptionally vivid in pattern or in hue. Thus when a patient looks at a lady wearing a brightly coloured frock, the colours may seemingly extend so as to involve the face, arms, legs, and even some distance beyond. This is *visuospatial perseveration* or *illusory visual spread.* Temporal factors do not apply, for when the stimulus has gone (as when the woman walks away) the colouring also fades and does not reappear. This type of visual perseveration is the rarest.

The foregoing phenomena have been specifically described by me in a series of publications since 1949. Previously, a few case reports had appeared in which something suggestive of visual perseveration was mentioned, but without arousing any special comment, and more recently the literature has contained a number of further case records. The circumstances under which the various types of visual perseveration have been described most commonly comprise parieto-occipital lesions; these may be either bilateral or unilateral, right-sided or left-sided. Epilepsy, states of toxaemia, and mescal delirium constitute less commonplace circumstances which may be accompanied by a visual perseveration. In at least one case no very obvious pathological process could be demonstrated other than a diffuse atrophy of the brain. In this chapter the topic of visual perseveration is briefly reviewed, and 4 additional cases recounted.

Case Reports

Case 1 (visual perseveration in space associated with the onset of an attack of migraine). Mrs. B., age 33, consulted me because of attacks of migraine. In the more severe attacks she would first of all experience flashes before her eyes like lightning. Sometimes, when at home, she would also notice all around her yellow blobs, which she eventually realised were actually an extension of the yellow checkered tiles on the floor of her kitchen. Thirty minutes later a severe headache would develop, accompanied by nausea.

Case 2 (optic alloesthesia with visual perseveration associated with a right parieto-occipital tumour). D. E., a medical man under the care of Prof. Morris Bender, had rather suddenly acquired a weakness of the left hand, associated with a homonymous hemianopia. When shown a two-digit number (15) printed on the wall, he missed the 1 but could see the 5. Thereafter, irrespective of the actual figure which was displayed, he kept seeing the 1; moreover, he continued to see it even after all visual targets had been removed. On another occasion he kept fancying that he could see a number of teddy bears and rabbits on the wall, which were actually an illusory elaboration of some bolts that were present in that situation. On the following day at breakfast, some Rice Krispies dropped from his plate on to his lap. He then imagined he could see them on the wall floating across from left to right. This illusion lasted 15 minutes.

Arteriography subsequently revealed a neoplasm in the right parieto-occipital region.

Case 3 (a right-sided parieto-occipital lesion associated with palinopsia). W. W., a 67-year-old man shown me by Prof. Morris Bender, had placed his spectacles on a dresser to the right, and a little later had picked them up. However, they still appeared as though they were lying on the dresser, and gradually they seemed to float downward and toward the left. A little later he was watching television and saw on the screen a woman smoothing her face. On glancing across at his wife he thought he saw her hands also moving over her face in a similar fashion, an action which went on for 10 minutes. Later a zebra appeared upon the screen. For the next 30 minutes he kept imagining he could see this animal, even when he was out of doors. On yet another occasion, when watching the traffic lights, the red seemed to continue for some minutes after it had been extinguished in favour of the green light.

Here again a carotid angiogram was abnormal, and suggested a mass in the right parieto-occipital region.

Case 4 (palinopsia in a patient severely paralysed with a Guillain-Barré syndrome). F. P. (A21911) was a patient under the care of Dr. C. J. Earl on account of an infective polyneuritis. Two months after the onset, and while he was still in the Respiratory Unit, he suddenly lost his sight for 24 hours. Vision returned, but for the next few days, a number of curious visual phenomena occurred: (1) illusory slow drifting of objects from right to left; (2) a recurring right-sided hemianopia; (3) a misshapen, distorted, and tilted appearance of objects; (4) patchy erythropsia; (5) episodic visual hallucinations; (6) dyslexia; and (7) visual perseveration. As regards the last-named, the perseveration occurred intermittently. Thus on the television screen, the scene which had actually faded would superimpose itself upon the succeeding frames. On another occasion a nurse walking across the room from right to left and out of the door, seemed almost immediately to walk out of this room again. This happened three or four times in succession. A third palinopsic incident occurred after the doctors had been testing his visual acuity by placing a Snellen's test card on the wall in front. After they had removed the card, the patient imagined the card was still there, and he almost called out to inform the doctors that they had forgotten it.

The explanation of the visual phenomena in this case is obscure. Some toxic, or at any rate anoxaemic, state would seem to be operative, or, alternatively, an embolism that had lodged temporarily in the basilar artery, afterward permanently occluding the left posterior cerebral artery.

The following case of mine has recently been published in the Soviet literature, but is not readily accessible.

Case 5 (palinopsia in a patient with cortical atrophy especially in the hind part of the brain). A healthy 54-year-old farm labourer showed little if any neurological deficit, and was an intelligent observer who was able to describe his own visual phenomena vividly. He was standing in his garden when suddenly he imagined he could see potatoes all around him. A month later while watching television he saw a program of a policeman urging a prisoner into a car. On turning his head to the right he discovered he could see the same incident depicted upon the wall of his sitting room.

Three weeks later he was casually looking in a shop window at a number of electric fires. Immediately afterward he continued to imagine he could see these objects wherever he directed his gaze. Once again, when seated before the burning coal fire in his sitting room, he fancied he could still see the fire both to the right and to the left of him.

The patient (A21911) was admitted to the National Hospital, Queen Square, where other episodes of visual perseveration took place. On one occasion he was gazing out of the ward window across the square at the Church of St. George-the-Martyr. On looking away he fancied he could still see, on the wall of the ward, the church in all its natural colours. This vision lasted about half a minute.

Two weeks later he was again standing at the window of his ward looking across Queen Square at the rooftops of the houses immediately in front. On turning his head to one side for a moment, he found he could still see the scene in front of him. So vivid were these perseveratory phenomena that the patient was able to make coloured sketches of these last two incidents (Figs. 1 to 4).

Full neurological investigation revealed no abnormality except an incomplete homonymous field defect to the left. Air studies, however,

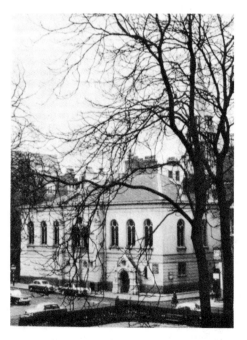

FIG. 1. The Church of St. George-the-Martyr, Queen Square, as viewed from the National Hospital.

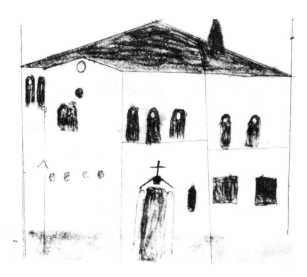

FIG. 2. The patient's drawing of the perseverating image of the church.

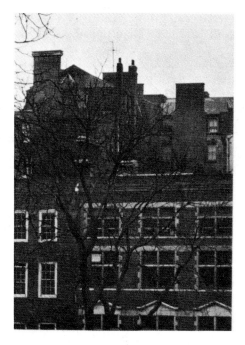

FIG. 3. Rooftops of the buildings immediately facing Queen Square, as seen through the Ward windows of the hospital.

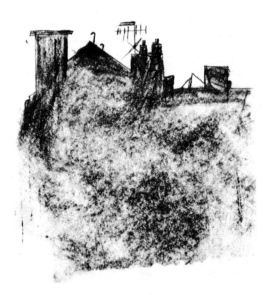

FIG. 4. The patient's sketch of the scene photographed in Figure 3 as appearing as a visual perseveration.

demonstrated a certain amount of cortical and central atrophy involving the left posterior lobe more than the right. There was no evidence of neoplasm.

Some time after the patient left hospital and went home, I learned from his ophthalmic specialist that on one occasion he was walking toward a river with his eyes fixed on a distant belt of trees. Suddenly he imagined that he could see nothing except those trees, and on that account he walked right into the river. He did not realise what had happened, or indeed even that he was wet, until the image of the trees had disappeared and he was able to realise where he was. Four or five other attacks of visual perseveration have occurred at irregular intervals during the past 12 months.

This last case report is reminiscent of the one described by Mooney et al. Theirs concerned a commercial artist, a 45-year-old man, who developed a parasagittal parieto-occipital meningioma on the left side. Shortly after its surgical removal, the patient began to experience recurring visual hallucinations and distortions of sight. The left eye of a nurse at the foot of his bed seemed to become fierce and staring, with the iris unnaturally blue and the sclera very brilliant. Although she left the ward, the eye remained vividly at a point where she had been standing. These perseveratory phenomena were depicted by the patient in water colours and were illustrated by the authors in their paper. Something reminiscent of illusory visual spread also took place when he noticed that a man in an adjacent bed seemed to have at least three arms instead of one resting outside the coverlet. There also occurred a number of other visual phenomena, part illusory, part metamorphopsic, and part hallucinatory, the patient's eyelids being either closed or open. Many of these experiences the patient was able to illustrate. Under medication with phenobarbital these manifestations soon disappeared, and the patient was able to return to his work.

Discussion*

The question may be posed why visual perseveratory phenomena are apparently so rare in clinical practice. Possibly the physician, ignorant of the literature, may miss the symptom altogether, or he may mistakenly ascribe it to a global intellectual loss, or even to a hysterical overlay. It is interesting to note how often the patient with visual perseveration retains a fairly clear, if not an intact, sensorium throughout his odd visual experiences. As a rule the patient is unable deliberately to provoke these manifestations. However, in a fourth case described in an earlier paper it was at times possible in the clinic to demonstrate the perseveration. The same applied to the two patients described by Kinsbourne and Warrington by dint of tachistoscopic techniques, as suggested as likely to happen in my paper of 1951. Perhaps it is not without interest how often these perseveratory illusions came on in the course of watching television, as incidentally was the case in the patient described by Bekény and Péter.

Lastly, I received a communication from one of my Nigerian postgraduate students which I already referred to in an earlier publication. Dr. Ilo told me of a piece of folklore among the Ibo-speaking natives of Eastern Nigeria. The gods rewarded a man for his lifelong piety with the gift of fortelling the future by dint of his vision. Objects which he looked at, and which remained in sight after they have gone, became endowed with special significance. He was consulted on all sides by people who would bring along some little articles for him to inspect. Thus barren women would bring green leaves. If the article or the leaves would fill the whole of his vision and thereafter persist, the omen was favourable. It was said that in later life the seer abused his divine gift and was punished by the gods with blindness and insanity.

Acknowledgments

I am grateful to Prof. Morris B. Bender and to Dr. Christopher J. Earl for allowing me to interview and to quote the patients under their care.

---

* Note added in proof: An important contribution by M. B. Bender, M. Feldman, and A. J. Sabin, entitled "Palinopsia," has appeared in *Brain* 91:321, 1968.
Reprinted from Critchley, M. (1969) : *Modern Neurology*. Little, Brown, & Co., Boston.

Modes of Reaction to Central Blindness

"Central" or "cortical" blindness is usually brought about as the result of bilateral occipital lesions. These may occur abruptly and simultaneously, the principal lesion being an occlusion of the basilar artery at its point of bifurcation. Less often the syndrome develops in two stages. That is to say a thrombosis of one posterior cerebral artery (leading to a hemianopia) may be followed some time later by an obstruction of the posterior cerebral artery on the other side.

The result is either a total amblyopia, or else an extreme limitation of the visual fields which are reduced to mere macular vision. In the latter case we meet with the rare syndrome of "tubular vision".

It is the more severe defect, however, which concerns us today, chiefly by reason of the diversity and unexpectedness of the psychological reaction. The sudden development of bilateral occipital dysfunction is likely to produce transient physical and psychical effects in which mental confusion may be prominent. It may be some days before the relatives, or the nursing staff, tumble to the fact that the patient has actually become sightless. This is not only because the patient ordinarily does not volunteer the information that he has become blind, but he furthermore misleads his entourage by behaving and talking as though he were sighted. Attention is aroused however when the patient is found to collide with pieces of furniture, to fall over objects, and to experience difficulty in finding his way around. He may try to walk through a wall or through a closed door on his way from one room to another. Suspicion is still further alerted when he begins to describe people and objects around him which, as a matter of fact, are not there at all.

Thus we have the twin symptoms of anosognosia (or lack of awareness of defect) and confabulation, the latter affecting both speech and behaviour.

While the patient is under observation further questioning may uncover other psychological aberrations. Thus if the patient with central blindness be directly taxed as to whether or not any visual trouble exists, he may give an outright denial of the fact. This is a reaction which goes far beyond a mere failure to complain of blindness. We neurologists have no agreed term to express this sheer rejection of disease, though the expression "noso-arnesia" or denial of disease has tentatively been put forward.

Another type of reaction may be traceable at times in patients with central blindness. Thus the patient does not volunteer any complaint but when asked about the state of his visual perception he may admit that objects appear dim. He projects the shortcomings on to the environment, however. Thus he may put the blame on inadequate lighting, or a failure to switch on the electricity or to pull back the curtains. This type of re-action was known 2,000 years ago, for we find among Seneca's letters to his friend Lucilius, the following: "You know Harpaste my wife's old nurse-maid: she has been kept on in my house, a burden wished on me through a legacy . . . . now she suddenly lost her sight. What I'm going to tell you sounds incredible, but I assure you that it's true. This silly woman doesn't even know she is blind. She keeps asking the housekeeper to change her living-quarters; she says her apartments are too dark."

There is yet another mode of reaction—one which is likely to come about after the patient has been in hospital for some time. The patient may now admit he has lost his sight, but he does so almost casually, or light-heartedly, as though it were something not very important. Unless directly prompted he does not allude to the subject, but retains an attitude of apathy or insouciance. Rarely if ever does he talk about it with his doctor. He does not enquire how serious the matter is; how long it is likely to last; and what are his prospects of getting back to work. He may even be mildly euphoric, exhibiting what Babinski called an "anosodiaphoria", or lack of concern about the presence of illness and its possible repercussions.

Yet again the patient will almost grudgingly admit to direct questioning that there may be something slightly amiss with his sight, almost as an after-thought. Pressed for further details the patient may respond as though it was merely a matter of short-sightedness or presbyopia or a need for stronger spectacles. The patient exhibits no distress whatsoever.

Allied to this attitude, is yet another mode of response, where the patient admits that he has become blind but only if directly taxed. An affect of despair is lacking, however, and the patient may not again spontaneously refer to his affliction, though he will admit it, if questioned.

Thus a woman of 75 suddenly went blind. At first she did not realise her plight and even denied it when questioned. Realisation of the blindness developed later, but she was not perturbed thereby. She was quite inaccurate as to the manner and the date of onset, claiming that her eyesight had been gradually failing over a matter of years. An elec-tric torch flashed into her eyes was not perceived. Asked if she could see anything at all, she peered around and finally said she was aware of a sort of "obstruction" to her left. She asserted that it was night-time though actually it was the morning. She was also disorientated in place.

Furthermore she had lost both her visual memory and her visual imagery. Although she said she could remember her doctor quite well, she could not make the slightest attempt to describe him. She could not call to mind her lodgings, nor her bedroom furniture, nor the view from her window. Asked the colour of a fire-engine she tentatively replied "greenish". She could not recollect the colours in the flags of Belgium or of France. Nor could she describe the facial appearances of Hitler, Goering, Winston Churchill, or King Edward VII. In contrast thereto she could promptly identify noises around her and she could recall and describe or even imitate the sounds made by a clock, a cuckoo, a cat, and a dog.

This case illustrates another common accompaniment of central blindness, namely the Charcot-Wilbrand syndrome of defective visual memory coupled with irreminiscence. Of course this syndrome may occur quite independently of loss of vision, and indeed in some of the recorded cases the organicity of the picture is open to serious doubt.

This woman also showed a bilateral astereognosis presumably because her occipital lesions were extensive in a forward direction. The association of defective tactile recognition of objects, with a central blindness, is by no means rare.

The foregoing catalogue of types of reaction to central blindness needs to be modified by the realisation that the patient often varies enormously in the character of his replies, not only from one day to another, but also from moment to moment. His reaction may also differ according to whether he is among doctors, or nurses, or relatives. Thus, in hospital the patient may stoutly deny that he is blind and yet in an inconsistent fashion he may allow the nursing staff to lead him around, feed him, and read and write letters on his behalf.

The following interview illustrates the characteristic inconsistency of such a patient:

Q. How is your sight?
A. I'd say it was good.
Q. Do you really mean that?
A. [No reply.]
Q. What's the matter with you?
A. My sight's not good.
Q. Can you see anything at all?
A. Oh yes, I can see some things.
Q. What's the colour of your pyjamas?
A. No sir.
Q. Do you complain of anything at all?
A. No.
Q. Why are you in hospital?
A. I'd have to enquire further.

Q. Haven't you any idea?
A. The answer's in the negative.
Q. What stops you getting up and going to work?
A. Nothing.
Q. Your work as a dental mechanic is pretty delicate: Do you think you could do it now?
A. Yes, Doctor.
Q. How would you get there?
A. On my bike.
Q. Could you find your way from here to your place of work on your bike?
A. Yes.

As an example of wild but unhesitating confabulation so typical of these cases of central blindness, particularly in the early stages, we may quote the following record:

Though utterly sightless she maintained she could see me standing at the bedside though her orientation was not accurate. She was quite incorrect in her description of what I was wearing. When I asked her to describe the appearance and dress of a woman by my side she did so without hesitation, *though no female whatsoever was in the room.* Questioned whether she had lately studied the newspapers, she replied that she had; but when a paper was given to her to read aloud she became merely distressed.

To this picture of unawareness or denial of blindness, coupled with loss of visual memory and imagery, and furthermore with erratic confabulation provoked by appropriate suggestion, there may also be added long periods of amnesia. The patient may even speak as though living in another decade. The psychiatric profile is very like that of a Korsakov syndrome.

The following record of an interview with a patient with a central blindness illustrates many of the vagaries which I have been describing:

Q. What does your wife look like?
A. A typical matron.
Q. Young or old?
A. About a year younger than I am. [Actually she was 48 and he was 60.]
Q. What does your house look like?
A. It stands on its own. [Actually they lived in a small basement flat.]
Q. How many bedrooms?
A. Seven.
Q. Can you remember the colour of the carpet in your living room?
A. Red. [Actually green.]
Q. Have you any pets at home?

A. A black cat called "Nigger". [Their cat had died 6 years before. It was ginger and white and had answered to the name "Whisky".]

Q. Do you keep chickens?

A. Yes, Rhode Island Reds. [He had not kept poultry for 6 years.]

Had one not checked the accuracy of these replies by enquiry of his wife, one might easily have been misled, for the patient never seemed to be in doubt and always gave his answers promptly and in a very plausible fashion.

A curious instance of "confabulatory pseudo-recognition" as we may term it is seen when a patient describes inaccurately the appearance of objects he has failed to identify. Thus shown an article he naturally fails to state what it is. When it is put into his hand he may now identify it, unless of course he has an associated astereognosis. But he proceeds to perpetrate two pathological modes of behaviour. Thus he now claims he can see it (when obviously he cannot) and he furthermore goes on to describe it—quite erroneously.

For example, a comb is held before the patient's eyes:

Q. Can you see this?

A. No.

Q. I'll put it in your hand; what is it?

A. It's a comb, Doctor.

Q. Now look hard at it. Can you see it now?

A. Yes.

Q. Really and truly?

A. Of course.

Q. What colour is it?

A. Brown and white. [Actually it was red.]

Unawareness of blindness and denial of blindness represent in the visual sphere what is more often encountered in cases of left hemiplegia. Anosognosia for paralysis is indeed a more familiar syndrome, and it is one which may be overlaid with the most fantastic aberrations in the domain of corporeal awareness, i.e. body-image. Some patients with central blindness also happen to be hemiplegic. Anosognosia can then occur either in the sphere of one modality but not the other, or in both.

Dr. Kremer has kindly allowed me to quote my findings upon one of his cases:

Q. Do you recognise me?

A. Yes.

Q. Can you see my beard?

A. Yes.

Q. What colour suit am I wearing?

A. Light grey.

Q. And my tie?
A. Red.
Q. Can you see the flower in my buttonhole?
A. Yes.
Q. What sort of flower is it?
A. A rose. [Not one of these replies was correct.]
Q. Is your eye-sight pretty good?
A. Yes.
Q. Can you move your arms and legs?
A. Yes.
Q. Is there anything amiss with your left hand?
A. Nothing special.
Q. Well squeeze my hand hard . . . . That's not a very good grip; why is that?
A. I don't want to hurt you. [Actually he had a left hemiplegia.]
Q. Can you see this? [Holding up an orange.]
A. No.
Q. Feel it: Now what is it?
A. It feels like a lemon.
Q. Can you see it?
A. No.
Q. Why not?
A. You do ask stupid questions.
Q. Look around you. Do you see any women here?
A. That looks like a young girl over there. [Not true.]
Q. Do you see any furniture about you?
A. No, there's a parting in the room.
Q. Parting? That's not a usual word.
A. It's not what I usually see.
Q. What have I got in my hand? [Holding up a bottle.]
A. I can see your hand, but not what you are holding.
Q. Well, take it in your left hand and feel it.
A. I've got a pain in my left hand today, and I can't move it.

The day-to-day inconsistency of this patient's replies was considerable. Note how his answers were at times tart, almost insolent.

This latter observation brings one to the very important factor of iatrogenicity. The inter-personal relationship as between doctor and patient may be important, even crucial, for these subjects are highly suggestible. Jaffé and Slote studied a series of ten patients using a double examination technique. Each patient was interviewed on separate occasions by two different neurologists. Each of these two prepared a set of questions identical in content, but slanted in diametrically opposite ways—i.e. a positive versus a negative direction. Thus one questioner would maximise the disability, the other minimising it, like *le médecin tant-pis and le médecin tant-mieux* in la Fontaine's fable. One doctor would say "feeling pretty poorly today?" while the other would ask "feeling pretty well today?" Another pair of contrasting questions would be: "Do you feel you're getting worse?" as opposed to "Do you feel you're getting better?" Doctor *Tant-Pis,* i.e. the maximiser, would present his questions in a grave, concerned, and somewhat depressing manner; while Doctor *Tant-Mieux,* in his enquiries, would exude a cheery, optimistic, and reassuring atmosphere. These two types of interview produced contrasting attitudes on the part of the patient. There was a general tendency for the patient to fall in with the suggestions subtly posed by the particular examiner. The patient's replies were marked on a 5-point scale ranging from total explicit denial; general optimism or minimising of illness short of complete denial; neutral, dispassionately objective, non-commital, or evasive replies; pessimism or depression, with the worst possible attitude towards illness; and finally, a catastrophic reaction.

The authors concluded—with a characteristic piece of psychiatric jargon —*that anosognosia represents a symbolic adaptive mechanism to be observed under the conditions of communicative interaction.*

Finally, let us enumerate the various theories that have been advanced to explain the odd behaviour of patients with central blindness, emphasising that these speculative ideas are not mutually exclusive.

(1) That the anosognosia for blindness is a specific manifestation of parietal involvement, particularly on the non-dominant side.

(2) That the unawareness is not a focal symptom but merely a striking instance of the "denial syndrome" which is inherent in every victim of brain-damage.

(3) That the lack of insight depends upon the personality of the patient prior to the onset of blindness.

(4) That visual anosognosia is largely an "artefact of the interview situation" and stems chiefly from the attitude of the doctors and relatives.

Let us recall that patients who have a gross and permanent disability often show a better adjustment than those with an incomplete and slowly altering dysfunction. Thus total blindness may often be ignored while incomplete loss of vision may be a source of bitter complaint.

Reprinted from Critchley, M. (1965) : *Czechoslovakian Neurologie,* Vol. 28.

Photisms in the Blind and in Those Without Eyes

May I at the outset briefly report two patients whom I had the opportunity of studying in some detail?

The first concerned a simple, relatively uneducated woman of 60, whose sight had progressively deteriorated since childhood and amounted to total blindness at the age of 57. A year after this happened she became troubled by a diversity of constantly changing visual hallucinations. An almost constant feature, however, was a centrally placed golden-yellow spot from which threads radiated like a spider's web. Occasionally this would be replaced by a golden horseshoe surrounded by coloured patches which continually changed in hue. To the left was jet blackness, above which lay a wasp-like pattern of alternating black and yellow stripes. These kaleidoscopic photisms would then temporarily merge to form elaborate scenes, like sailors with yellow faces, their bodies cut off at waist level; yellow flowers on a blue table; a desert scene with a deep blue sky above. Such visions were most oppressive and distressing. They persisted despite the instillation of her optic nerves with alcohol. An injection of mescaline produced a temporary sense of depersonalisation and derealisation but did not materially alter the hallucinations. A prefrontal leucotomy relieved her preoccupation with the visual symptoms, which, however, persisted. She now complained of feeling shut in as if her head were encased within a helmet or swathed round and round with a blanket. The phantasms altered somewhat so as to take the form of perpetually changing colours which occasionally would coalesce to constitute the shape of ladies' faces.

I continued to see this woman for several years. Since her leucotomy she had become more serene, but the visions still obsessed her and indeed over the years had become more obtrusive. From a spatial point of view they seemed to her as though they were painted upon the back of her eyeballs.

An occipital leucotomy was seriously considered but the idea was rejected because of the risk of her losing the ability to read Braille. We were also afraid that her so-called sixth sense or awareness of obstacles might suffer.

My second patient was of a very different type. He was an American male, aged 42 years, a university professor of Philosophy. He had lost sight first in one eye and then in the other, and because of intractable pain it became necessary to remove surgically both eyeballs. Thereafter he became plagued by distressing and almost continual visual hallucinations which took various forms such as a glare, flashes of light, and billowing multi-coloured clouds. Towards nightfall, when feeling drowsy, he would see myriad stars of many colours. So uncomfortable and so depressing were all these phantasms that he had submitted to an alcohol-injection of the stumps of both optic nerves but without any resulting benefit. His symptoms continued despite medication with chlorpromazine and other nerve-sedatives. A leucotomy was considered, but a decision was deferred.

Here then was a case where hallucinations occurred in a blind subject who was without any retinal receptor organs.

A neurologist may well ask his ophthalmic colleagues about the nature of the subjective visual experiences of the totally blind. Does a sightless person ordinarily experience an environment of utter blackness, by night as well as by day, and whether the eyelids are open or shut? Maybe the situation differs from case to case, but surely some statistics must be available as to how many blinded live in a world of darkness, and how many experience a sort of colour-filter, or a veil of erythropsia, or luminosity, or some other positive manifestations.

Over 50 years ago, Col. Elliot discussed this very matter and he drew attention to what he termed the "memory-sight" of the blind. He emphasised that not only can the visual experiences be positive rather than negative, but they may often be something quite elaborate, pleasurable, and evocative. One patient of his, though totally blind, would sit at a window and describe details of the scenic environment with which he had long been familiar. If one interprets the author correctly, one suspects this phenomenon to have occupied a place halfway between an actual hallucinatory percept, and a vivid visual concept. Perhaps this judgment also applies to another of his blind patients who took pleasure in her subjective sensations of light and her comforting phantasmagoria which were to some extent controllable, for she could make herself see objects and persons around her. Thus she could perceive every stitch of the knitting in her hands, just as she did in the days when she had her sight. Yet another of his patients, who was not only blind but also devoid of the organs of sight, was constantly aware of glowing white mist as if illuminated from behind him. Furthermore he could see pieces of furniture in the room so vividly that he would carefully walk around them. Whether these objects were there in actuality is not clear from the author's text.

In my practice, I have been struck by the frequency with which the blind describe photisms or hallucinations, either habitually or occasionally. In my patients it was neither a case of "memory sight" nor of vivid imagery, but of actual phantasms. When one turns to the literature, however, one often finds the records muddled if not ambiguous.

Hallucinations have been reported in patients with cataract, but it is not always explicit whether vision was entirely lost or merely much reduced and thereby distorted. Some patients did not experience hallucinations until their cataracts had been extracted, when presumably some glimmer of perception was present. Others again were hallucinated before their operations at a stage when sight was not wholly lost. For this reason, the cases described by Flournoy in 1902 and 1923, Naville in 1909, and Brunerei and Coche are suspect. Some other blind patients reported as being visually hallucinated happened to be frankly psychotic, and here belong two of the cases of Brunerei and Coche and also the case of Daumezon.

But neither confusional insanity, nor dim vision, nor even vivid imagery can explain some of the instances which one encounters. Visions amounting even to elaborate phantasmagoria of persons and landscapes may take place whether the victim is in the dark or in bright sunlight, whether his eyes are open or shut. How often such hallucinations occur is uncertain, for reticence and diffidence may inhibit the sightless person from referring to his unexpected symptoms. We are grateful, therefore, for those personal descriptions afforded us by blind physicians, such as, for example, Truman Abell. Writing in 1846, he described his own spectral illusions as being threefold in nature. First he might experience, over a matter of days, a luminous or "lighted up" impression of whiteness which would provoke so much vertigo as to interfere with his balance. Then quite abruptly this brilliance might be replaced by a sense of utter blackness. Occasionally intermediate phases would occur, agreeable in nature, and comparable but not identical with a state of dreaming associated, as Abell put it, with "mesmeric" sleep.

A scrutiny of the cases in my series and in the literature suggests that the presence or absence of hallucinations may be determined by a number of variables, occurring singly or in combination. Most important, perhaps, is the question of age. In the majority of cases the subjects have been in their 8th, 9th, or even 10th decade, even though no intellectual shortcomings are evident. A second possible role is that played by the degree of abruptness with which vision was lost. Allied to this is the factor of pathology, and the morbid circumstances responsible for the sightlessness. The frequency with which cataracts are mentioned, and less often macular degeneration, raises the suspicion that dysfunction of the receptor organs may conceivably derange the perceptual impulses in such a way as to lead to misinterpretation of stimuli or to false sense-data. This notion falls down, however, when one encounters florid hallucinations in persons with no peripheral organs of sight, i.e. in those who have undergone surgical removal of the eyeballs. The occurrence of brilliant photisms and visions in such persons immediately conjures up the analogy of those bizarre phantom-sensations experienced by an amputee, as in the patient I mentioned earlier.

Other circumstances which may influence the phantasms, even if they do not provoke them, are such physiological states as fatigue, proximity to sleep, and even the time of day.

Still more important are endogenous determinants independent of age.

The intellectual rank of the patient may well be significant. His educational status and his degree of introversion may be operative. One must not overlook the basic affective state, whether it be one of depression or its opposite. We must not forget, furthermore, such personality traits as the aesthetic standing of the blind subject, and his power of imagery prior to the onset of blindness.

In conclusion one must mention those cases of colour-hearing, or synaesthesia induced by sound or even by thinking-processes, occurring in blind subjects. Voss has written a fascinating monograph upon *"Das Farben-hören bei Erblindeten"*. Such phenomena also occur, let us remember, in certain sighted individuals, particularly those of sensitive, introspective, and artistic temperament, but the synaesthesia rarely attains the same degree of intensity. In very many blind subjects, on the other hand, noises abrupt or prolonged, musical notes, even melodic and harmonic stimuli, may evoke an image—sometimes even a photism—specific in its shape, its brilliance, and its hue. That is to say, the visual phenomenon may change according to the pitch or intensity of the acoustic stimulus, while remaining constant and distinctive for a particular note or musical phrase.

Let us admit that in any discussion of hallucinations, whether in the sighted or the blind, we cannot avoid referring to the topic of *visionaries*. These are individuals, lying within the ambit of normality, to whom hallucinations or visions are liable to occur either as an isolated phenomenon, or on frequent occasions. Some of these individuals are gifted with a power of such vivid visualisation that a mental image elaborates itself so as to constitute an actual percept or visual sense-datum. This endowment is referred to as "eidetic imagery". Certain circumstances or environmental factors facilitate such phenomena. Goethe, for example, was an *Eidetiker*, and by closing his eyelids could evoke a realistic hallucination of a rose. Others belonging to this class include William Blake, Emanuel Swedenborg, Carl Jung, and a large number of so-called mystics. The factor of auto-suggestion is raised when one recalls that Jakob Boehme needed to peer into a shining pewter vessel, and Loyola had to gaze at running water. "Faces in the fire" are a common manifestation of an eidetic propensity, especially in children. Crystal-gazing (or scrying) is the best known and perhaps the most potent means of stimulating hallucinations, and it has been estimated that one person in 20 claims the ability to see visions within a crystal ball after concentrating long enough.

The factor of blindness constitutes a potent enhancement of any such latent tendencies, and leads us back to my original enquiry: "How often do such visual phenomena occur in the blind, both those born with sight and those who have lost their vision, gradually or abruptly."

The Syndrome of Periodic Hypersomnia and Megaphagia in Adolescent Males (Kleine-Levin): What Is Its Nature?

In 1925 Kleine collected from the clinic of Professor Kleist in Frankfurt a series of five patients with episodic drowsiness of diverse aetiology. Four years later Levin, a psychiatrist in New York, writing on the topic of narcolepsy, specifically drew attention to one very atypical case where periodic somnolency happened to be combined with excessive appetite. In 1936, Levin re-published this case and now for the first time suggested that a "syndrome of periodic somnolence and morbid hunger" represented a novel and specific entity. Within this group he included one of the cases described by Kleine, as well as some other isolated case-reports which he discovered in the literature.

During my war-time service in the Royal Navy I came across two striking examples which I published in association with Surgeon Lieutenant-Commander Hoffman. The eponymous term "Kleine-Levin syndrome" was for the first time applied by us, and this expression has since passed into the nomenclature of neurology and psychiatry. A number of case-reports have subsequently appeared, and it has been my good fortune to have met with no fewer than 14 or 15 such cases. In my paper in *Brain,* written in 1962, I drew attention to some additional clinical points: (1) limitation to the male sex; (2) an age-incidence which usually lay between 15 and 25 years of age; and (3) the presence of schizoid-like symptoms. I furthermore stated that, in some patients at least, the excessive intake of food was not so much a question of bulimia or exaggerated hunger, but rather a compulsive eating. Lastly I made the observation that these patients seemed spontaneously to lose their disability in the course of time. It was for these reasons that I proposed as a title for this syndrome "periodic hypersomnia and megaphagia in adolescent males", rather than the Kleine-Levin syndrome. Whether the two conditions are identical, or not, I could not be sure, nor am I confident even today.

Arising out of the foregoing, a number of questions come up for discussion:

(1) *The role of increased intake of food.* This symptom has been present in many of the patients, but certainly not in all. There have been patients who have shown somnolency and excessive eating in some attacks, but nothing except somnolency in others. Periodic food-intake in excessive amounts does not seem to occur in isolation, however. In one or two of the patients who have been closely studied in hospital, it has been found that the patient—though he ate to excess—was not strictly speaking hungry. He did not demand food. If a meal was put before him he would eat it up, greedily and wolfishly. If more food was brought he would eat that too. Should the patient not be strictly confined to bed, he might make his way to the kitchen or pantry and devour every article of food within sight. Whether this feature applied to all cases previously described in the literature, I cannot say. It was for this reason that I deliberately avoided both the terms bulimia and hunger, and spoke of "megaphagia", meaning by that an excessive ingestion of food.

Inordinate eating is the symptom which is most apt to be missing from the syndrome of periodic somnolency in adolescents, with agitation, petulance, fantasy-formation, and schizoid-like features. In some patients indeed the periodic attacks may, to begin with, show the complete syndrome, but later the excessive eating may cease to occur. Among many other cases in my series, this was so. This was also so with the patient published by Garland et al. This young man eventually left Leeds for London, and in his subsequent attacks came under the care of Professor Gilliatt who kindly invited me to see him.

(2) *The nature of the disturbance of consciousness.* In a recent paper Oswald has criticised me for stating that patients in the throes of an attack of so-called Kleine-Levin syndrome exhibit a state of "sleep" which does not differ from the normal pattern except for its immoderate duration, the ordinary appearances of sleep being present. Oswald objected that without the evidence of a characteristic E.E.G., a rise of electric skin-resistance, pupillary constriction, and slowing of the heart, one was not justified in using the term "sleep" in this context.

This strikes me as smacking of pedantry, and it suggests strongly that Oswald has never had the opportunity of witnessing a patient with this disorder in the throes of one of his attacks. When in a railway carriage I observe the passenger opposite me to close his eyelids, nod, slump limply, and then snore, I do not need the assistance of electroencephalography, or of skin-resistance tests to tell me that he has fallen asleep. Nor do I feel it incumbent upon me to feel my fellow-passenger's pulse, or to lift his eyelids in order to observe the size of his pupils.

No; like all others who have described such cases, I submit that it is not possible to deny that the patient with the Kleine-Levin syndrome "sleeps" too much. I will however concede the point that, in *addition* to the hypersomnia, the patient also shows, for some hours during the day, a qualitative change in his waking state which cannot strictly speaking be called "sleep". Nevertheless he is certainly not alert; he may be depersonalised, and a prey to vivid fantasies often with a violent or sexual colouring; his behaviour or comportment may be odd or uninhibited; he may be mildly confused, irritable, or even aggressive, especially when interfered with. This irascibility is a feature which appears over and over again throughout the case-histories recorded in the literature.

The argument that these day-time phenomena are not genuine manifestations of sleep should not be exaggerated. The point is that the patient with hypersomnia, who may have slept unduly long or unduly heavily at night-time, might be doing his best during the day to keep awake, and to comport himself in a normal fashion. Subjective depersonalisation and overt truculence are not too surprising in a patient bemused with overpowering sleepiness, who tries to keep alert but with dubious success.

This naturally leads us to a consideration of those patients *whose behaviour is so abnormal during the attacks as to raise suspicions of a recurring schizophrenic illness.* Oswald spoke of the "schizo-affective disorders" described by Crammer or alternatively of the "cycloid psychoses" reported by Leonhard. These two conditions are not identical and it behoves Oswald to make a choice. The soldier-patient described in 1951 by Robinson and McQuillan was depicted as being uninhibited, creating a disturbance, laughing, and shouting. He was untidy and unkempt, off-hand, casual, and uninterested. He smiled fatuously and was vague. Later he indecently exposed himself, masturbated, and made lewd overtures to the nursing staff. This type of behaviour is but an extreme instance of what has been recorded in other patients, who—by force of circumstances—cannot indulge their compulsive desire for sleep.

In my paper of 1962 I quoted many statements made by the patients themselves particularizing their curious disorder of thinking or of mood. It was obvious that many could not sharply distinguish between dreams in sleep and vivid fantasies during a semi-wakeful state, which—after all—is nothing more than an exaggeration of what a normal light sleeper experiences.

May we now take up the question as to *whether the Kleine-Levin syndrome, or the more circumscribed syndrome of periodic hypersomnia and megaphagia which I have described, can ever occur in females?*

From the literature a few cases can be isolated for discussion. We recall the example described by Castello del Pino involving a girl of seven years. I rejected this case, and a personal communication from the author concerning the follow-up study leads me to the confident conclusion that I was justified. Sagripanti in 1952 described two cases of lethargy occurring in females of 33 and 66 years—but both these cases were actually very unlike the instances under consideration. Two patients recorded by Roth concerned a women of 48 and a girl of 14 but these cases which I regard as entirely "unconvincing". Similar reservations are attached to the cases described by Ortez de Zarate where a mother and son were similarly afflicted.

A very typical case has also been reported by Duffy and Davison in a girl of 20 years.

In my own clinical experience I have encountered only one case which comes up for really serious consideration. This concerned a young and world-famous horsewoman of 20 years who, six weeks after a concussion, began to suffer episodes of drowsiness, which would come on abruptly. She would feel sleepy and take every opportunity to retire to bed. However she could always rouse herself, though her motor coordination was impaired as evidenced by her poor performance in equestrian show-jumping and in swimming. In this patient's case there was absolutely no increase in food-intake.

In considering the possibility of a Kleine-Levin-Critchley syndrome occurring in females, I am inclined to the opinion that there exists a sort of physiological continuum in women, ranging from an undue drowsiness (or alternatively bulimia) at one end of the scale, to a syndrome of lethargy together with excessive eating at the other. This latter end may be encountered in patients after severe head-injuries. Somewhere in the middle of this spectrum lie those not infrequent cases of young women, who, in their mid-menstrual cycle and at the time of ovulation, develop a sort of syndrome comprising ravenous appetite, inordinate torpor, excessive thirst, and motor clumsiness.

But the cases which occur in adolescent males are rather different. The association with over-eating is too intimate. Oswald has argued that the cases in the literature show a considerable heterogeneity, and that the true nature of such disorders is obscure. I agree with the latter statement, but would ask: Is this a psychiatric affection, that is to say one which is psychologically determined? I submit that it is not: but that it is an organic affection of obscure origin. Jaffee in 1967 has published a psychopathological analysis of an isolated case of this kind, but her observations are unconvincing arguments in favour of a psychogenesis in this particular syndrome. I believe that it would be unwise to jump to the conclusion that these episodic disorders were psychiatric in nature or psychologically determined. The phenomenology of narcolepsy and more particularly of temporal epilepsy are just as replete with mental aberrations, and just as diverse from one case to another, and yet we do not hesitate to ascribe them to purely organic influences.

In my experience of neurological practise there exist manifold cases wherein either somnolency, or megaphagia, periodic or continual, can occur. At present many of these are quite obscure in nature, and will no doubt eventually yield their secret to future neurological study. But today, in 1979, there is, I submit, a very real entity of periodic megaphagia and somnolency which, though psychiatric in its trappings, is actually organic in nature.

Let us then conclude by attempting a present-day assessment of what might perhaps be called the Kleine-Levin-Critchley syndrome: A periodic disorder occurring chiefly in adolescent males, with schizophrenic-like mental symptoms, associated with diverse autonomic disorders, in nature organic but wholly mysterious.

Reprinted from Critchley, M. (1967): *Revue Neurologique (Paris)*.

Observations upon *les Idiots Savants*

The discovery of special abilities, especially of an intellectual order, and which stand out conspicuously against the general background of defect, is a striking phenomenon which rarely fails to arouse interest among psychologists and doctors.

Many years ago in a paper entitled "Genius and Mental Defect" I described four personal instances of these so-called "brain athletes", and I made a rough classification along the following lines:

(1) *Superlative technical skill.* A notorious case in point was *James Pullen, the* "Genius of Earlswood". *Pullen* was an imbecile deaf-mute who had been for 50 years an inmate of the Royal Earlswood Colony for the mentally retarded. He was an adept in the construction of model ships, one of which was awarded a medal. At 26 years he built an elaborate barge symbolising the universe.

Some cases of unusual musical talent also belong here. A blind and severely retarded boy described by Kerr had the faculty of absolute pitch. Not only could he identify any note struck upon a piano but he could also pick out the individual components of a chord even though ten notes were being sounded simultaneously. Once the chapel organ went out of order, and when a particular stop was pulled several notes were sounded together. No one except the patient could identify the notes concerned.

(2) The commonest group is made up of patients with *hypermnesia* or *exaltation of memory.* Milder instances are not too rare in institutions or colonies. Barr described an epileptic illiterate girl of 22 years with a mental age of 5. None the less she could recall the dates of every visit she had been paid, as well as the names of her visitors, extending back for many years. She could repeat verbatim popular songs, mimicking the words, intonation of voice, and the gestures of the speaker, even when the language was unfamiliar. Witzmann's patient knew by heart the date of Easter in every year from 1000 to 2000, and also the patron saint of every day throughout the year.

One patient shown to me by the late Dr. R. M. Stewart was an imbecile of 29 years who had been cared for in the Leavesden Mental Hospital since the age of 17. He was stunted in stature, with a high arched palate, severe myopia, and a squint. His memory was exceptional in certain particulars. He was able to describe the colours of every well-known football club. In addition he could recall the results of local cricket matches, the scores of each batsman, and the bowling averages. His special *forte,* however, lay in his knowledge of the church hymnal. Given the number of a hymn, he could at once recite the corresponding first line.

My second patient, also from Leavesden, was a diminutive, docile, microcephalic imbecile of 72 years who had been an inmate since he was 16. He too was able to correlate the number of a hymn with its first line, and usually in fact with the complete text. Moreover he was able to give the dates of arrival and of departure of the hospital staff who had come and gone over his fifty-seven years' experience.

A patient seen in the Hawthorn Center near Detroit can be quoted through the courtesy of Dr. Ralph Rabinowitch:

R. J. male aged 13 years and 10 months. No perinatal anomaly had occurred. As a baby at 6 months he could sit up unsupported, though he did not walk until 20 months. Speech developed rather early, and as the result of the mother's tuition the child could read and spell at the precocious age of 3 years thus illustrating the rare syndrome of hyperlexia. He was hyperactive, and rocked in his crib, sucked his thumb, and pounded his head. For some years he was enuretic. At 5 he was so restless, boisterous, and unmanageable that he was expelled from his kindergarten school. He could not adhere for long to any one idea, and became increasingly irritable, negativistic, and explosive. Contemptuous of toys, he became obsessed with books, papers, and magazines, which he hoarded in such a way as to make the home intolerable for his father.

At the age of 5 the boy was psychologically tested, and upon the WISC scale gave a verbal I.Q. of 91 and a performance I.Q. of 115. These figures were probably an underestimate of his abilities, owing in part to his lack of cooperation. At this chronological age, he was able to memorise a large number of telephone numbers, and to reel off lists of automobile dealers with their addresses. When he was 9 years of age his psychometric tests were repeated, yielding a verbal I.Q. of 100 and a performance I.Q. of 99.

His present special abilities began to show themselves in an intense preoccupation with the New York Stock Exchange. He continued to collect thousands of magazines which he perused chiefly for their financial news. The boy was able to reel off the top 500 North American Industrials in appropriate order: he could recite from memory their assets, turnover, dividends, share prices, the chief periodic fluctuations, the president of each company, and the main as well as the subsidiary interests of the company, so often concealed beneath a proprietary name or set of initials.

The boy's personality remained odd, even schizoid. Various rituals had appeared, such as edging backwards out of a doorway when leaving a room, and a tic-like movement of the face and trunk. He did not mix with other boys who seemed to shun his company, for he was too conceited and aggressive. Of late he had developed uninhibited masturbatory habits which he did not bother to conceal.

(3) Within a special class belong the *calculating idiots* where an apparent superlative arithmetical skill rises conspicuously above the lowly level of general intelligence.

Thus the literature holds a record of the case of *Sabine*, a Polish postencephalitic dement of 22 years. Her mood varied between a noisy mania and a severe depression. Her speech was badly articulated, and was made up of a barely intelligible gibberish full of rhymes and klang associations. She had two main topics—her persecutory ideas and her calculations. Thus she could solve problems of mental arithmetic with amazing speed and accuracy, especially multiplication. The products of 17×18 and of 16×37 were given instantaneously. To multiply 56×16 took her one second; 99×16 two seconds; and 36×16 three seconds. It was noticeable that she was particularly adept at dividing and multiplying when 16 or a multiple of 16 was one of the factors. Another peculiarity was found at times: thus asked to multiply 23×23 she replied "529", and then went on to say "this is the same as $33 \times 16 + 1$". In like manner she gave the result of 36×36 as "1,296, or 81×16"; 14×14 as "196, or $12 \times 16 + 4$". Again, in monetary manipulations when reckoning the number of kopecs or groschen in so many roubles, she always replied in terms of 16. It was as though she possessed two numerical systems, one the ordinary decimal type and another with 16 as the key number.

The case of *Fleury* was more remarkable still. A blind, intractable, destructive imbecile, he was restless and betrayed tic-like movements. Bored with inactivity, he began to indulge in mental calculations. The meaning of a "square of a number" was explained to him, and he immediately gave the squares of numbers made up of 3 or 4 digits. A few days later he began to work out the square roots of figures in a matter of a few seconds. Later his prowess grew. He produced the cube-root of $465,484,375$ ($= 775$) in thirteen seconds. To multiply 287×341 took him ten seconds. On one occasion he was asked how many grains of corn would there be in any one of 64 bins if one grain was placed in the first, two in the second, four in the third, and so on. He gave the correct answers instantaneously for the 14th bin (8,192); the 18th (131,072); and the 24th (8,388,608). *Fleury* was afforded special coaching at the hands of a university professor, and he learned to solve algebraic problems with great rapidity. He was incapable, however, of grasping even the rudiments of geometry.

(4) Within a special class lie the *calendar artists* who are able to name the day of the week corresponding with any given date.

Thus another personally observed case comprised a megalencephalic idiot.

He was tetraplegic, and suffered periodic epileptic fits. His speech was lalling and he frequently laughed in a vacuous fashion.

He had an astonishing memory for dates. For example, he could recall when attendants first came to the ward and when they were transferred; and the dates when various of his fellow-patients died.

His chief ability lay in the correct naming of the day of the week upon which a given date fell. Thus if any date, past or future, were named, he would state correctly the corresponding day of the week. Replies as to dates within the past 10 to 15 years were given almost immediately. Dates in the remote past, or distant future, were forthcoming only after an interval, and not always correctly. It seemed likely that some process of mental calculation was entailed, and not pure hypermnesia.

Within a special category belongs the case of the mnemonist S who was studied over many years and eventually written up in detail by A. R. Luria. S excelled by virtue of his phenomenal memory which required only a few minutes of intense concentration for its establishment. Once rooted, the data could be recapitulated exactly, decades later, and without any intervening practise or recapitulation. S was not a calculator, but a pure hypermnesist. He could recall written works even if they were in an unfamiliar language, or even if the data was a medley of nonsense material, literal or numerical. Complicated mathematical formulae could be memorised and recalled even though S had no basic acquaintance with this science. Luria analysed the mental mechanics of his subject's talent, his imagery, and the oddities and deficiencies of his personality. His subject was not an oligophrenic and therefore does not belong to the category of the *idiot savant*. As with other "memory men", S relied upon vivid visual imagery, in his case supplemented by important colour-taste-tactile synaesthesiae, and a linkage with bygone topographical scenes. Again, as is typical of other similar memory-artists, one of the greatest problems is not that of remembering, but of forgetting. Employing divers mental tricks, S went to elaborate pains to forget, to wipe the slate clean so as to ensure that his cerebration was not cluttered up with the obtrusion of a thousand and one trivia.

Some of these features were very obvious in my personal experience of K, a chess master and a mnemonist. One of K's extravaganzas was to gaze for three minutes at a large blackboard divided into 64 squares. Into each of these he would chalk a name, number, cipher, a series of letters—meaningful or not—anything indeed which was asked of him. After three minutes, the board was removed from K's sight but not that of his audience, and he was given to start with, one of the items written in any square at random. K would then make a mental four-fold "Knight's move" and proclaim the contents of the four squares which lay obliquely around the given square. From that start, he proceeded to memorise and announce every single item occupying the whole 64 squares. In the course of this astonishing performance I noted that *K* hesitated in identifying correctly the cipher which occupied one square only. On looking at the model blackboard I noticed that this square had been slightly smeared by *K's* sleeve accidentally brushing the chalk-marks. Consequently this was the least clear-cut of all the 64 models, and presumably gave rise to a less vivid image.

Like Luria's subject *S, K* told me that his principal difficulty lay in deliberately forgetting, a ritual which he had to go through at the end of each day before retiring. *K* assured me that his memory was not all that good; he was often in trouble with his wife who would upbraid him for his forgetfulness when she sent him out shopping.

The topic of *idiots savants* has little or no tie up with the subject of musical prodigies. These constitute a well documented chapter in neuromusicology. Another is the correlation of musical ability with psychiatric illness. The records, however, hold little or nothing concerning the existence of musical genius with mental defect.

Discussion

Inaccessibility of the subjects within the foregoing categories of *idiots savants* is apt to preclude accurate knowledge of the operative psychological processes. However, there are available those studies which have been made upon certain mathematical geniuses and lightning calculators of normal intellectual calibre. For instance, there are the autobiographical accounts of the elder *Bidder,* and of *Dase.* Scripture and also Mitchell have contributed to this topic. Most important of all has been the classic monograph by Alfred Binet entitled *"Le Psychologie des Grands Calculateurs et Joueurs d'Echecs"* written in 1894. Binet was privileged to investigate in detail two famous professional calculators, *Pericles Diamandi* and *Jacques Inaudi,* both of whom had for years toured the music halls of Europe. He drew attention to certain features which he described as the marks of a well-defined *famille naturelle* wherein the arithmetical prodigies belonged. Some of these criteria hold true for the *idiots savants.*

(a) In most instances *the mental imagery is not visual in type. Sabine,* for instance, was an auditive. The blind *Fleury* possessed a tactile imagery and thought, and calculated in terms of the projections of the Braille type.

(b) Both the *idiot savant* and the mathematical genius show a conspicuous *singleness of purpose.* In the mentally defective this is evidenced by a poverty of ideation which permits an astonishing concentration of effort. This restriction of the intellectual horizon is further enhanced when there is some special sense deprivation like blindness or deafness.

(c) The *idiot savant* and perhaps also the mathematical genius usually betrays an *obsessional preoccupation* with his special abilities. *Sabine* for instance had no interests except in collecting coins and buttons, which she would arrange in groups. *Buxton,* when in church, paid no heed to the sermon, except to count the number of words spoken. *Pullen,* in order to protect his model ships, erected in his workshop elaborate mantraps to kill any would-be intruder.

(d) Furthermore the *idiot savant* is characteristically *conceited, vain, and even boastful* where his particular aptitudes are concerned.

(e) The relative part played by arithmetical prowess as opposed to sheer memory, is an interesting source of debate. Broadly speaking the enactment is the outcome of *enhanced memory rather than mathematical skill.* It has been clearly shown that even when calculation seems to be operative the subject may actually be resorting to feats of memory. There may be an extended multiplication table. Thus *Fleury* memorised the products of all numbers up to 100×100. When *Inaudi* was asked the number of seconds in 39 years, 3 months, and twelve hours, and gave the correct reply in 3 seconds, it must be realised that he knew beforehand how many seconds made up a year, a month, and so on. More than one key-system of numeration may be accessible. The calculating idiot may employ mnemonics, "tips", cross-multiplications, and various simple short-cuts. None the less he is usually unwilling to admit what he owes to pure memory, preferring to allow his accomplishments to be put down to some esoteric process of rapid calculation.

Even in the case of the calendar artist, memory is more important than reckoning. The subject has probably committed to heart some key-date like Christmas day or the following first of January. These dates fall on the same week-day, which in turn corresponds with February 5th, March 5th, April 2nd, May 7th, June 4th, July 2nd, . . . and so on—except in a Leap Year.

In drawing the foregoing generalisations it is necessary to realise their limitations. We must agree with the conclusions arrived at by Mitchell, who recognised at least three psychological categories:

(1) the *"calculating" prodigies*—who may be persons of inferior intellectual calibre and who rely upon ingenious short cuts;

(2) *arithmetical prodigies* like *Colburn,* and *Dase,* with a moderately well-developed knowledge of arithmetic; and

(3) *mathematical geniuses,* such as the elder *Bidder.* These are endowed with exceptional abilities, and their knowledge of pure mathematics is profound.

Luria's patient S belongs elsewhere, for he is to be looked upon as a pure mnemonist and no *idiot savant.*

Reprinted from Critchley, M. (1968) : *Ideggógyászati Szemle,* Vol. 21.

The Training of a Neurologist

The life of a vestal virgin was divided into three portions; in the first of which she learned the duties of her profession, in the second she practised them, and in the third she taught them to others.

This is no bad model for the life of a neurologist.

His training is both arduous and all-demanding. Such is the penalty for the choice of a career which makes one of a small coterie within the medical profession, dedicated and highly selected. To paraphrase a saying of Lloyd George, you cannot make a first-rate neurologist out of a third-rate scholar, a fifth-rate teacher, a no-rate scientist, and an irate doctor. In other words, the neurologist is a rather exceptional person. When he has gained acceptance among his colleagues, the young neurologist will find that his future functions are three-fold:

(1) the diagnosis and care of the neurological sick within the community;

(2) the teaching of students, both undergraduate and post-graduate; and

(3) research.

The relative importance of these three functions will differ from one individual neurologist to another, being in part a question of opportunity, and in part a matter of personal choice and expertise.

Furthermore the training of a neurologist will probably differ widely according to the country in which the student resides. University career-structures are far from identical over the world or even within English-speaking areas. The following suggestions refer particularly to the British scene.

Early in the student career the trainee neurologist will probably have already decided that his future will lie within the territory of the nervous system, whose mysteries and allure will have exercised their subtle fascination. Less often the young doctor merely slips into a neurological career through motives of opportunism. Although he has already set up for himself a goal in neurology, the undergraduate in his student-career will serve exactly the same apprenticeship as any other would-be doctor.

There is, however, one exception. He must make it his business during his student days to acquire a working knowledge of both the French and German languages. Years hence it may be necessary for him to be able to read Russian as well, but that time has not yet come. In order to learn

French and German the student may find it necessary to take special evening-classes, and to sacrifice some of his social or sporting activities. This, however, would merely be a foretaste of what is likely to happen to him in his future career over and over again.

We now arrive at the point when our would-be neurologist officially qualifies by way of his final examinations. In Great Britain a compulsory year's work in hospital must elapse before he can get his name placed upon the official Medical Register. This period of internship must be spent at an approved hospital, and it must be carried out in the division of general medicine, or of general surgery, or of obstetrics and gynaecology. Special departments other than the foregoing are not recognised for this purpose. The young doctor may, if he chooses, do six months in two of these subjects, or twelve months in one. Neurology will not suffer in the slightest because of the fact that a year has been spent in the practise of surgery or gynaecology.

Sometime during this statutory year's apprenticeship, the future neurologist would be well advised to try and secure for himself a voluntary, part-time, "clinical assistantship" in ophthalmology. In this way he will acquire a dexterity in the use of the ophthalmoscope and other technical armamentaria; a familiarity with the fundus oculi in health and disease; and a facility in testing ocular movements and visual fields.

We now come to the first real step in a neurologist's career—one which still lies outside the province of the nervous system. Nonetheless it is fundamental, and inescapable. I refer to an eighteen-month senior internship in general medicine. We in England believe that neurology is an aspect of internal medicine—not of psychiatry, nor of surgery—and that no neurologist will ever attain full stature who has not built his edifice upon a firm foundation of internal medicine. We deprecate strongly any premature attempts at specialisation. This period is hallmarked by the successful attainment of the examination for the membership of the Royal College of Physicians.

After this all-important novitiate, the future neurologist should now leave the hospital wards where hitherto he has been devoting the whole of his time and energies. He must now serve another apprenticeship, this time over a period of eighteen months, in the basic sciences. The first six months should be devoted to the two academic subjects of genetics and medical statistics. Never again will the neurologist have the chance to secure a competency in these two difficult but vital disciplines. A familiarity with the grammar of genetics and statistics will not only mould his mind into the framework of scientific thinking, but it will furnish him with a background of knowledge that will support him throughout his professional life.

Next follows a twelve-months term in a laboratory, and here I suggest that the future neurologist can for the first time exercise a choice in subject but in each case with a neurological orientation. Thus he may decide to spend a year at neuro-anatomy; or neuro-physiology; or morbid anatomy or clinical pathology; or biochemistry; or epidemiology. The young neurologist now has the opportunity of satisfying his professional inclinations, by picking upon the particular subject to which he is most powerfully attracted. He should select only *one* of these topics that I have mentioned, and not dissipate his year's laboratory experience among two or more academic pursuits. His choice may include the intimate study of such special methods as the E.E.G., the computerised scintiscan, and the electromyogram, though it is the interpretation rather than the technical refinement which is all important. If in doubt as to which of these topics to select, he would do well to be guided—not so much by the intrinsic nature of the particular discipline—as by the personality of the professor in charge. In other words he should go for the man rather than the subject.

After these important preliminaries—clinical and academic—the young neurologist must return to the bedside, and now for the first time he will be really achieving his ambition. A four-year period of clinical neurology is now necessary, most of this time being spent as a resident doctor. In this crucial period he now advances from the amateur to the professional status. He must learn to know his diseases not as a zoologist knows his species and his genera and his orders—by descriptions of comparative characters—but as a hunter knows his lions and tigers. At last he begins to familiarise himself with all manner of clinical problems, major and minor, chronic and acute, including the catastrophic emergencies of neurological practise. Thus he becomes conversant with the art of history-taking; of bedside clinical examination; and of special techniques. He will now realise the help which can be afforded by neuro-radiology, electroencephalography, and electromyography, even though it may not be necessary for him to master the actual details of the technique.

This four-year clinical training—following as it does the 18 months in basic sciences and 18 months in internal medicine—is the high point of his career. But even now his education is not ended.

At this juncture, I recommend a year's study abroad, in a laboratory devoted to one of the basic sciences and preferably not the academic subject at which he had already worked four years before. Thus, if he has already put in a year at neuro-physiology, he could now do a year in neuro-pathology. If he elects to do this part of his study in Europe he could with advantage choose one of the German-speaking countries. In this way he would not only perfect his modest knowledge of written German, but he would make contacts and friendships which are likely to be of the greatest significance to him throughout the rest of his life. It is during this foreign *Wanderjahr* that he might profitably select psychology as one of the optional academic subjects, rather than anatomy, pathology, or physiology.

Then comes the ninth and final year of the neurologist's lengthy apprenticeship. This is marked by a return to clinical neurology, again in some centre outside one's *alma mater,* and preferably abroad. A year's clinical neurology in France or the States would afford the young man a new look in neurology with an opportunity of seeing fresh faces, different techniques, and novel ways of thinking. Once again he will have the inestimable advantage of meeting other neurologists, and learning to evaluate them at first hand.

Our neurologist's training is at last complete. With such education and experience he cannot fail to attain a university post. Presumably now he will be undertaking the instruction of juniors. Somewhere along the path, therefore, he should be given the chance of learning the art and technique of teaching. This is a common gap in training. Someone should give him a few lessons on how to lecture clearly; how to master voice-production; and how to avoid the irritating mannerisms of speech and movement which so often mar the performance of even quite distinguished personages. We have already referred to the acquisition of French and German. The fully-fledged neurologist should also be taught finally to manipulate the Queen's English in an elegant prose-style, clear, crisp, and unambiguous. He should now be able to write scientific papers without slipping into jargon, journalese, gobbledygook, or waffle. This is anything but simple. He will then find himself in a rarified atmosphere which he shares with but few indeed of his medical colleagues. Let us bear in mind what F. L. Lucas has written . . .

A research student may turn his life into a concentration camp; he may amass in his own field an erudition which is staggering; but he cannot write. And where the words are so muddled, I suspect that the mind is muddled too.

You will observe that throughout this 9-year apprenticeship I have said nothing about psychiatry. This has been deliberate because I believe that service in a psychiatric hospital is of relatively minor importance, compared with what I have already outlined. Of course, if the young neurologist could fit in a spell as a part-time clinical assistant in a psychiatric clinic sometime during his 4-year neurological residency, so much the better. Personally I do not believe that neurology should be orientated too closely towards psychiatry, but rather towards internal medicine; or if one prefers, psychology. A neuropsychologist is far less of an anomaly than a neuropsychiatrist.

Perhaps I should have said a word about the school-days of the future neurologist. Unfortunately a schoolboy nowadays may have to specialise at a very early age, and to make up his mind whether to switch to the modern or the classical side of the school. This decision may need to be taken long before the boy has any clear idea as to what his future is likely to be. In the case of the neurologist he will obviously have to take biology at school, but it would be a thousand pities if by so doing he were to neglect the humanities. It may sound old fashioned, but I am convinced that every member of a learned profession like that of medicine is a better man for having been well educated, and by that term I mean having been brought up in an atmosphere of culture with a knowledge of literature, Latin, and even Greek. "Time given to a study of the humanities is like that which a soldier spends on making his armour shine."

Let us interpose a quotation slightly modified from Bacon.

> The men of experiment are like the ant; they only collect to use: the reasoners resemble spiders, who make cobwebs out of their own substance. But the bee takes a middle course, it gathers its material from the flowers of the garden and of the field, but transforms and digests it by a power of its own. Not unlike this is the true business of neurology. . . .

The gloom of this disconcerting narrative of sloggery may perhaps be relieved if not dispelled by indicating the fitting culmination or goal. One of the wisest physicians of this century expressed the objective to which the student should aspire, in the form of a prayer:

> From an inability to let well alone; from too much zeal for what is new and contempt for what is old; from putting Knowledge before Wisdom, Science before Art, and cleverness before commonsense; from treating patients as cases; and from making the cure of the disease more grievous than its endurance; Good Lord, deliver us.

When the neurologist is ready to accept these beatitudes, he can consider himself to be adequately trained.

Reprinted from Critchley, M. (1975): *International Journal of Neurology*, Vol. 9.

"All the King's Horses . . ."*

Since its inception at Portugal Street in 1840 King's College Hospital has been notorious for the quality of its medical and surgical staff, many of whom have achieved international repute. Indeed at that time its consulting staff was said to be the most distinguished of any hospital in London. One of the most conspicuous features of the history of the hospital has been the early institution of special departments. This was due to the foresight of the Board, the Dean, and the staff immediately before and shortly after the First World War. It is not perhaps realised today what a dramatic innovation it was which came about, not without a certain opposition and much to the astonishment of many other of the teaching hospitals in London and elsewhere. However, I would like to select as a theme those King's men who have been particularly distinguished in the field of neurology. Here is where "all the King's horses" come in, for each of them was of respectable blood-stock, from the best stables; all of them starters, most of them runners. Some of them were graceful Arabians, others stately shires or percherons, but all were thoroughbreds with clean hocks, thick withers, and powerful quarters. Long before the First World War and before a pure strain of neurologist had been bred, our hospital was notorious for the accomplishments of some of our medical staff in a study of nervous diseases —a discipline which we speak of today as neurology.

First in time was *Robert Bentley Todd* (1809–1860). He was actually a contemporary of Charcot of Paris, the first Professor of Neurology ever to be appointed. Bentley Todd was, of course, a general physician, and the eponymous term Todd's cirrhosis was applied to his work on hepatic disease. He was born and qualified in Dublin, one of 16 siblings, his father's other occupation being that of a surgeon in that city. Robert Bentley Todd in due course had been appointed Professor of Physiology and Morbid Anatomy at King's College in the Strand in 1836, and when the hospital was instituted he was elected to the staff and was the first clinical Dean in 1842.

His principal interests and most of his practise concerned patients with diseases of the nervous system. In retrospect, it seems highly probable that he was responsible for the first description in the world's literature of locomotor ataxia, later to be known as tabes dorsalis. It is true that his

* An address to the students and staff of King's College Hospital, London.

original mention of this disease was not particularly detailed, and in most countries outside of Great Britain credit is given either to Romberg of Berlin, or to Duchenne (formerly of Boulogne, later of Paris) who certainly afforded us a pioneer detailed account of this important and, from a clinical point of view, protean disorder. But Todd's paper was published four years before that of Romberg and 11 years before Duchenne's.

Robert Bentley Todd also made important contributions to the topic of peripheral neuritis due to lead intoxication. The name "Todd's paralysis" is still in use to describe the transient hemiparesis which may follow a fit.

It was regrettable in more ways than one that he died comparatively young. In the first place, his demise was avoidable at the time because Todd was a firm believer in the therapeutic merits of hard liquor—a belief which he practised to the full in his own case. He was in the habit of prescribing alcohol in the treatment of most of his cases irrespective of the diagnosis. Students took a delight in associating his name with *"toddy"*, a term traditionally applied to a measure of rum. Indeed he was destined to perish from the condition he had described so well, alcoholic cirrhosis of the liver.

It is regrettable too that Todd's death synchronised with the institution of the National Hospital for the Paralysed and Epileptic in Queen Square, Bloomsbury. This hospital, destined to become world-famous, started in 1860 with a staff of two physicians. Had Bentley Todd lived, he would undoubtedly have been invited to join the staff and would have taken his place among such pioneers as Brown-Séquard, Hughlings Jackson, and William Gowers. Oddly enough Todd had been associated with another institution in Queen Square, situated immediately opposite the National Hospital and alongside the notorious examination hall of today. I refer to *St. John's House* where Florence Nightingale accommodated her band of ladies who not only constituted the first respectable members of a nursing staff, but also saw active service in the Crimea. Today St. John's House belongs to the National Hospital and houses its matron.

Todd was in great favour at the Royal College of Physicians and in addition carried on a fashionable private practice from Brook Street. Though said to be frequently fuddled, he was immensely popular with his clientèle. Perhaps he devoted more attention to them than he should, for in 1850 he was courteously but firmly invited to retire from the staff of King's College Hospital.

In discussing the topic of my choice, I find it impossible to avoid mentioning *William Bowman* (1816–1892). Although he was not a neurologist but an eye-specialist of great distinction, he was one of the first of those we may term neuro-ophthalmologists—a specialty which since his time has been followed at King's with considerable distinction. Bowman was born in Nantwich and in due course was appointed to King's College as Professor of Physiology. In 1839 he was made assistant surgeon to King's College

Hospital. When he joined the staff at Moorfields in 1846 he became increasingly dedicated to ophthalmology, and eventually retired from general surgery at King's in 1863. I will not retail his contributions to his specialty but will merely mention that his name today is principally associated with the biennial Bowman Lecture, an honour which has fallen to quite a number of distinguished neurologists over the past century, including Hughlings Jackson, William Gowers, Gordon Holmes, Francis Walshe, C. P. Symonds, and Lord Brain.

Another physician, not quite contemporary with Bowman and with Todd, was *Dr. Edward Liveing* (1832–1919). The Royal College of Physicians remembers him as a worthy Registrar, an appointment that he held for 20 years dating from 1889. Neurologists hold him in high respect for his magnificent pioneer monograph on *Megrim and Allied Disorders*. This book, published in 1873, is a collector's piece today for it contains a wealth of clinical detail to which but little can be added except things emanating from the pharmacological laboratory.

Though strictly speaking *Sir William Fergusson Bt.* (1808–1877) was not a neurologist, he was not only on the staff of King's but also of the National Hospital, Queen Square. In 1839 he had left Edinburgh to accept the Chair of Surgery at King's. Thereafter his career was dazzling and was not held back by his pronounced Scottish accent. He became surgeon to Queen Victoria and to the Prince Consort and was appointed President of the Royal College of Surgeons in 1870. On the institution of the National Hospital, Queen Square, in 1860 he became its consulting surgeon and his name added considerably to the social standing of that hospital. He was a remarkable man, "with the eye of an eagle, the heart of a lion, and the hand of a lady", as someone said. As Royal Surgeon, his services were in great demand among the quality. I once unearthed in the Royal College of Physicians the case-notes he made when he was discreetly summoned to Paris in 1856 to report upon the health of the Emperor Napoleon III. A faint pencilled note at the end of the dossier was a brief "3,000 guineas"— his fee I presume.

We come next to *Sir David Ferrier* (1843–1928). He was an Aberdonian who studied psychology at Heidelberg and then received his medical training at the University of Edinburgh. It so happened that his chief in medicine was Thomas Laycock, who himself had been interested in the nervous system. When Marshall Hall brought out his unorthodox concepts of reflex function, he received at first scant recognition and indeed was snubbed by the Royal Society. Thomas Laycock, however, keenly supported these pioneer views. Before he attained the Chair of Medicine at Edinburgh, Laycock had been on the staff of the now defunct medical school of York, and was indeed the teacher of Hughlings Jackson in his undergraduate days.

After qualification David Ferrier—like so many good Scots—travelled the highway south, and entered general practice in Bury St. Edmunds. Later he was appointed lecturer in physiology at the Middlesex Hospital. Perhaps it is not altogether surprising that when a vacancy arose at King's College Hospital he made a change and first worked there in the department of physiology. At the age of 29 he was, oddly enough, appointed Professor of Forensic Medicine. This was a temporary gesture for he became, in succession, Physician to the West London Hospital; The Hospital for Epilepsy and Paralysis, Maida Vale; and assistant Physician to King's in 1874. In 1880 he was appointed to the National Hospital, Queen Square. He was, both a neuro-clinician and a pioneer neurophysiologist. Although his approach to the subject was quite different from that of Hughlings Jackson, Ferrier's practical experimental work supported the philosophic speculations of Jackson. His researches were carried out partly at King's and partly at Wakefield Asylum. His name will be forever linked with that of Fritz and Hitzig, for the first two were able to demonstrate by galvanic stimulation of the cortex localised centres controlling motility. Ferrier did the same with faradism. People still talk about the notorious debate which took place in London in 1881 between Ferrier and Goltz on the topic of cerebral localisation. It was the far-seeing work of Jackson which stimulated Ferrier, and between them they can be regarded as the ancestors of neurosurgery. Ferrier insisted that there was nothing sacrosanct about the dural coverings of the brain, and that it should be quite possible for a skilled surgeon to deal successfully with circumscribed tumours of the cortex such as came to light only in the post-mortem room. It is not surprising, therefore, to learn that on 25th November, 1884, Ferrier, after consultation with Jackson, persuaded Rickman Godlee, a surgeon at University College Hospital, and nephew of our own Lord Lister, to perform a craniotomy and to remove successfully a sharply demarcated growth involving the precentral cortex of a patient. This was done at the Regent's Park Hospital for Epilepsy and Paralysis (now the Maida Vale branch of the National Hospital, Queen Square). Ferrier went even further, for he also persuaded Professor Rose, also on the surgical staff at King's, to remove for the first time ever the Gasserian ganglion in a patient with trigeminal neuralgia.

Somehow Ferrier contrived to cope with the burden of a fashionable practise over and above his work in the laboratory. He was well known for his treatment of patients with multiple sclerosis by the use of *aurii bromide*, which became known throughout the West End of London as Ferrier's Golden Drops.

Ferrier (Fig. 1) was on the staff of the National Hospital, Queen Square, between 1880 and 1907. After his retirement he lived another 21 years, and continued to visit that hospital from time to time, being conspicuous for the fact that he always wore his silk hat when walking the wards at Queen Square. I myself remember him vividly.

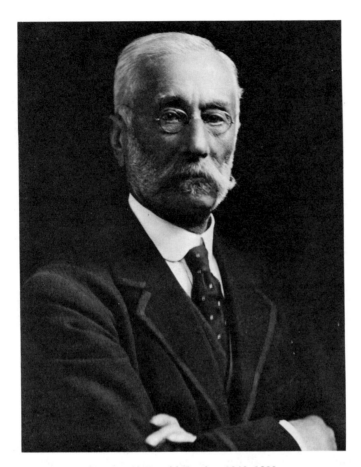

FIG. 1. Sir David Ferrier, 1843–1928.

Sir David was undoubtedly a highly successful neurologist, a pioneer, whose monograph on "Functions of the Brain" published in 1876 constitutes an important landmark in the literature of our discipline. Despite his extensive practise he did not shine as a clinician. Personally he was a perky, even cocky, little individual, not much taller than 5 ft., dapper and dandified in his dress, and admired rather than liked by his colleagues.

When he died, an obiturist wrote: "Ferrier did not have Jackson's breadth of patience and painstaking clinical scrutiny, but he had notable mental vigilance, and a consuming desire for information."

In his laboratory work Ferrier was assisted first by Sherrington, but more especially by *William Aldren Turner* (1864–1945) who was elected to the staff of King's College Hospital in 1899. Aldren Turner belonged to a distinguished family. His father was Sir William Turner, a very well known Professor of Anatomy at the University of Edinburgh. Sir William had two sons, one of whom, Logan Turner, was appointed Consulting Laryngologist to Edinburgh Royal Infirmary, while William Aldren Turner followed the well-worn trail to London. As a clinical neurologist, Aldren Turner was a simple, dignified, and rather self-effacing man. He is particularly remembered for his clinical monograph on the subject of epilepsy and for his modest *Textbook of Neurology*, written in collaboration with Grainger Stewart. At the National Hospital, Queen Square, to which he was appointed in 1900, he stood out as a very great gentleman, modest to an unusual degree among the caucus of brilliant egocentrics by whom he was surrounded. I had the privilege of being his last House Physician at Queen Square, and recall with affection his many kindnesses to me personally. Indeed, one of my first contributions to neurological literature was carried out in collaboration with my chief, Aldren Turner, stimulated by the curious respiratory complications of the epidemic of encephalitis lethargica which was raging at that particular time. Every year during my three year stint at the National, I was invited to his house on Christmas day for a family luncheon party.

Aldren Turner had no time whatsoever for medical politics nor for the neurological rat-race, and no one was surprised when he retired somewhat prematurely from the staffs of both King's College Hospital and the National Hospital, Queen Square.

Incidentally, it was on his retirement that I was privileged and lucky enough to be his successor in 1928 at both these hospitals within a space of three weeks.

Shortly before the outbreak of World War II, Aldren Turner's son—John Aldren Turner—became my House Physician at the National Hospital, and he has only recently retired from the position of neurologist at St. Bartholomew's Hospital, where at one time he was Dean of the Medical School.

We come now to that brilliant and well remembered figure, *S. A. Kinnier Wilson* (1878–1937) (Fig. 2). Like two of his predecessors, he was a Scotsman who contrived to be born in Cedarville, New Jersey, but left the United States at the age of a few days when his father was appointed Presbyterian Minister at Co. Monaghan in Ireland. Later the family moved to Edinburgh and he entered the University, qualifying in 1902. One of his first resident appointments was to Professor Byrom Bramwell, a distinguished exponent of diseases of the nervous system. Wilson's next residency was in Paris on the service of Professor Pierre Marie, then at the Bicêtre. This year moulded his subsequent thinking in an indelible fashion, besides giving him an intimate acquaintance with the principal figures in French neurology, including Babinski, Foix, and Souques, and incidentally a working knowledge of the French language. Before returning to this country he put in some time at Leipzig. Back in Great Britain he joined the National Hospital, Queen Square, as resident Medical Officer. His

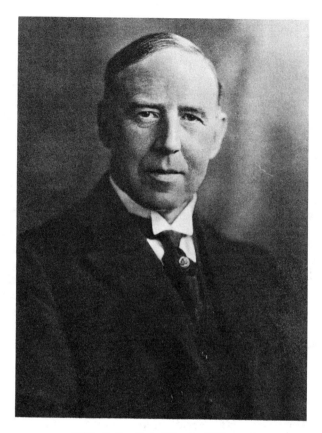

FIG. 2. Dr. S. A. Kinnier Wilson.

fellow resident was the well-known Foster Kennedy, who afterwards left Great Britain to win fame and fortune in New York. Kinnier Wilson proceeded to the appointment of Registrar, and during this period he was fortunate in having access to a handful of very strange cases, some of them members of the same family, most of whom succumbed and became available for post-mortem histological examination. The results constituted a landmark in neurological endeavour, for the pathological findings were striking and indeed unique. Each caudate nucleus showed localised softening. This explained the symptoms the patients had presented during life, namely a universal extra-pyramidal rigidity; crude involuntary movements; a typical facies with a conspicuous wide silly grin; and a dysarthria. Already, for many years, neurologists had been talking vaguely about the basal ganglia and had been making timid speculations as to their clinical significance. Wilson's discovery established beyond all question the association between striatal disease and its clinical counterpart. At a stroke, what had hitherto been wild guesswork now became an established fact. Wilson's pathological investigation, however, went one step further, by demonstrating in a most unexpected manner the co-existence of a finding which up till then had been quite unforeseen. I refer to the presence of a multi-lobular cirrhosis of the liver. This was an odd association indeed, and presumably it held some significance, although it was difficult at that time to discover its meaning.

In the prosecution of his researches, the young Kinnier Wilson was dedicated, hard-working, and enthusiastic to a degree which would shock and astonish the Junior Hospital doctors of today. After the discharge from hospital of one or two of these patients he kept a close watch on their movements, and, like a vulture, lay in waiting for their demise. To his great annoyance, one of these patients under surveillance took it in his head to leave England and to perish in Switzerland. However, the local doctor was cooperative and sent Wilson a telegram announcing the patient's demise. Wilson did not hesitate. He rapidly totted up his financial resources and found that he was just able to count out ten golden sovereigns into his purse. Right away he took a train to Zürich. Permission had been given for an autopsy and Wilson subsequently told us of what transpired. That he would find bilateral naked-eye degeneration of the caudate nuclei he had no doubt, and so it happened. What really was at stake was whether this patient, too, would turn out to have liver-disease for, like the others, the patient had shown during life no suggestive hepatic symptoms. Wilson deliberately left to the last the examination of the abdominal contents. He made the appropriate incision and put his hand inside the peritoneal cavity, but he did not do so immediately. Overcome with the most poignant emotion, as he afterwards told us, he waited for a moment or two, for the whole crunch or nub of his discovery turned on the presence or absence of a cirrhosis. Eventually he steeled himself to insert his hand and palpate the liver-surface. To his relief he realised that the surface of the shrunken liver was nodular, indicating an advanced degree of cirrhosis. For quite a while he was so overcome by emotion that he could not proceed.

These original observations, clinical as well as pathological, were the basis of a bulky thesis which earned for him not only the Doctorate of Medicine at the University of Edinburgh with a gold medal, but international fame. So we find him at the age of 33, still Registrar at the National Hospital, but a household name throughout the neurological clinics of the world. The discovery of what became universally known as "Wilson's disease" (which he diffidently had termed "progressive lenticular degeneration") stimulated a vast amount of work throughout the world, good, bad, and indifferent, on the presumed nature and functional activity of the basal ganglia. In reality Wilson never was a modest man and he soon was referring to his own syndrome as "Wilson's disease", like everybody else. At the same time he poured bitter scorn upon the vague entity "pseudosclerosis" which had been described by Westphal and Strümpell, and which sat far too close to his discovery to be comfortable.

Wilson's foot was securely set upon the ladder of neurological fame. Shortly after this work had been published, he was appointed Assistant Physician to the National Hospital. A little later he was made Assistant Physician to the Westminster Hospital. He continued his research work, which was now more clinical than pathological, and he set up his plate at what was then considered to be the "better end" of Harley Street, i.e. near Cavendish Square. In the laboratory he scorned any technical assistance and he carried out his own fixing and staining of specimens and their subsequent microphotography.

With the wind of change which blew like a gust through King's College Hospital just after the First World War, Wilson was offered the post of Physician in charge of a neurological department. He was, of course, junior to Aldren Turner, who continued to rank as general physician but with neurological leanings. It is not easy to realise nowadays just how important this step turned out to be. Wilson's appointment actually was to the first department of pure neurology in any medical school within the United Kingdom. Rival schools and hospitals were at first askance if not shocked, but one by one they followed suit, so that neurology—which incidentally had always been regarded with awe coupled with a certain jealousy by the general physicians—became a respectable discipline, worthy of standing on its own feet. Neurologists became a race apart even though they continued to constitute a sort of *corps d'élite* among their colleagues in general medicine like racehorses in a stable. I think it is true to say that every medical school in London and probably now everywhere else in the United Kingdom has its own special department of neurology. Neurologists were responsible for more Fellows of the Royal Society than any other discipline in medicine. Incidentally, Wilson's alma mater, the University of Edinburgh, was one of the last to fall into line and form a neurological department or division.

Wilson's professional accomplishments were formidable both in quantity and quality. He was a consecrated worker who devoted little or no time to leisurely pursuits or recreations, physical, cultural, or intellectual. He was an assiduous writer and he founded the *Journal of Neurology and Psychopathology,* now known irreverently as the Green Rag. His literary style was uneasy and idiosyncratic. Like most neurologists he was vain about his ability to put pen to paper, but it is doubtful whether his prose was really as distinguished as he thought it was. Certainly it was unusual, for he had a liking for curious words, unexpected turns of phrase, and he larded his flamboyant text with French, German, and Latin words, phrases, and sentences to an extent which was mannered and irritating to a purist.

There are no two opinions about his teaching abilities. His lectures and

clinical demonstrations were arresting and histrionic in a way surpassed by
few. To his junior colleagues and students he was particularly stimulating.
In many ways he was a lazy man, at least as far as *physical* exertion went.
Rarely did he examine a patient with the customary thoroughness. More
often he sat back in his chair with his eyes half closed and listened intently
to what the patient had to say, interrupting now and again with a probing
question or comment. Then beneath his hooded eyelids his piercing gaze
would light upon some particular feature which had caught his eye—a
pupillary inequality; a twitching of a lip; a wasted hand-muscle; an odd
posture; or a slight anomaly of speech. Piecing together the patient's story
with these minor objective anomalies, he would weave in a romantic fashion
a fabulous pattern of thinking aloud on the problem before him. Always
he would be asking . . . why? for he was never content with simple observation and diagnosis. What was the mechanism behind the inequality of
the pupils? What was the physiological explanation of the involuntary
movements? Did they represent some obscure irritation, somewhere deep in
the neuraxis, or were they the result of the letting up of some inhibitory
process? Why did the patient walk or talk in the way he did? Aside from the
diagnosis—which was a simple matter which any other neurologist could
cope with—why, why was the pattern of behaviour conforming in this way
rather than another? For the common neurological literary contribution he
had contempt, dubbing such a paper as merely descriptive and devoid of
penetrating ideas.

His junior colleagues often came to him with their problems, much to
Wilson's delight. Their questions set him off musing and cogitating aloud
and speculating in a fashion which always threw light from some quite
unexpected angle on to the clinical problem, however banal and straightforward it had appeared at first sight. As Johnson said, his imagination
would place things in such a view as they are not commonly seen in. It is
not surprising to learn that Wilson was a worshipper at the shrine of
Hughlings Jackson. Indeed, I rather suspect that Jackson was the only man
in neurology he ever really respected. Wilson was one of Jackson's last
house physicians, and he continued to attend upon his master during the
latter's periodic visits to Queen Square which took place for long after his
retirement. In a precious and closely guarded notebook, Wilson recorded
verbatim his periodic conversations with Jackson and acted as Boswell to
the neurological Dr. Samuel Johnson. I only wish I knew what has happened to this record of which he was so proud and which he permitted me
to peep at from time to time. Incidentally, Wilson also kept another note-
book in which he recorded jokes and witticisms, mostly salacious, and all of
them rather jejeune.

It is difficult to narrate *in extenso* all of Wilson's contributions to neurology. He had a huge collection of medical volumes and the four walls
of his study were lined with books from floor to ceiling. He was able to

read well enough, but perhaps not too accurately, many European languages, which enabled him to be conversant with the world's literature to an extent which was unusual. His contributions were diverse and numerous indeed. He described mesencephalitis syphilitica. He wrote a detailed monograph on that newly discovered entity narcolepsy, but was furious because he was beaten to the post by his junior colleague, W. J. Adie, whose monograph on the same subject appeared a month or two before his. Wilson, incidentally, was the first physician ever to witness an actual attack of narcoleptic cataplexy, and I was fortunate enough to be there in the room at the same time, and could confirm the transitory appearance of extensor plantar responses.

Like others of his distinguished colleagues—Hughlings Jackson, Gowers, for example—Wilson avoided medical committee meetings like the plague.

Wilson was not popular. His colleagues never warmed to him, and he was touchy and opinionated. I have already spoken of his vanity which was almost childish. He lapped up praise like a sponge. "Dr. Brown", I have heard him say "is a very sound man—he thinks a lot of me".

His private practice was small, for he was cold towards some of his patients and offhand towards the referring practitioners. His clientèle numbered Ronald True, the notorious murderer, and also Charlie Chaplin with whom he was on terms of friendship. Indeed on one of his American lecture tours he stayed a couple of days with Chaplin in his Hollywood home, an experience which he often regaled me with. Another quirk was his meanness. He was said to possess an automobile but no one ever saw it. In his visits to and from King's he used to cadge lifts from his colleagues, particularly Sir Lenthal Cheatle.

I could continue with tale after tale, but this is a historical and not an anecdotal society, and I think I have said too much.

Inborn Indifference or Insensitivity to Pain

Admittedly this topic constitutes a rare clinical phenomena. But every practising doctor knows well that his patients react very differently to pain-stimuli which, as far as can be determined, are equal in intensity. There would appear to exist a kind of spectrum at one end of which are those staid phlegmatic individuals who tolerate pain with equanimity, even indifference. At the other extreme are those who react excessively and shrink from painful eventualities. Whether this over-reaction represents an actual perceptual hypersensitivity in the physio-philosophical sense, or merely an exaggerated fear of pain-bearing stimuli, is open to argument. In this chapter I am more interested in the individuals who represent the non-sensitives. Is their apparent stoicism merely a complacency due to psychological traits of hardihood? Or are such subjects endowed with a perceptual peculiarity, a veritable hyposensitivity to stimuli, which to anyone else would be uncomfortable in the extreme, if not agonising? There are two distinct problems here, but I wish, if I may, to concentrate on the latter. These are the individuals otherwise physically and mentally normal, who do not belong to the category of those who have been acclimatised to pain. In fact, never since birth have they been endowed with the normal experience of physical pain.

Such cases are without doubt extremely rare and yet, from the evidence of the literature, their existence is indubitable. Perhaps all of us have encountered in our clinical experience what we may call "partial" cases of this type. I am referring not to an insensitivity, which is relative in degree, but rather a total insensitivity which is localised. Here perhaps belong those individuals—otherwise unremarkable—who have never known what it is to suffer a headache. Such a state of affairs is not rare, and yet it has been glossed over by clinicians, even by migrainologists, and no explanation—anatomical, physiological, or chemical—has ever been advanced. Less common are those patients, and I expect we have all encountered them, who have undergone such catastrophic disasters as a cardiac infarction, or even a perforation of a peptic ulcer, without any warning signal of localised pain.

But the cases to be discussed now are even more bizarre and, despite their infrequency, they offer important and even intriguing problems of biological as well as philosophical nature. I refer to those individuals, otherwise normal and non-conspicuous, who go from the cradle to the grave without ever having known the sensation of pain. And yet they are not anaesthetic or analgesic. Pricked with a pinprick they are aware of what has happened. They can distinguish a sharp jab from a gentle touch; they can differentiate between the head of a pin and its point. With their hands or body immersed in water they can tell the difference between hot and cold and even various degrees of temperature (as in the Hardy-Wolff technique of testing). And yet one of these "patients"—if one can term them such— would often pick up glowing coals which had fallen from the fireplace and replace them. Another reported patient, in the course of his work was often splashed with molten lead (T. 800°F) without feeling any discomfort. Cuts, bruises, burns, scalds, fractures, surgical interventions are painless. As a rule the subjects do not understand what is meant by visceral pain, head-ache, toothache, or earache. Menstrual periods occur without suffering and even childbirth may prove painless.

Nowadays these individuals with pain-insensitivity are recognised in early childhood and, by the time the youngster is brought before the doctor as a kind of medical curiosity, his body may bear a diversity of scars. Fingers may be the seat of whitlows or purulent paronychia. Or the distal phalanges may be eroded. One child showed macerated and deformed feet the result of displaying his ability to jump from considerable heights. One little girl was taken to the doctor, because while seated in a bath-tub she had turned on the boiling water and remained there for half-an-hour. In a rather older age-group the joints may be the seat of painful hypertrophic-atrophic de-rangement, similar to the Charcot arthropathies of tabetics and patients with syringomyelia.

One little boy aged 7 years, in trying to jump over some iron railings, had impaled himself on a large iron spike between his legs. After being lifted off, he walked home a distance of 2½ miles, bleeding profusely. Thirteen stitches were needed. The boy felt no pain either from the injury or from the surgical treatment.

Probing the clinical circumstances more deeply, one finds that these in-dividuals are neither hysterical nor feeble-minded. Their physical habitus is unremarkable: in other words the pain-insensitivity is not the manifesta-tion of any unusual toughness such as one associated with heavy-weight boxers, paratroopers, or marine commandos. Physical examination, in-cluding intimate neurological testing, is negative. Not only are all tendon reflexes present in the ordinary way, but even the corneal reflexes, which are often regarded as belonging to the category of a pain-response, are usually intact. This is interesting because the presence in the normal cornea of nerve-endings for touch, as opposed to pain receptors, has been denied.

There is some variation, as judged by the cases recorded in the literature, as to the matter of sweating. In some instances it does not occur, while in others it is normally present.

A complete investigation of such cases calls for many clinico-physiological procedures. Thus a number of putative pain-producing interventions may be made, but in every case with negative results. Thus no pain follows from intradermal injections of histamine; from the artificial production of muscle ischaemia; or from strong electric shocks. In one recorded case a "vitalometer" was attached to the teeth conveying a current of 60 milliamps, 5,000 cycles per second, but without pain resulting. The cilio-spinal reflex is usually unobtainable. Psychogalvanic responses do not occur. The cold pressor test of Hines-Brown is also negative.

Skin-biopsies—performed incidentally without local anaesthesia—have always given a normal histological picture as regards neurofibrils and nerve-endings.

Ramos and Schmidt produced skin-blisters in patients of this sort and the fluid when analysed proved to be normal in that it contained the ordinary pain-producing chemical factors.

It is of particular interest to enquire as to whether any uncomfortable cutaneous or visceral sensations occur, short of pain. For example the phenomenon of itching, which has been spoken of as a "slow-pain", may probably occur in some cases, though possibly not in all. Thus this experience was unknown to the patient described by G. A. McMurray. Hunger and thirst are certainly not foreign to the experience of some of the individuals, nor are the specific sensations of a distended bladder and a loaded rectum. There may also be some blunting of the sense of taste or of smell, but not invariably so.

That some strange subjective sensory experiences are operative in these cases, uncomfortable perhaps or annoying, is suggested by the fact that many of these non-sensitive children practise a veritable self-mutilation. Often children with pain-insensitivity are found to chew their lips or tongue to the extent of producing serious trophic wounds; or to gnaw at their fingers; or pick their noses to the point of producing ulceration. For example, one little girl described by D. A. Boyd, Jnr., and L. W. Nie would often deliberately burn herself on a hot stove, proclaiming that "it felt good". She would pick her nose till it bled "because it tickled". Another child reported in the literature seemed to indicate that potentially painful stimuli were merely amusing. Whether these activities are directed towards *allaying* an unpleasant dysaesthesia, or to producing a subjective experience which is pleasurable, is uncertain.

A relative insensitivity to various tastes and smells has occasionally—but not always—been noted, as in the patient reported by P. C. Gautier-Smith.

These various observations must surely be regarded as something quite remarkable. It is perhaps of even greater interest to pass to another consideration, namely to see what the other side of the coin displays. In other words, is there also a comparable insensitivity towards feelings and sensations that are usually regarded as pleasurable? We have seen that the phenomenon of itching may be in abeyance in these cases; what about tickle? is this also lost? Do these children with congenital insensitivity to pain respond like other children to such overtures as kissing, caressing, cuddling, and cosy warmth? At a later age do they find enjoyment in muscular activity, running around, dancing, and playing games? Still later do we find a loss of libido, or even of gentler sexual feelings and sentiments? These are questions that are easy to ask, but unfortunately the handful of cases in the literature have not been adequately studied, or followed up longitudinally far enough into adult life for us to be able to say with confidence whether, side by side with this indifference towards or insensitivity to pain, there also occurs an anhedonia or lack of pleasurable feelings.

There is some suggestion that this innate indifference to pain does not invariably confer an immunity to pain following every intercurrent illness. One of the best studied patients in the literature developed a severe head-ache after a lumbar puncture. Again there is a certain indication that in some cases at any rate, the insensitivity to pain lessens as the subject grows older. This is not invariably so, however.

Just what these inconsistencies mean is as yet impossible to say.

The history of this remarkable syndrome is interesting and it does not actually go back very far. Some time during the latter part of the 19th century, Dr. Weir-Mitchell described a case of this character which, as a matter of fact, occurred in an attorney who was a friend of his. Throughout his 56 years of life he had never known what it was to suffer pain, despite the fact that he had undergone many injuries. His finger had been crushed in the course of a dispute over politics and, because it incommoded him, he bit it off. For three years he had a painless ulcer on one toe. Once a severe abscess developed on his hand and spreading to the forearm en-dangered his life. No pain was felt, however, not even when the arm was lanced. He actually underwent an operation for the extraction of a cataract from each eye without the use of a local anaesthetic. Only on his death-bed did this gentleman suffer a little discomfort.

Probably the next case reported in the literature was in 1932 when Dear-born recorded the case of a well-known vaudeville artist, Edward Gibson, "The Human Pincushion". This man had suffered an occasional headache, but these were the only truly painful experiences throughout his life. Numerous accidents had befallen him during the fifty-four years of his life. He had been struck in the face with a pick-axe; his head had been laid open with a hatchet; a revolver bullet had passed right through a finger; his fibula had been fractured; his nose broken; his hand burned when he unwittingly rested it on a hot gas-stove, noticing nothing until he became aware of the stench of charred flesh. An important observation is that in some of the more serious traumata, he had sustained a certain degree of surgical shock but no pain. He had suffered acute otitis media, double pneumonia, and typhoid, each illness running its normal course but in a painless fashion. In his vaudeville act, he would appear in appropriate undress, and invite members of the audience to come up onto the stage and stick pins deeply into him anywhere except the abdomen and the groin. At any single performance perhaps as many as sixty pins would be driven in right up to their heads. He offered the sum of five thousand dollars to any doctor who could discern in him any evidence of pain. His professional career culminated when on one occasion, he elected to be crucified on the stage. Four gold-plated spikes with needle-sharp points were prepared and a wooden cross was erected. A man from the audience hammered one of the nails through the palm of Gibson's hand, and would have gone on with the other extremities had not the performance been broken up at this point by the collapse of some of the audience.

I think the next case to be recorded was actually one of mine in 1934 when I observed, in the out-patients clinic at King's College Hospital in London, a weedy-looking individual who had been referred to me from the cardiological department, because of the patient's chance observation that never in his life had he known what it was to suffer pain. He did not wince when I drove a pin hard into him, proclaiming it "nothing very much". Like the cases described by Dearborn and Weir-Mitchell, this man, too, had had numerous accidents and injuries which one would have expected to have been attended by pain. In the course of an argument someone had broken an umbrella over his head without hurting him at all. All his teeth had been extracted, and a whitlow had been lanced, without any anaesthetic. I found that this man was typical in that he could feel, identify, and recognise the intensity of various painful stimuli but without suffering discomfort.

In the last thirty years quite a succession of cases has been recorded, principally in the British and American neurological literature, and we have now available the experience of a couple of post-mortems, to be described later.

In discussing these cases, the question of terminology is of some importance. Some have spoken of "congenital analgia" but this is not a satisfactory term. The words "indifference to pain" and "insensitivity to pain" have been used more or less inter-changeably. Likewise, "congenital" or else "constitutional" have been prefixed at random. Dr. Kunkle has, however, written a strong plea for the dropping of the term "indifference to pain" in favour of "insensitivity to pain", pointing out that these individuals do not actually *appreciate* pain at all. "One cannot be indifferent to a message one does not receive"—as he put it. Another physician, Pacella, has argued "if the patient has never experienced pain, how can he experience the *absence* of pain?" I have compromised by speaking of "inborn indifference to or insensitivity to pain", but I must confess that the perfect term still eludes us. The question of differential diagnosis is important. We are all familiar with a relative state of analgesia in some psychotic patients and also some gross mental defectives.

Elsewhere I have described some of these cases: "Idiots and imbeciles often cause self-injury by biting or pummelling themselves, or beating their heads against a wall. Psychotics have been known to burn or scald themselves severely, to chew broken glass, and to perform all manner of terrible auto-mutilations. Goodhard described a girl who avulsed her eyeballs. Conn's patient fractured her phalanges, dislocated her thumbs, and tore off one of her ears. Weatherley's patient was a woman who had made many attempts upon her life. On one occasion she was discovered in flames: she had torn out her eyes and had placed flaming hot coals in her vagina, anus, and armpits. At the same time she was roaring with laughter and cried exultingly: 'Now I've got you, you devils!' "

The explanation of this sort of behavior is problematical, and may indeed vary from one case to another. In mental defectives, the pain-sensation may possibly be incorrectly interpreted. Perhaps in most cases the self-infliction of pain represents an effort to appease a sense of guilt or to atone for a misdeed, real or imaginary.

Obviously the cases we are discussing do not fall into either of those groups. There is, however, another type of psychiatric patient which comes up when discussing differential diagnosis, namely cases of hysteria. Patches of analgesia or anaesthesia are banal, but less familiar to modern medicine are those patients in whom the lack of pain-sensation is universally distributed. Undoubtedly, the whole pattern of hysteria has changed in character over the last few generations, but in the older literature there are many such cases on record. One of the first of these cases is that written up by Daniel Ludwig of Weimar in 1672, who referred to a youth of 18 who woke one day speechless and devoid of pain-sensations. Ludwig said that he pricked him on the head, the nape of the neck, the shoulder-blades, and in the back. In the fleshier parts the pin was thrust in half its length, but without registering any attention or pain. Turning him round, he was similarly pricked in the stomach, chest and arms . . . but the subject merely laughed "either by the singularity of the case, or as if he was being well-treated". This case was dramatically cured.

Turning from psychiatric problems to organic neurological states, there are three or four conditions which may to some extent mimic the syndrome under discussion. I refer to the rare cases of *lumbar syringomyelia,* where the therm-analgesia may be unusually widely distributed, but in such cases there are naturally many organic neurological physical signs which betray the diagnosis. Secondly, in advanced cases of *tabes dorsalis* there may be a more or less generalised blunting to pinprick, though not necessarily to light touch. Here again no real difficulty in diagnosis should occur, as the tabetic has so many other physical manifestations which are unmistakable.

Perhaps the greatest difficulty in differential diagnosis is met with in the child. The rare condition of *sensory radicular neuropathy,* either progressive or non-progressive, familial or non-familial, associated at times with nerve-deafness, is an obscure neurological condition brought about by widespread pathological changes in the sensory roots of the spinal cord.

Reference must also be made to a rare condition which is said to follow lesions of the parietal lobe, usually on the left side. This is the so-called *asymboly for pain* described originally by Schilder and by Stengel. The patient—who was said to be usually middle-aged if not elderly—sustains a lesion of the brain—vascular or neoplastic, sometimes traumatic—and thereafter shows a universal loss of pain-discomfort even though he is not analgesic. The syndrome is said furthermore to be accompanied by a morbid, introspective interest in sensory stimulation, whereby the patient may endeavour to produce painful sensations by pricking himself with a needle. I must confess that I have never seen a case of pain-asymboly even in quite a large experience of lesions of the parietal lobe, and I am consequently a little dubious as to whether this condition really exists.

Another odd syndrome in children has been described which to some extent resembles our cases of constitutional inborn indifference to pain. I refer to the *Riley-Day syndrome of familial dysautonomia.* It occurs in very young children and is commoner in Jews. The clinical features comprise instability of temperature, blotching of the skin, excessive sweating, but diminished secretion of tears, corneal insensitivity, sluggish tendon jerks with hypotonia and incoordination, chronic chest disease, delayed attainment of developmental milestones, often some degree of mental defect, and —most important of all for our purpose—constitutional indifference to pain. Personally I, again, have never seen one of these patients, but experienced paediatricians inform me that the syndrome does exist even though it be one of excessive rarity, in Great Britain at any rate.

The Nature and Aetiology of Cases of Inborn Insensitivity to Pain

Discussion has largely resolved itself into two main questions. Are we dealing with some inborn anatomical anomaly of the pain-pathways somewhere in their extent? If the latter notion is favoured, the further question arises as to whether a psychogenic disorder is envisaged.

It has already been mentioned that skin biopsies have yielded a perfectly normal picture of nerve-endings and neurofibrils. This negative finding supports the contention that there is no inborn defect of the pain-pathways at a peripheral level.

That there might be a structural anomaly at a thalamic level has been suggested from time to time.

Many writers have drawn an analogy with the attitude toward pain which lobotomised patients so often display. This has in turn led to the conception of some possible defect located at the highest level, and in particular within the fronto-thalamic connections.

In most of the cases where clinico-physiological methods of investigation have been carried out, the results seem to have suggested a relatively high-level defect, the local axon-reflexes having been demonstrably intact in all cases available for quotation.

The most remarkable feature in this syndrome is a typical lack of conformity between the feeling of pain as a *discriminative* quality of sensation, and the registration of distress, either overtly or autonomically. This discrepancy is reminiscent of what may follow the operation of lobotomy, and also of the "pain asymboly" of Schilder and Stengel; it differs from these conditions, however, in that they also entail a defect of the second component, i.e. the specific pain-feeling. This component may or may not be intact in cases of congenital insensitivity to pain.

The term "agnosia for pain" has been used by some and disapproved of by others who have preferred to visualise an inherent disturbance in the emotional capacity to react to pain. I dislike this term and, for that matter, the imprecision of the underlying conception.

Yet another line of argument avoids the invocation of structural lesions within the neuraxis. It is pointed out that in normal individuals there is a sort of spectrum of pain-experience which extends from those who are relatively tolerant of uncomfortable somatic sensations, to the other end of the scale occupied by the "sensitives". Whether these extremes represent differences in the intensity of the crude feelings of pain, or only in the feeling-tone of displeasure, or of both, is uncertain. Expressed differently, it is debatable whether the scale comprises a difference between the cognitive and the affective factors, or some combination of the two.

Can it be that the victims of congenital indifference to pain represent those otherwise normal persons who happen to lie at one extremity of this spectrum—being offset by those who are constitutional hypersensitives?

To look upon these cases as occupying the tip of the natural scale or gamut of sensitivity does not necessarily entail any morphological defect. An analogy with congenital word-blindness (dyslexia) or with Daltonism has been suggested, or, even better, the possession of a "musical ear" with its apogee in the faculty of absolute pitch.

Perhaps the weightiest argument against this "natural" hypothesis is the extreme nature of the indifference towards pain. In ordinary experience, the scale of natural variation in sensitivity would seem to be a rather restricted one, and falls short of the production of severe trophic lesions. Whether this argument is sufficient to upset the hypothesis must, for the time being, remain open.

As has been said, we are now in possession of two reports of autopsies carried out in cases of constitutional or inborn indifference to pain. Suffice it to say that in one of them absolutely no abnormality was found in the central nervous system, even after the most scrupulous investigation. In the other case however there was a minor peculiarity detected in the brain, a relative reduction in the number of myelinated fibres in the subcallosal fasciculus. This is a structure which, as far as we know, does not participate in the reception, conduction, or perception of pain, and it may well be that the pathological finding in this particular case is non-significant.

My final remarks concern what little we know about the personality of these individuals after they have attained adult age.

The fact that the well-nigh universal experience of pain has been something quite outside the experience of these persons must surely lead to certain qualitative inadequacies in their personality. We are reminded of the congenitally blind who find it impossible to comprehend what others mean by colours, or by a reflection in a looking-glass. Some of these patients with indifference to pain are also said to demonstrate indifference to danger, to threatening gestures, and the like. As individuals they must be incomplete—possibly liable to betray callousness or lack of interest as regards the sufferings of others. They are said to have unsympathetic "flat" personalities, with a corresponding poverty in their vocabulary and their use of language. However we really do not know enough about these patients to be sure. We need experience of more cases; more thorough physiological and psychological investigations; and more satisfactory follow-up studies.

This fascinating subject may turn out to be an even more intriguing problem for the philosopher than the physician.

Reprinted from Critchley, M. (1956): Congenital indifference to pain. In: *Annals of Internal Medicine*, 45:737–747.

Five Illustrious Neuroluetics

Contemporary neuropsychiatry is fortunately spared the calamitous phenomena which used to darken our clinical practice, namely the manifestations of syphilis of the nervous system. This grave social scourge was all the more distressing when it struck down men in their fifth or sixth decades at the peak of a successful career in the arts or sciences, or in the business or political worlds. Medical historians recognise many instances where persons of repute have been victims of a rapidly advancing general paralysis, or of that lingering affliction, locomotor ataxia.

Today I will select from this band of talented unfortunates five examples where the diagnosis of neurolues would seem, in retrospect, to be as definite as any clinical evaluation can ever be, short of the serological confirmation which, of course, was not then possible.

The first of these is *Heinrich Heine* (1797–1856) (Fig. 1). To quote an anonymous critic of a century ago ". . . I will write of Heine; of the poet whose genius has torn up the treaties of Vienna, and carried the boundaries of France to the Rhine; of that tearful trifler, that sardonic sentimentalist, that strange, sad, significant fellow, who laughs at old legends over his wine, and shudders beneath the black Lurlei-rocks in the twilights. I will write of him, not only because he is strange, sad and significant, nor because he tears up treaties, and quizzes Kaiser and Vaterland, and parodies the songs of Israel by the waters of the Seine—but because the music of his melodies 'beats time to nothing in my brain' today; because, in this sweet Rhenish weather, I have first learned how exquisite is his singing, how subtle and how true is the rhythm of his genius."

Although Heine has at times been suspected of being afflicted by multiple sclerosis, I submit that the more likely explanation of what he called his *Matratzengruft* ("mattress grave") is actually a tabes dorsalis. His symptoms began about 1840 and continued until his death 16 years later, though they were preceded for years by recurrent depression. About 1831, he met the beautiful scatter-brained grisette Mathilde Mirat, whom he married *au troizième arrondissement*—that is to say with whom he shared an apartment. In 1837 Heine developed violent ocular pain, and mention was made of incipient optic atrophy. The sight failed in the left eye, and he developed a ptosis first one side, then the other. He had to prop up his eyelids with his fingers in order to scrutinise an object. His heart felt "bound as by an iron frost". Everything he ate tasted like dirt. Later his lips became in-

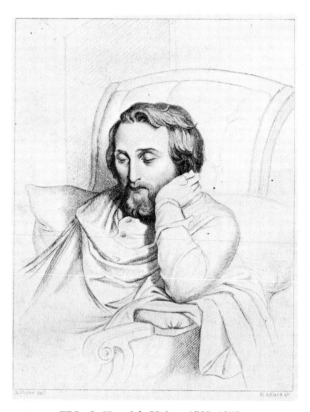

FIG. 1. Henrich Heine, 1797–1856.

sensitive, so that kissing was devoid of feeling. With his wife he would sit for hours in utter silence—"German small-talk" as she called it. Early in 1846, Heine was speaking of his "paralysis, which like an iron band pressed into the chest". He likened himself to a flower which was drooping and parched, though not yet completely withered. His finger-tips became numb and he took to a walking cane because of lameness. "Mysterious pains" steadily increased, and as a biographer put it—"something more terrible than paralysis had taken possession of his enfeebled frame". But the brilliance of his intellect if anything grew brighter—"like that fantastic flower of Borneo which displays its richest blossoms as the stem rots slowly to the root". By 1847 he was virtually incapacitated, because of what the doctors called "consumption of the spinal marrow". Eagerly he studied every medical treatise he could get hold of, in order that when he reached Heaven he might be able to lecture upon the futility of earthly doctors confronted with spinal complaints.

His biographer, William Sharp, has told us that "the sufferings of the poet became terrible: the fire of an undying fever scorched his veins, the frosts of a living death cramped his muscles, 'unborn agonies' took possession of his racked nerves. With bent body, half-blind, lame, without senses of smell or taste, with hands unable to guide the pen save for a few roughly-scrawled lines, with lips unable to respond to his wife's kisses, with ears painfully alert to any discordant sound, in straits of poverty, misunderstood, maligned, deceived, and defrauded, his was indeed a pitiable case." In January 1848 he entered a private clinic where he became caught up in the current revolution, and his carriage was upended to make a street barricade. In May he took his final painful stroll, and, defeated by fatigue, he took refuge in the Louvre, where he came to a halt in front of the Venus de Milo. "Overcome, agitated, stricken through, almost terrified at her aspect, the sick man staggered back till he sank on a seat, and tears, hot and bitter, streamed down his cheeks". Many years of sickness went by. His pains worsened and called for large doses of opium. His wasted legs felt like cottonwool. Periodically his cramped and twisted spine was cauterised by a negress in attendance. As he wrote in one of the last of his *Lieder:*

> . . . . I am but cinder,
> Mere matter, rubbish, rotten tinder,
> Losing the shape we took at birth,
> Mouldering again to earth in earth.

Lying on the garret floor he received, as in a fashionable salon, a succession of visitors like Béranger, Dumas père, Gautier, Gérard de Nerval, Taillendier, and Berlioz. In 1849 the Hungarian physician, Dr. Gruby, the first to diagnose Heine's complaint, took over the treatment, with some temporary benefit. It was at this period that Heine wrote his Romancero poems, the *Letzte Gedichte,* and also the "Confessions". Despite his sufferings he was able to laugh at himself. "I am no more a Divine biped . . . the high-priest of the Germans . . . the great heathen . . . a Hellene of jovial life and portly person, laughing cheerfully down on dismal Nazarenes; only a poor death-sick Jew."

When his poems were translated into Japanese, Heine grumbled "Alas, fame, once sweet as sugared pineapple, and flattery, has for a long time been nauseous to me; it tastes as bitter to me now as wormwood. . . . The bowl stands filled before me, but I lack a spoon. What does it avail me that at banquets my health is pledged in choicest wines, and drunk from golden goblets, when I, myself, severed from all that makes life pleasant, may only wet my lips with an insipid potion? What does it avail me that enthusiastic youths and maidens crown my marble bust with laurel wreaths, if meanwhile the shrivelled fingers of an aged nurse press a blister of Spanish flies behind the ears of my actual body? Of what avail is it that all the roses of Shiraz so tenderly glow and bloom for me . . . when in the dreary solitude of my sickroom, I have nothing to smell, unless it be the perfume of warmed napkins."

Among his last poems was *Leib und Siele* (Body and Soul), where, anticipating Oscar Wilde, he wrote that he had "two rooms: the one I die in, and the grave".

Later Heine and his wife moved to a fifth floor apartment in the Avenue Matignon with its balcony overlooking the Champs Elysées. Here he was repeatedly visited by that mysterious frail and beautiful young lady whose pen-name was Camille Seldon, but whom Heine spoke of as his "Lotus-flower", or, more often, as *La Mouche* because of the fly engraved upon her signet ring. She had answered Heine's advertisement for someone to come and read to him, a role which was beyond the capacity of his wife Mathilde. She too had known a neurological incapacity. She had been temporarily paralysed and for a time had been immured in a mental hospital in London. "The last flower of my mournful autumn", as he called her, charmed him with her manner, her voice, her fluency in German, and, above all, by her electric sympathy, and intellectual insight. His passion for her was beyond control.

One of Heine's finest poems, composed shortly before his death, was *Die Passionblume* dedicated to *La Mouche*. May I quote Mrs. Pfeiffer's translation?

> We did not speak; but oh, I could perceive
> The inmost secret of your spirit clearly;
> The spoken word is shameless, may deceive,
> Love's pure unopened flower is silence merely.
> Voiceless communing! Who could ever deem
> That time could fly as in my happy dream
> That summer night so full of joy and fear?
> What we then said, oh, ask it of me never!
> Ask of the glow-worm what it says in shining;
> Ask what the wavelet whispers to the river;
> Question the west wind of its soft repining,
> Ask the carbuncle of its fiery gleam;
> Ask what coy sweets the violet is betraying;
> But ask not what beneath the moon's sad beam
> The passion flower and her dead are saying.

Everyone remembers Heine's deathbed irony—how an officious friend asked him if he had made his peace with God. "Don't bother yourself", Heine replied. "God will forgive me—that's what he's there for."

Let us now turn to the history of *Jules de Goncourt* (1830–1870) (Fig. 2). This is the story, not of tabes, but of general paralysis of the insane. The *Goncourt Diary*—that fabulous storehouse of backstair scandal —contains a vivid account of the fulminating illness, written by the elder brother, Edmond. Early in 1870 Jules had the premonition that his working days were numbered. In March his brother detected a very subtle change in personality, coupled with a somewhat babyish mode of articulation, as though he were reverting to the cruel egoism of childhood. Then came days when he lapsed into an obstinate silence, staring before him and averting his gaze from the passing scene, with straw hat tilted over his eyes. Proper names eluded him, and sometimes he did not recognise familiar streets. As his powers of concentration waned, his features changed into what his brother called the "haggard mask of imbecility". Increasing defect in intellectual vigour went hand in hand with an affective change, a moodiness, and lack of warmth towards those close to him. In despair Edmond became a prey to morbid ideas of destroying his ailing brother and himself. A deterioration in table-manners began to show itself, causing embarrassment in restaurants. He emptied the salt-

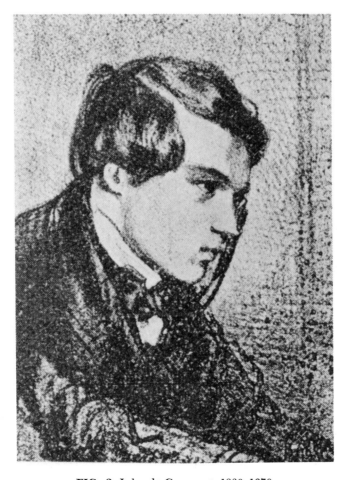

FIG. 2. Jules de Goncourt, 1830–1870.

cellar over his fish and clutched his dinner-fork with both hands. Conversation became laboured, and Edmond had to repeat himself three or four times before an answer was forthcoming. An increasing poverty of speech caused his brother to fear *une paralysie de la parole*. There were days when nothing escaped his trembling lips save an infrequent "yes" or "no", with the latter soon dominating the conversational scene. He began to fidget, crumbling and fumbling objects in a destructive fashion. By mid-June his speech had disintegrated to mere fragmentary phrases, truncated words, and half-formulated syllables, which he would angrily reiterate.

At this period of his illness one or two odd episodes took place. He would often throw back his head and let out a raucous, guttural, terrifying scream. His handsome face would become convulsed, terrible spasms jerking his arms, twisting them in their sockets. From his ravaged mouth trickled a blood-flecked foam. Attack followed attack, gradually leading to a delirious calm. Like the flapping of a wounded bird, he would agitate himself. Bloodshot eyes, violet lips, half-open eyelids gave him the sub-human appearance of a veiled and mysterious da Vinci. Often he would cower beneath the sheets in terror as if from an apparition at which he would hurl incoherent cries. Once he pointed a frightened finger and was heard to scream "go away". Sometimes a kind of occupational delirium would manifest itself, and he would go over the make-believe actions of his everyday life, screwing in his monocle, exercising his dumb-bells, and plying his literary craft.

The end came abruptly in the morning of Monday, 20th June, after 48 hours of coma in which he lay like a little child asleep.

More important to us today is the case of *Alphonse Daudet* (1840–1897) (Fig. 3), in that we possess a valuable document in the form of a detailed personal record of the subjective experiences, sufferings, and incapacities due to his chronic tabes dorsalis.

Daudet admitted to the Goncourts that he had contracted chancres and pox from a lady of high rank. Perhaps he was being snobbish, for Daudet—despite his exquisite sensitivity and his warm domesticity—had been an incorrigible sensualist since the age of 12. His long liaison with the *Chien Vert*, or Marie Rien, may have been significant. She, of course, was the one he immortalised in his novel *Sapho*.

At the age of 44 the earliest tabetic symptoms appeared, and continued until his death in 1897, thirteen years later. Daudet kept a diary which was not published until 35 years after his death, which he entitled *La Doulu*, the Provençal word for "pain" or "suffering". As we might expect from a writer of Daudet's calibre, the writing is of a superlative order, though florid perhaps by our present-day standards. Witness the description of his lightning pains ". . . Great tracks of flame slashing and lighting up my carcase"; "Contractures in the foot, with burning as high as the flanks. All the pluckings of the strings of the human orchestra tuning

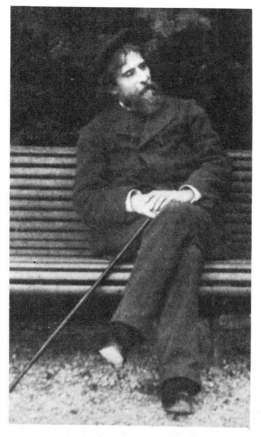

FIG. 3. Alphonse Daudet, 1840–1897.

its instruments . . . the human orchestra of pain." The characteristic girdle-sensation was particularly troublesome. "The 'cuirass' . . . months during which it penned me, so that I could not unfasten it or breathe . . . my everlasting belt with its holes of pain . . . veritable armour, cruelly clasping my loins with steel buckles—and tongues of burning coal, sharp as needles."

The manifold dysaesthesiae of tabes were evidenced by numbness and burning in the feet. Daudet referred to "the mythological sensation, the insensitivity and hardening of the torso encased within a sheath of wood or stone, and as the paralysis creeps upwards, the victim changing himself little by little into a tree, a rock, like the nymph of the Metamorphoses".

The diary contains many references to increasing difficulty with walking. "A feeling as if the legs were sliding away, and slipping lifelessly . . . the legs spreading themselves, and the arms outstretched, seeking support. . . . Inability to go downstairs without stumbling, or to walk on a polished parquet floor. . . . In order to reach my armchair, as much effort and ingenuity as Stanley in an African forest."

Charcot sent Daudet to Lamalou-les-Bains (Fig. 4) for treatment. Here he underwent the traction therapy then in vogue. According to Edmond de Goncourt "for this mysterious operation, they wait in baths until everyone has gone and then go furtively to a poorly lighted room full of shadows. There, the hanging takes place, a hanging which lasts a minute, a long, long minute, a minute made up of sixty seconds. Then they unhook you, and you find yourself back on the ground with a dreadful pain in the neck. That hanging in the half-light is something quite indescribable . . . a real Goya."

Lamalou was distasteful to the sensitive Daudet, who loathed the con-

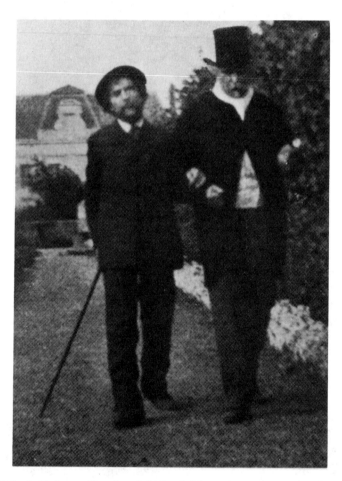

FIG. 4. Alphonse Daudet (*left*) and Edmond de Goncourt (*right*).

tact with other victims of ataxia and pain. As he wrote ". . . Never before had my sad nerves suffered from the promiscuity of the hotel. To
watch my neighbours eat was odious: their toothless mouths, their dis-
eased gums, tooth-picks in their crumbling molars, and those who could
eat only with the side of their mouths, those who ruminated, the chewers
and the devourers of flesh! Human bestiality! Jaws in action; their glut-
tonous, haggard eyes never raised from their plates, their furious glances
at the dish that was late in coming; it sickened me and put me off my
meals.

"And the painful digestions, the two W.C.s at the end of the corridor,
side by side, lit by the same gas-jet, so that one could hear all the groans
of constipation, the splash of excess and the rustling of paper. Horrible!
. . . the horrors of living!"

In May 1891 Goncourt made an entry in his diary regarding Daudet ". . .
How he suffers! I saw him today breaking off in the middle of a conversation, twisting his body about, painfully stretching his legs—and all
the time looking so terribly ill! And during the three hours, the poor
fellow gave himself three injections of morphine."

Daudet's diary ceased in 1894, but he continued to work in his apartment in the rue de Bellechasse, up to a few weeks before his sudden death
from a stroke.

His young friend, Marcel Proust, had written a tribute a few months
before. For ten years he had heard, so he said ". . . of the continuity of
his atrocious pains, of the daily necessity of ever more dangerous sedatives,
and how each evening the suffering of his body as soon as he lay down,
becoming intolerable, forced him to take a bottle of chloral in order to
go to sleep". Proust spoke of Daudet's spirit as being purified and refined
by disease. . . . "I saw this handsome invalid beautified by suffering, the
poet whose approach turned pain into poetry, as iron is magnetised when
brought near a magnet—this poet detached from himself and entirely devoted to us all, absorbed in *my* future and the future of other friends,
smiting us and glorifying happiness and love."

The next striking example of an illustrious neuroluetic is *Guy de
Maupassant* (Fig. 5). In this particular case we have striking evidence of
a premorbid eccentricity and unorthodox personality. In early adulthood
he contracted syphilis. He was always preoccupied by physical prowess,
especially in the amatory field. As an inveterate womaniser he collected
mistresses as others collect birds' eggs or stamps. In his role as a bedroom
Hercules he sneered at Casanova's Monsieur Six-fois as a puerile and
amateurish performer. He became that most boring of bistro boasters who
claimed he could attain a physical climax twenty times in short succession. It was not enough to boast, he had to show off his erotic accomplishments before witnesses, and he used to demonstrate that he

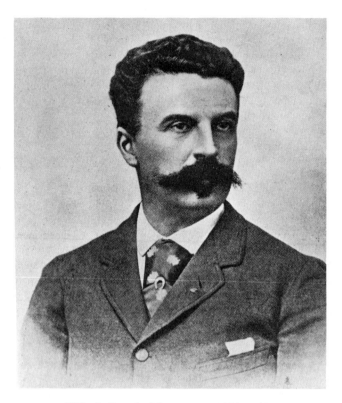

FIG. 5. Guy de Maupassant, 1850–1893.

could produce at will visual proof of his potency. In later life he became
a victim to drugs, and more particularly to ether.

Macabre ideas of a parapsychical sort always appealed to him, and he
asserted that at times he experienced heautoscopy or specular hallucinosis. Perhaps these strange notions and ideas inspired him to write that
bizarre story "Le Horla", a document of a haunted man. There is no
good evidence that he was mentally deranged at that time, but the stage
was set, and soon afterwards strange ideas developed. The dates are important. Maupassant was 37 years of age when he published "Le Horla"
in 1887. This piece of phantastica demonstrates his morbid interest in
the abnormal. As Maupassant wrote ". . . most critics will think I have
gone mad, but you'll know better. I'm perfectly sane, but the story interested me strangely." Two years later came odd symptoms such as extreme feelings of coldness, neuralgia, intolerance to noise, insomnia, and
pains in the limbs. He fancied he could see spiders. Later he complained
of "that hideous evil, headache, which tortures as no torments have ever

been able to torture, which grinds the head into atoms, and which makes
one go mad".

There are many contemporary records of Maupassant's terminal mental
decay. Let us select Frank Harris despite his inherent unreliability.

> Three or four years before the end, Maupassant knew that the path
> of self-indulgence for him led directly to madness and untimely death.
> . . . Even in his creative work he was warned after every excess and in
> fifty different ways. First, an orgy brought on fits of partial blindness,
> then acute neuralgic pains and periods of sleeplessness, while his writ-
> ing showed terrifying fears. . . . Then came desperate long-continued
> depression broken by occasional exaltations and excitements; during
> which his mind wandered and which he recalled afterwards with hu-
> miliation and shame; and always, always the indescribable mental
> agony he spoke of as *indicible malaise*. Finally he lost control of his
> limbs, saw phantoms on the highway and was terrified by visions that
> gave him the certainty of madness. . . .

Maupassant's last days recall those of Heine. Regular visits by a mysterious Madame X were always followed by obvious physical and mental
weakening. With a certain amount of awareness, Maupassant wrote ". . .
There are whole days on which I feel I am done for, finished, blind, my
brain used up and yet still alive. . . . I have not a single idea that is con-
secutive to the one before it, and my hallucinations, and my pains, tear
me to pieces." After an abortive attempt at cutting his throat, he was
immured within a mental hospital at Passy. This was in 1892. Ideas of
grandeur included delusions of immense wealth. He proclaimed that he
was the younger son of the Virgin Mary. He planted twigs into the soil
of the gardens around the clinic believing they would flourish as little
Maupassants. He would howl like a dog and lick the walls of his cell.
Curious obsessions concerned his bladder-function. He deliberately practised retention, saying his urine was "all diamonds . . . all jewels. . . ."

Dr. August Marie has left us the following account of his bizarre delusions:

> In his moments of delirium, he fancied his thoughts had escaped
> from his head, and searched anxiously for them, asking everybody:
> "You haven't seen my thoughts anywhere, have you?" Then suddenly
> he fancied he saw them, he had found them again and seemed radiant
> with happiness. There they were all around him and he saw them in
> the form of butterflies, infinitely varied and coloured according to their
> subjects: "Black thoughts for sadness, pink thoughts for merriment,
> golden butterflies for glory." And then suddenly he would cry out: "Oh
> what a fine shade of red: it is the purple of sanguinary adulteries." He
> seemed to follow the butterflies in their flight, and made gestures as
> though trying to catch them as they flitted near.

His last days were violent, necessitating mechanical restraint. He died in July 1893, at the age of 43, his last words being *"des ténèbres . . . des ténèbres".* (darkness . . . darkness).

Striking a homelier note we finally turn to one who was born in 1860, in St. Pancras, London. Today his humble birthplace is perpetuated by a preposterous railway terminal. I refer to that most brilliant of music-hall comics, *Dan Leno* (Fig. 6).

Dan Leno's first stage appearance was at the age of 4, at the Cosmotheca Hall in Paddington, where he was billed as "Little George, the Infant Wonder, Contortionist and Posturer". Thereafter he toured the provinces with his mother and step-father, acting in public houses, smoking concerts, singing rooms, and free-and-easies. He taught himself tap-dancing, and at Oldham in 1883 he won a championship belt and was proclaimed the greatest clog-walloper of the world. During the first twenty years of his professional life, he "did the smalls"—that is to say, he played outside London and his act was principally made up of uncannily intricate dancing to the conventional la-tum-tiddle type of orchestration. His friend Hickory Wood has recalled the scene ". . . I fancy I see him now, a slim

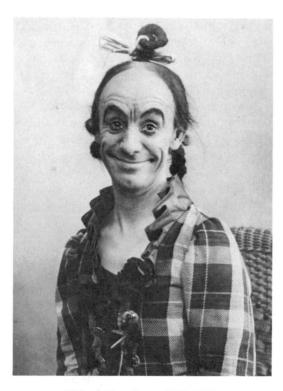

FIG. 6. Dan Leno, 1860–1904.

youth, standing on the stage of a Manchester music hall, wearing his championship belt in demure silence. . . . Then the belt was removed . . . and Dan danced. He danced on the stage; he danced on a pedestal; he danced on a slab of slate; he was encored over and over again; but throughout his performance he never uttered a word."

In 1885, Dan Leno went to London to work, his first appearance being at the Forester's Music Hall. Metropolitan audiences cared less for his dancing than for his comical singing, and especially his patter.

Known as the King's Jester or the "funniest man on earth", he became the most beloved exponent of vaudeville in its heyday. His secret lay in his simplicity, his humanity, and his likeness to the ordinary man in the street. Understandably he was not comprehended in the States. His songs and his patter were always homely and beautifully timed, compounding the ridiculous with the wistful with uncanny skill. Who can forget his account of how the domestic geyser exploded and blew his mother and father through the roof—the first time in years that he had known them to go out together?

As a comedian he was meticulous in choosing his songs, and then in working them up to determine precisely the most telling presentation. In show-business this is the hallmark of a true professional. When he was studying a new number, his favourite technique was to take long walks at night in the rain, and as he trotted along, he would keep time with his feet to the melody.

A contemporary writer had this to say about him:

> Beginning as a champion of one of the most diabolic forms of human expertness—clog-dancing, Mr. Leno has moved on to become a master of twenty-minute, cheerful, happily-inspired, pleasing exhibitions of ditty and monologue. He is grotesque without seeming to be hideous; he is unkempt without seeming to be pediculous. He is often farcical in the very extreme, often outrageous beyond measure; but he is always acceptable. He can make you laugh every time: you cannot resist him. He can keep you fixed in your seat till he has finished: you cannot wish to be otherwhere. His gasp of surprise at seeing you laugh, alternated with his own merriment in regard of some fictitious person's nonsense, is a thing to be up-gathered and stored against a barren day of rain and depression. Women assert that he is "so silly"; but, at his domestic allusions and feminine personalities, they laugh as approvingly as loudly. Men assert that he is wonderfully entertaining and amusing; and they are quite right. And so long as Mr. Leno does not try to put his humour between two book-covers, but is content to exhibit the same from behind the guard of the foot-lights, for just so long will he be recognised as a comedian who never fails—as a comedian who is not only comic, but funny—as a comedian who not only makes caricatures, but presents characters.

Increasing deafness became something of a professional handicap but at the age of 43 his mind gave way. Constance Collier, leading lady in Beerbohm Tree's company, has described him at this period. He told her in tremulous tones how his father had been a Marquess. He begged for a contract to play in Shakespeare. In his hand he was clutching a valuable diamond which on the way home he gave to a barmaid.

Another early symptom comprised unpredictable flashes of temper usually directed against his closest and dearest friends. As a rule he would afterwards be most contrite, but sometimes his memory of the outburst was a blank. Eventually he was admitted to Camberwell House for treatment. On one or two occasions Dan Leno escaped by diddling the nursing attendants, as he put it. As time went by, it became necessary to cast the next pantomime at Drury Lane. Ordinarily Dan Leno would have topped the bill, for as a critic of great experience has said, he was incomparably the greatest Dame of all time. But he was still a sick man in the mental hospital. The manager, Arthur Collins, took expert advice as to prognosis from the well-known psychiatrist Dr. Savage, and was told that there was a 50% prospect of a temporary remission. Consequently Dan Leno was earmarked in his absence to play Queen Sprightly in Humpty Dumpty and his name appeared upon the billboards. If, however, Dan Leno was still too ill to appear it was arranged that his star role was to be played by Herbert Campbell. But if Dan Leno was well enough then Herbert Campbell was to take on the role of King Sollumm—a part especially written in for him.

As events turned out, Dan Leno had his hoped-for remission near the end of December. News of this ambiguous state of affairs must have leaked out for, when the opening night came, the audience reacted enthusiastically. As Dan Leno made his dramatic entrance gorgeously arrayed as the comic Queen descending the Palace steps, the audience rose in their seats and cheered and cheered for over five minutes. Dan Leno was overcome and faltered in his diction. After a while he rallied and all went well. Or relatively so. He fluffed his words and missed his cues. Few except his fellow players realised this, for Dan Leno was a master of improvisation. His quips came readily if appropriately fed, but the others were often disconcerted not knowing what Dan Leno was going to say. Often the orchestra was equally at sea. Harry Randall who played the role of Cook would come to the rescue by feeding his friend with well-worn gags taken from earlier shows in which they had played together. Humpty Dumpty was a different performance each night. There were occasions when Dan Leno sulked in his dressing-room and refused to go on, until talked into his costume by his old friend Randall.

The pantomime ran for three months and then Dan Leno went to the London Pavilion. It was now obvious that his memory had completely failed, and his appearances were pathetic to witness. One night at the conclusion of a performance a four-wheeler was waiting at the stage-door to take Dan Leno back to Camberwell House where, on October 31st 1904, he perished.

A certain amount of insight into his failing memory must have been retained during these painful days, for on the last night of Humpty Dumpty he presented Randall with a large portrait of himself inscribed "To Harry, from Dan . . . with many thanks".

Reprinted from Critchley, M. (1969) : *Proc. Roy. Soc. Med.,* Vol. 62.

A Medical Commentary upon Napoléon III and His Son

I beg my audience here in Paris not to be shocked when I confess that I am perhaps the only subscribing Bonapartist in Great Britain. My interests, I hasten to add, are historical and literary; anything but political, and certainly not territorial. To most students the career of the first Emperor is paramount. To me, however, the social history of the Second Empire is more fascinating, and the characteristics of this period pivot around the personality of Napoléon III, a man whom I believe to be a rather misjudged and underestimated figure. Perhaps one day history will rehabilitate him. As a neurologist I naturally focus my attention upon his medical record, as well as that of his son, the Prince Imperial.

Prince Louis-Napoléon (afterwards the third Emperor), born in 1808, was the grandson and also the nephew of Bonaparte, his father having been King Louis of Holland, while his mother was Hortense, the daughter of Josephine. Scandal also had it that the Prince was Napoléon Bonaparte's son. Be that as it may, the mother and her sons lived after the battle of Waterloo as exiles in the Swiss town of Arenenberg. The elder survivor of the three brothers died on 17 March 1831 of measles complicated by pneumonia as confirmed by autopsy, leaving the third—Prince Louis-Napoléon—the sole claimant of the Bonapartist faction. It was at this juncture that Queen Hortense risked a secret return to France under the pseudonym of Mrs. Hamilton. Reaching Paris on 23 April, the party put up at the Hotel de Hollande, 16 rue de la Paix. Already the young Prince was feverish, and it was clear that he too had contracted the measles from his late brother.

The hotel proprietor demanded that a doctor should be called, and recommended an English medical man in the belief that this was the nationality of Mrs. Hamilton. Fearing that this step might betray her illegal entry into the country, Hortense insisted that the doctor must be a Frenchman and a Dr. Balancier was summoned. The identity of the visitors nonetheless came to light, and the authorities ordered the Prince and his mother immediately to leave the country. Perhaps the urgency was because the anniversary of the death of Napoléon I ten years before was due to be celebrated on the 5th of May in the nearby Place Vendôme. On 6 May the party left for London. By this time the Prince was jaundiced, which raises the possibility of an infective hepatitis. Perhaps the ensuing period of apathy and depression put an end to all immediate ideas of any attempt to snatch the throne of France.

The next entry in the medical dossier is in 1840. Prince Louis-Napoléon was now 32 years of age. Arrested after the fiasco of the *attentat* at Boulogne, he was now prisoner in the fortress of Ham, not far from St. Quentin. His incarceration was anything but rigorous, for he was afforded a suite of rooms—even if damp and dilapidated—books, writing-material, servants, and even a personal physician, Dr. Conneau. Nor was he denied the gentler comforts, for the affectionate solace of the laundry-maid Eleonore Vergeot—*la belle sabotière*—was to hand. Indeed she bore him two sons. It would be interesting to know more of these. The elder, we believe, was created le Vicomte d'Orx, married a Belgian, and died in 1910 in his Chateau des Castets, St. André-de-Seignaux, leaving three children. The younger went to Mexico, and on his return was made Comte de Labenne and Receveur des Finances. He died in 1881 in the rue de Miromesnil, his son surviving him by only two years.

During his incarceration, Louis-Napoléon also had a liaison with the gaoler's daughter. Their son was Leon Masse, who eventually lived in Paris in the rue Gaillon.

While in Ham he wrote various monographs, ranging in theme from Napoleonic philosophy, the use of artillery, to a project for an artificial waterway through Central America, thus anticipating the Panama Canal.

Despite all these activities the Prince fretted and lost weight. He became low-spirited, and suffered from neuralgia and rheumatism which caused him to limp. His depression did not entail apathy, however, and he began to make plans to escape. This was difficult, for the Governor's routine was to visit the Prince four times daily. On 25 May 1846, Dr. Conneau did the trick. That morning he reported that the prisoner was not well, that he had been given castor oil, and was not to be disturbed. To lend verisimilitude the bold doctor swallowed the purgative himself, but with-out the expected effect. Compelled to produce a repellant stench within the bedroom, he and conspirators burned a concoction of coffee, crusts of bread, and nitric acid. The smell must have been unconvincing, for the Governor became more and more suspicious. Refusing to be put off any longer, he brushed the doctor aside, entered the bedroom, and dis-covered a dummy in the bed. The Prince had walked out of the fortress disguised as a workman carrying a plank.

The rest of the story is well-known. In 1848 he was elected Prince-Président, and in 1852 came the *coup d'état* when he proclaimed himself Emperor Napoléon III (Fig. 1).

Something of his habits and personality are known to us. Though ab-stemious, he smoked heavily. His chief indulgence, however, was in the direction of womanising. His notorious conquests included the wealthy

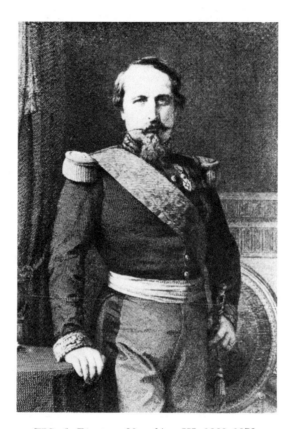

FIG. 1. Emperor Napoléon III, 1808–1873.

Englishwoman Miss Howard, the well-born Italian Comtesse de Castiglione, and also la Comptesse de Mercy-Argenteau. By la Castiglione he
had a son who, it is believed, studied medicine and eventually became the
personal physician to the Empress Eugènie up to the time of her death in
1920, aged 94 years. But his favours also included such *cocodettes* as his
peasant mistress from Brittany Marguerite Bellanger. Even the notorious
Cora Pearl had her name coupled with his, perhaps unfairly so, for she
was really the perquisite of his half-brother, the Duc de Morny.

Napoleon III was perhaps the first representative of the Common
Market. As Guérard put it ". . . Creole and Corsican, a Dutch prime
through a brief whim of fate, a Southern German by education, he was to
find himself perfectly at home among the British aristocracy, and he married a Spaniard. But next to France, his country was Italy."

Although the Emperor's many vilifiers did not shrink from hinting at
venereal disease, supporting evidence is lacking. Nevertheless one cannot
refrain from the reflection how often Fate strikes the individual in his

most vulnerable faculty. "A book opens most easily at the most read page." Just as Beethoven was afflicted in his faculty of hearing, and Baudelaire in the sphere of language, so the Emperor was ironically destined to be victimised within the urogenital sphere.

In 1856 the faithful Dr. Conneau, worried over his Emperor's ill-health, thought fit to call into consultation a foreign doctor, and Sir William Fergusson (President of the Royal College of Surgeons of England, and Surgeon to Queen Victoria) was discreetly summoned to Paris. Symptoms such as aching and hypersensitivity of the legs; dyspepsia; lassitude; irritability; poor sleep; anorexia; haemorrhoids; and sexual inadequacy were ascribed to over-work and lack of exercise. The day after the consultation the Emperor was said to have looked unwell, pale, and wan. He had woken in the night confused and shaky, with pain and oppression in his chest. He had unconsciously voided urine in bed, an accident which had happened at least once before. Sir William spoke of the malady as being on the "verge of an epilepsy".

In 1865 we first hear mention of the diagnosis of a stone in the bladder, diagnosed by Baron Larrey. Next year at Vichy he developed retention of urine, and was catheterised by Dr. Guillon. A consultation followed with Dr. Rayer and Professor Nélaton, the administrations of the latter being rough and uncomfortable. In 1869 two other specialists came on the scene, namely Dr. Fauvel and Dr. Ricord; he was also seen by a German surgeon, Dr. Chelius. Just before the Franco-Prussian war broke out, Professor Sée and Dr. Corvisart met in consultation, for the Emperor had been having hematuria. A lengthy session took place on 1 July 1870 in the rooms of Dr. Conneau. Professor Sée confidently diagnosed a stone; Corvisart spoke of a "cold"; Fauvel of an abscess. A wordy document was drawn up and signed by Professor Sée, in which mention was made of cystitis due to a calculus; flatulency, piles, anaemia, and "neuro-muscular hyperaesthesia" of the lower limbs. It was never shown to the Empress Eugènie, and no action was taken. After Dr. Conneau's death this report was found in his desk, sealed and unopened.

Three days later war broke out, and Napoléon's sufferings were much intensified by long hours in the saddle or in a jolting carriage. During the campaign the Emperor more than once was seen clinging in agony to a tree-trunk blanched and drenched in sweat.

After the tragedy the battle of Sedan, Napoléon joined his wife into exile in England. They resided in Camden Place, Chislehurst, near London. Two years later his symptoms returned. Dr. Conneau and Dr. Corvisart, who had faithfully followed their Emperor, met in consultation Sir William Gull (physician to Queen Victoria) and Sir Henry Thompson the urologist. Napoléon was a pigheaded patient, and refused to undergo an examination of the bladder, or to take opiates.

Dr. Thomas Evans, the American dentist to the Imperial household, found the ex-Emperor pale and puffy in the face, slower in movement, and dispirited. Sir James Paget met the other doctors in consultation, but urged conservative measures. But the ex-Emperor worsened, and on 26 December Sir Henry Thompson passed a sound into the bladder and found a stone the size of a large date. On 2 January the calculus was crushed with a lithotrite. The post-operative course was stormy, and a second and difficult operation was needed to dislodge a fragment which was impacted in the neck of the bladder. Uraemia supervened, and Napoléon perished on 9 January 1873.

As Dr. Guillon's son put it in a letter written in 1890 ". . . . *Vous savez que Napoléon 1ᵉʳ souffrait d'une rétention d'urine a Waterloo . . . singulière coincidence et conclusion: Napoléon 1ᵉʳ et Napoléon IIIᵐᵉ ont perdu leur trône par le fait d'une maladie des voies urinaires!"*

Afterwards differences of opinion were expressed in the press by the doctors concerned, Sir William Gull, as usual, being obstructive. In France an atmosphere of excitement arose. At the house of M. Rouher the Bonapartist opposition made wild statements to the effect that the surgeons had rejected the sage advice of Sir James Paget for political motives, asserting that the Emperor had wished to be fit enough to re-enter Paris in triumph on a horse. Some said he had been given too much chloral, or perhaps it was too much chloroform. Eventually the tactful intervention of the Prince of Wales became necessary to silence the critics.

Meanwhile the left-wing cartoonists in *Le Grelot, Le Sifflet,* and so on made merry with the dead Emperor and his weaknesses. Certain themes repeated themselves over and over in these caricatures. Napoléon was often depicted as a dressed-up pig, or as a prematurely aged cigarette-smoking pantaloon with exaggerated mustachios, clutching an enema syringe, a bottle of copaiba or some other urinary disinfectant, crutches, and a mangy eagle. Sometimes he was crowned with horns, a reference to Eugènie's friendship with Olivier. Often he was surrounded by champagne bottles and houris *en déshabillé*. Such scurrilities continued for some years after Napoléon's death, and the cartoonists invented a top-hatted figure as a symbol of Bonapartism, adorned as always with an imperial beard and mustache, as well as with the badges of urinary and intestinal malaise (Fig. 2).

Gradually the Bonapartist movement dwindled. As an anonymous informant reported to Rothschild in 1873 ". . . Complete indifference amongst most of the population; sincere regret amongst the small group which was personally attached to him; disappointment among the senators, deputies, and civil servants of the Second Empire, who still cling to the belief that the regime could be reinstated; despondency amongst the men who were plotting for his return."

May we now turn to the son, Prince Louis-Napoléon—or "Lou-Lou"

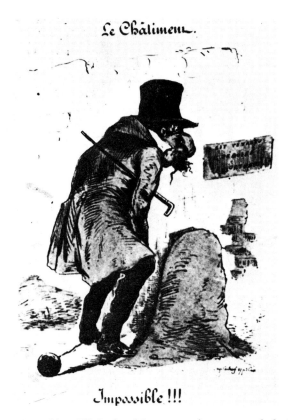

Le Châtiment.

Impossible !!!

FIG. 2. Emperor Napoléon III depicted by cartoonists as a symbol of Bonapartism.

(Fig. 3) as he was often called? Born in March 1856, he proved to be a nervous and difficult child. Nowadays we would call him hyperkinetic: at that time they referred to him as a *"bougillon"* on account of his fidgeti-ness and inability to sustain attention. He was not allowed to go to school, being spoiled by his father though not by Eugènie. *"Papa dit toujours oui; Mama dit toujours non, et je finis toujours par obtenir ce que je veux."*

Napoléon doted upon his son, looking to him to maintain the Bona-partist legend. But disappointment and difficulties soon arose. In charge of the Prince was the strict General Frossard with three other high-ranking *aides-de-camp*, whom Lou-Lou called "mes quatre-z-officiers". After a false start, the education became the responsibility of the young tutor, Augustin Filon, who was brought to the Tuiléries from his lycée in Grenoble. Filon found a problem-youngster on his hands. Neither the capacity nor the willingness to learn was apparent. Filon entertained doubts as to the intellectual future of his pupil. In addition he was moody, restless, un-

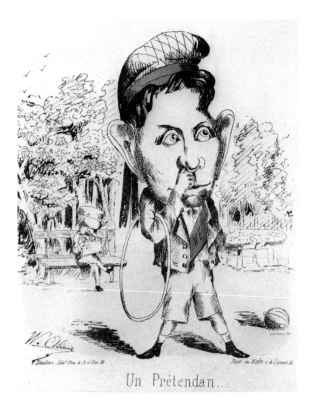

Un Prétendan....

FIG. 3. The Emperor's son, Louis Napoléon. A cartoon from a contemporary anti-imperial periodical.

controlled, and irritable. His nights were disturbed, and at times there was sleep-walking. Was he really stupid—it was asked—or merely inaccessible? He never seemed to listen: *"il était ailleurs"*. He seemed to have every good and charming quality, except brains. Reading, writing, and spelling were his worst subjects. And yet by way of contrast, he was proficient at the piano and at singing, at history and political science. And when it came to sketching and drawing he actually excelled, and showed a competency well beyond his years.

Indeed Filon thought that this artistic talent was a detriment, and a handicap to spelling. "When a word was pronounced to him, he saw it in his mind's eye—the man or the thing—and not the printed word." Words called up images instead of alphabetical formulae.

Filon asked himself "did he observe? did he reflect? did he enter into relation with ideas or objects by swift intuition? We never knew. . . ."

As yet between the ages of 16 and 18 there was an extraordinary

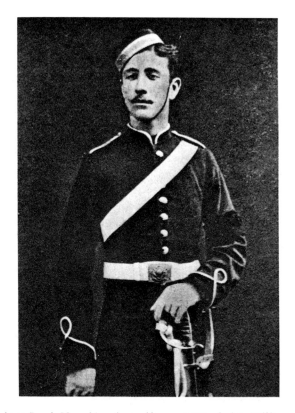

FIG. 4. Prince Louis-Napoléon in uniform at Woolwich Military Academy.

blooming, and we know that in exile the Prince Imperial entered Woolwich Military Academy (Fig. 4), was commissioned in the Artillery, saw active service in South Africa, and was killed in an ambush during the Zulu war on 1 June 1879 at Itelezi.

These medico-psychological fragments suggest strongly the diagnosis of a reading-retardation, in all probability due to a veritable developmental dyslexia. This diagnosis is supported by two or three pieces of evidence:

(1) The poor penmanship and spelling obvious in his letters. This is shown in the note he penned to Marshal Bazaine congratulating him on the capture of Pueblo in the Mexican adventure. This was written in 1863 when the Prince was seven. Caught up in the Franco-Prussian War, the Prince wrote to his tutor from the front, and asked him to overlook the numerous errors in spelling (Fig. 5). The Prince was then fourteen years of age.

(2) Most significant of all is the piece of evidence which good fortune placed in my hands. This is an apparatus constructed by Filon in order to

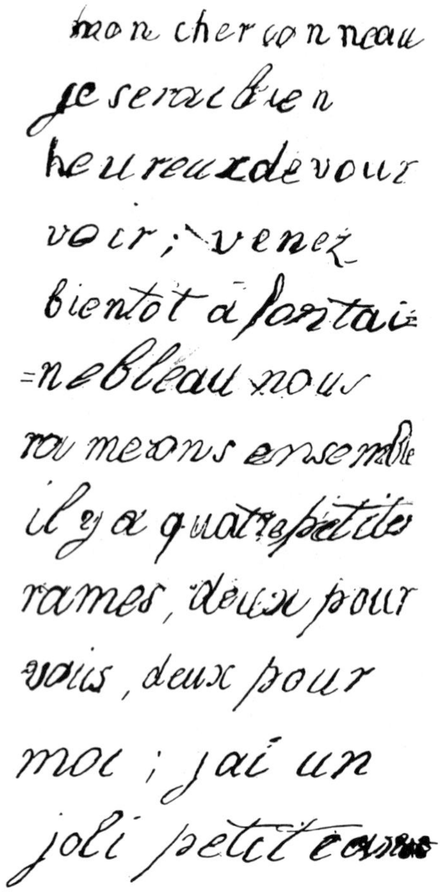
mon cher conneau
je serai bien
heureux de vous
voir; venez
bientôt à fontai=
=nebleau nous
ramerons ensemble
il y a quatre petites
rames, deux pour
vous, deux pour
moi; jai un
joli petit canot

FIG. 5. Letter written by Prince Louis-Napoléon.

teach his pupil to read (Fig. 6). This—probably the first reading-machine ever to be constructed—is now in my possession. By turning various knobs, different letters of the alphabet are displayed, as well as simple phrases broken up into syllables.

If I am correct in thinking that young Lou-Lou was dyslexic, I recall he was not the only royal personage to be so afflicted. Karl XI, one of Sweden's wisest kings, never learned to read properly. Relying upon his quick wit and his fine memory he would speak from documents, only too often open at the wrong page or even held upside down.

On January 1973, I was privileged to attend the memorial mass commemorating the centenary of the death of Napoléon III. It was held at the Convent at Farnborough where the widowed Empress Eugènie had

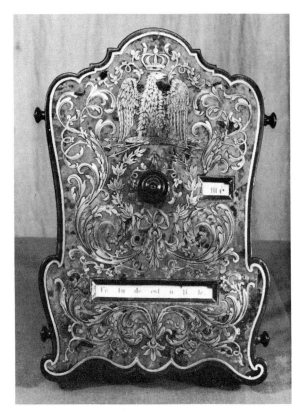

FIG. 6. A second Empire "reading machine" constructed in buhl and vermilion lacquer, measuring $16 \times 11 \times 2\frac{1}{2}$ in., decorated with imperial badge of Napoléon III. This was used by Prince Louis-Napoléon, under the supervision of his tutor, M. Augustin Filon.

lived for the last years of her long life. The body of the Emperor lies in the crypt of the Convent Church. In attendance at the memorial service were the contemporary Prince Napoléon and his wife, the Prince and Princess Murat, as well as representatives from the French embassy and from the British Foreign Office.

Gordon Holmes: The Man and the Neurologist*

It must have been in 1923 when I first met Gordon Holmes (Fig. 1). He was at that time 47 years of age, but to me he might have been any age for he seemed ageless, an institution, a living legend. Our first meeting was on the occasion of my joining the house staff of the National Hospital, Queen Square, which I found to be something like entering the Valley of the Kings at Luxor. I seemed to be surrounded by the ghosts of such monumental figures as Brown-Séquard, David Ferrier, Bastian, Beevor, Batten, William Fergusson, Marcus Gunn, Charles Ballance, and Felix Semon.

And yet some of the dead seemed still to be alive. For example, Hughlings Jackson, Gowers, and Victor Horsley. It was an eerie, awesome feeling, as though they were looking over one's shoulder.

But here the metaphor ceases; in the Valley of the Kings they were still striding through the halls, very much alive and in the flesh, giants, High Priests, and Pharoahs. Chief among these was that Colossus, physical as well as intellectual, of Gordon Holmes who shone brightest among the galaxy of stars surrounding him.

For at least two years it was my privilege to have been his house physician which implies that I was his apprentice, his disciple, his oblate, and his maid of all work.

I had previously been warned by one of my Chiefs at Great Ormond Street that I would find Gordon Holmes to be a man who was "tempestuous . . . volcanic". I did.

He was surrounded by a cluster of brilliant post-graduate students mainly from Canada, the United States of America, and Australia, some of whom are here today, and all of whom were destined to become pioneers of clinical neurology in their own countries.

A big man in stature, brusque, demanding, Gordon Holmes trained us like a sergeant major in the Brigade of Guards or the Royal Marines, and we were keen and willing recruits.

He made exorbitant demands upon us. He exacted the utmost accuracy and dedication and he got it willingly. How junior hospital doctors of to-

---

* Paper read in 1977 on the occasion of the celebration marking the centenary of the birth of Sir Gordon Holmes.

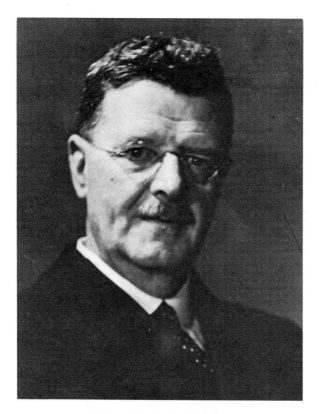

FIG. 1. Sir Gordon Holmes.

day would have fared, I tremble to think. Probably they would have been flung out. We were expected to be on duty for twenty-four hours a day. Our work might entail travel into the remote parts of the field to follow cases in which the chief had been particularly interested. I recall a case of pituitary basophilism—long before Cushing described it—and I had to visit the patient in his home in the Midlands after he had left hospital. Once, Gordon Holmes ordered me to a remote farmhouse in rural Essex to perform a drawing-room autopsy on a patient of his with a brain tumour. Often I was despatched to libraries to look up obscure references, chiefly in German. All these chores we took in our stride, for we were only too proud to carry out the master's wishes.

Like so many myopics, Gordon Holmes was a meticulous, obsessional observer. All who worked with him recall the mannerism whereby he would abruptly remove his glasses on one side only in order to peer closely at a sheet of paper. Moreover, he was a scrupulous recorder of observed data. He had no time for woolly thinking, airy speculation, or high-faluting notions. He examined every patient from top to toe, taking no short cuts. Even a Parkinsonian was subjected to the most rigorous sensory testing, though the diagnosis had been obvious to him right from the start. Only once did I know him make a spot diagnosis, when to his disgust he identified in a flash a so-called syringomyelic whom I had spent many hours in working up, as a leper, as indeed she was.

His clinical technique was thorough, and many would have said rough, even terrifying, and yet he was so warm hearted that he never could understand why he was regarded as a bully, as indeed he was. Not to the patient, not for a moment—who was just bewildered—but to any student or house physician guilty of slipshod work. I have known him tear up the case-notes and scatter them across the ward; and throw on the deck his percussion hammer or his king-size tuning fork.

He could coax physical signs out of a patient like a Paganini on the violin. Perhaps it is still not yet generally realised that every neurologist alive today—wherever he works—is unconsciously utilising the routine clinical examination propagated, perfected, and perpetuated by Gordon Holmes.

It was a sheer delight to watch him evoking one physical sign after another in a patient with, say, tabes—a common disorder in my young days. Like some violent conjuror, he would demonstrate the typical zones of hypalgesia, and we used to say that one of the hallmarks of a tabetic was Holmes's pin left in situ, at the tip of the nose of an uncomplaining patient, perhaps with an adjacent tiny trickle of blood.

As a colleague, Holmes was exciting. He rarely put in an appearance at medical committees. His few angry attendances were like war-drums announcing an impending battle over some issue which evoked his tornado-like feelings.

He was not endowed with wit, nor any broad sense of humour. Rarely did he smile, and I cannot recall him giving vent to anything like a belly-laugh. Towards the other members of the staff he had mixed feelings. Some, he just brushed aside as though they did not exist. A few of them blossomed in the warmth of his affection and esteem. Among those few were the neuropathologist, Godwin Greenfield, who was, incidentally, the most likeable man in neurology. Here too was his dapper neuro-surgical colleague, Sir Percy Sargent—"pretty Percy"—as he was called at St. Thomas's. Sargent had worked side-by-side with Holmes behind the front line in France during the First World War, and mutual respect had grown up. Percy Sargent was the only one who could pull Holmes's leg and tease him and Holmes would take it. At the same time Sargent would never venture to operate without Holmes standing over him and indicating on the skull with his finger-tip the precise site of the underlying tumour. F. M. R. Walshe, a junior colleague, was a younger man whom Holmes admired and respected, and to whom he would always listen seriously.

The one-sided feud with Kinnier Wilson cannot be glossed over. Students who came to Queen Square found themselves in a modern Verona, with the Montagues and Capulets at war. They had to align themselves either with the Kinnier Wilson clique or with the followers of Holmes. Never could they do both. Wilson was a vain and touchy man, jealous of Holmes, and he would ostracise anyone who strayed into the other camp. Holmes for his part could not care less, and simply ignored his colleague.

Outside Queen Square, Holmes had a number of good friends, like Bolton, the gastro-enterologist; the centenarian, Sir Thomas Barlow, who had been Queen Victoria's doctor, and Hume of Newcastle, whose son became the Abbot of Ampleforth and who is now the Cardinal–Archbishop of Westminster.

Abroad, Holmes's favourites included Wilder Penfield, Patrick of Chicago, Otto Foerster, and, in particular, Brouwer of Amsterdam—a giant of a man, very like Holmes in many respects. He had an admiration for Dandy, but certainly none for Cushing.

I have referred to his apparent lack of humour; perhaps I should qualify this. He used to tell me how, when he worked on cortical sensory impairment with Henry Head (a most unlikely alliance, by the way) experience taught him that two types of patient had to be rejected as test-subjects: (1) school-teachers, who would never give a plain "yes" or "no" but only rambling, parenthetical, introspective, wordy replies; and (2) Scotsmen who too could never answer "yea" or "nay" . . . suspecting that there might be a catch in the questions.

When I ceased to be his house physician and was either the Registrar or his junior colleague, I would often come face to face with him and his cortège in the corridor. He would always halt, seize me violently by the collar or by the shoulder, and bellow at me "what are you doing these days? What are you working at? If only you would go out less often at night and keep away from the cinemas, you might get somewhere." This was his form of blustering, benevolent, humorous encouragement.

Others will be speaking about Holmes's major contributions to our neurological lore, visual, sensory, or cerebellar. Visual, including the cortical representation of the macula, and the subtler concepts of visual inattention and visual disorientation. As to the sensory system, Holmes never referred to epicritic or protopathic. He always alluded to the instrumentalities—like touch, pinprick, two-point discrimination, the localisation of touch. The rich symptomatology of cerebellar defect was Holmes's very own province.

Holmes came to Queen Square from the laboratories of Edinger and Weigert, fluent in German, and highly conversant with the intricate anatomy of the nervous systems. These were two valuable qualifications which today are not fashionable. He fitted perfectly into the heady atmosphere of Queen Square, where he developed abounding and perpetual admiration for his chiefs, especially Jackson and Gowers. Goodness knows, the latter was an oddity for, despite his genius, he was an indifferent judge of character or of aptitudes. He advised Purves Stewart to take up skins and become a dermatologist, Wilfrid Harris to be a surgeon, and Stanley Barnes to get lost in the provinces. Not content with this, he urged Holmes to devote himself to academic anatomy. Perhaps Gowers did not welcome such a powerful figure close to the throne.

Though a very great man, conscious of his qualities, Holmes was modest to a fault. Accorded the distinction of many academic prizes of the Royal College of Physicians, he was not concerned with the inner workings of the College. He was one of the last of the clinicians to be elected to the Royal Society. There again many awards fell to him. He did not, however, receive public recognition until late in life, for he was never one to tread the corridors of power or to defer to the High Priests of dispensation. He was not a diner-out, or a fashionable physician. Some of us junior colleagues were bold enough more than once to beard the panjandrums of patronage in their dens in protest. We were told gently but firmly what indeed we had already guessed: Holmes had never guarded his tongue, nor had he gone out of his way to refrain from treading on the toes of the touchy. All came right in the end, however.

The time came, too, when we mooted the idea of a portrait. There was no dearth of eager subscribers from all over the world. The snag was, could we ever get Holmes, the unassuming elder statesman, to agree and, even if he did, would he have the patience to sit still and refrain from fidgeting? Again, all came right in the end.

Our only regret is that the portrait was not painted earlier. When he was my chief he was a heavily built, robust man but a victim of flatulent dyspepsia. He carried round with him a box of sodamints, into which he would periodically dip, with benefit, benefit that was obvious and audible to us all. Not long afterwards he became afflicted with a severe gastric problem. He must have lost forty or fifty pounds in weight. Though he changed considerably in build, he did not change his tailor, and thereafter his clothes hung on him like the skin of an elephant.

My remarks so far have been anecdotal. Perhaps so, but they are not the data which a future historian will find embodied in formal obituaries and appreciations, and for this reason I think they are worthwhile, for they give some idea of a great man in his entirety. Havelock Ellis put this over well when he said, "To describe the birth and growth of a great man as he was in his real nature, physical and psychical, as a grape-cluster on the tree of life, and not as a drop of alcohol in the vat of civilisation—*that* is biography. The biographer is the biologist of this new life, to whom we come to learn the origin of this tremendous energy, the forces that gave it impetus, and that drove it from one channel rather than another."

Holmes was one of the past generation of clinicians who advanced knowledge in their chosen subject without any outside assistance, financial or otherwise. Not only did he never have a department, he was not even afforded the privacy of a room or office in the hospital. Head, Gowers, Jackson were in the same predicament. His researches had to be carried out in the open wards, and at home in his own time working far into the night. Apart from his original Stewart research scholarship to Germany from Trinity College, Dublin, he never received a penny for his work. This is not to say he was not afforded opportunities. Although the University of London did not recognise his hospitals, he received, to my knowledge, offers of Chairs at Johns Hopkins, and also one of the Regius Chairs in Physic, both of which he turned down.

May I speak of him as Editor of *Brain?* His approach was unusual, and, I am grateful to say, stimulating. You sent him a paper. Later you would be invited to his house and, after dinner, he would go over the whole text with you, sentence by sentence, word by word. With his ruthless blue pencil, he would erase every adjective which was merely decorative; every "very", every "etc."—terms which he so rightly said had no place in scientific papers. When he came to a lengthy complicated sentence, allusive and abstract in nature, he would jerk to a halt and demand "Just what are you trying to say?" When you replied, aggrieved, in a word or two, giving him the gist of your nebulous thinking, he would say at once, "Why the devil don't you say so?" and out would go your purple patch, your flight of fancy, your probing into the higher ether. He was just as ruthless with your illustrations. Ruler in hand, he would demand what the microphotograph was really intended to show. With diffident forefinger you would point to a sorry-looking astrocyte in the centre, and out would go the pictorial background leaving the offending structure conspicuous but naked as Godiva. I learned so much at his Editorial Chair that I can truthfully say that whatever command I possess of the Queen's English is due to my one and only teacher of style, Gordon Holmes.

In his down-to-earth attitude Holmes had no time for neurotics and hysterics, and less than none for the pagan gods of psycho-analysis. When Holmes took over the beds from Aldren Turner, Senior, on his retirement, I became his house physician. In the ward there was a blonde bombshell of twenty-one with mild tension headaches. She was as pretty as a picture, plump as a partridge, who the previous year had been the *Daily Mirror* Bathing Beauty Queen. The first time I took Holmes round, he stopped at the foot of the bed and said "Who is this woman?" I explained, whereupon he jerked his thumb towards the door and said "Get rid of her." Of course I did nothing of the sort, for she was useful in keeping up the morale of us house officers. A week later he came round and said "I thought I told you to get that woman out of here?" Yet another week passed. On this occasion I got the Sister of the ward to hide the patient in the bathroom during the ward round. Standing at the foot of the empty bed, Holmes paused, then said to me "Look here, my boy, either she leaves the hospital or you do—and I don't care which."

If so far I have given you an impression of Gordon Holmes as a kind of ogre, I have failed to depict the man in all his plentitude. To paraphrase something which Penfield wrote, "although he appeared to be a martinet, he possessed a heart of Irish gold". If he liked you he would go to great lengths to help you. It was a delight to see him at his home with his gentle, charming lady wife. At Christmas he would visit the ward along with his three lovely, boisterous, dimpling daughters, whom I am delighted to see here today. He was devoted to them and most proud when all three joined Womens' Forces during the War.

Outside neurology, Holmes had three main passionate interests, hard-hitting golf, vigorous gardening, and a considerable knowledge of Gothic architecture. As far as I can determine he was not interested in painting, the theatre, or music, and only to a limited extent in literature—in this way resembling Hughlings Jackson.

I have said little enough about Holmes as a neurologist. The subject is too vast, but others will complete the picture. It is a conventional habit to finish a talk such as this with a quotation, and I have sought something appropriate from one who in many ways strongly resembled Gordon Holmes. I refer to Dr. Samuel Johnson, also a big man, a great man, a legendary figure. Holmes had none of his eccentricities or multiple tics, but he was very, very reminiscent of Johnson who, in 1759, wrote, "The life that is devoted to knowledge passes silently, and is very little diversified by events. To talk in public, to think in solitude, to read and to hear, to inquire and to answer inquiries, is the business of a scholar. He wanders about the world without pomp, and is neither known nor valued but by men like himself."

God and the Brain:
Medicine's Debt to Phrenology

Definition and Nature of Phrenology

Phrenology—a theory of brain-function promulgated by Gall—began, like Truth, as a heresy and ended as a superstition. His followers, Spurzheim, George and Andrew Combe, Vimont, the Fowlers, Caldwell, and others elaborated and later debased his doctrines. As originally put forward there were four cardinal premises, namely that: (1) the brain is the material instrument through which the mind holds intercourse with the outer world; (2) the mind entails a congeries of discrete mental faculties each with its own specific cerebral centre or organ;* (3) the size of each organ corresponds with the functional efficiency of each faculty; and (4) the development of these organs is reflected in the shape, size, and irregularities of the encompassing cranium.

Inevitably this theory of neuro-physiology expanded so as to constitute an aspect of moral philosophy. It differed from most other schools of metaphysics in that it was derived from direct observation of Nature rather than introspective reflection. Gall's slogan "God and the Brain; nothing but God and the Brain" symbolised the almost religious nature of his thinking. One follower deemed it a system of theology devoid of fraud and imposition, being furnished by Nature itself. But eventually phrenology deteriorated from a claim to establish the physiology of the brain into a technique of prognostication, allegedly divining personality and intelligence. Thus philosophy and pseudo-science became intermingled, the latter finally acquiring domination.

Predecessors of Gall

Gall's first dogma equating the brain and the organ of mind was already more or less established at the end of the 18th century, the earliest thinkers to single out the cerebrum rather than any other viscus as the seat of the

---

* Some of the later phrenologists like Mattieu Williams were of the opinion that "organ" was perhaps an unfortunate term, and that it would have been better to speak of a "centre" in this connection.

personality or the soul being Pythagorus and Plato. Hippocrates had regarded the brain as the "messenger and interpreter of intelligence and
wisdom". Much later the idea gradually grew up that there was some rough
distribution of function within the brain (Erasistratus, Herophilus), and
also of some relationship between the dimensions of the head and the
intellect (Averrhoes, Rhazes, Avicenna, Thomas Aquinas). More specifically, Albertus Magnus divided the brain from before backwards into
three regions, subserving judgement, imagination, and memory respectively;
or, to use the terminology of Bernard Gordon in 1296, commonsense,
phantasie, and memory. Indeed, pre-phrenological cranial models had been
designed by the Bishop of Ratisbon (Albertus Magnus) in the 13th century; by Petrus Montagnana in 1491; and by Lodovico Dolce in 1562. Most
mediaeval anatomists, however, played down the role of the cortex and
localised vital functions of the soul within such unlikely parts of the
nervous system as the meninges (Schabtai-Donolo), pons (Lotze), ventricles (Gordon), nerve-roots (Meyer), corpus callosum (Lancisi), cerebellum (Dorincourt), or the pineal (Descartes). Though Thomas Willis
was inclined to upgrade the importance of the corpus striatum, he also
submitted that sensory impressions might be stored in the brain "as in
little boxes or jars, cells or repositories". These then were the remote ancestors of phrenology. Of more immediate significance was Lavater. His
system of physiognomy claimed to divine character and temperament
("inner power") by a shrewd appraisal of physical characteristics including stature, stance, attitude, and facial delineaments.

Another immediate antecedant of Gall was Prochaska. Thus in his 1784
Dissertation on the Functions of the Nervous System he wrote . . . "it
is . . . by no means improbable that each division of the intellect has
its allotted organ in the brain, so that there is one for the perceptions, another for the understanding, probably others also for the will and imagination, and memory. . . ." And according to Professor Gordon, the Edinburgh anatomist, Gall owed much to Reil. These were important works of
anticipation because the climate of opinion at the end of the 18th century
was more inclined to a holistic view of brain-function. Thus we find Cullen
in his *Practice of Physic* (1776–1784) asserting "nor have we been able to
perceive that any particular part of the brain has more concern in the operations of our intellect than any other. Nor have we attained any knowledge of what share the several parts of the brain have in that operation."

Gall, however, would never acknowledge these influences. It was always
claimed that his system was born out of original inspiration nurtured by
way of observation, experience, and induction. In more modest vein Gall
wrote in 1796 ". . . they call me craniologist, and the science which I
have discovered, craniology. I rather think that the wise men have baptized
the child before it was born. The object of my researches is the brain. . . ."

"Phrenology," be it noted, was not an expression used by Gall, who al-

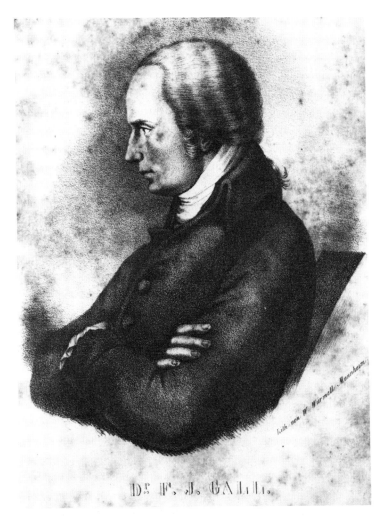

FIG. 1. Dr. Franz Josef Gall, b. 1757. A lithographic print by W. Würmell.

ways spoke merely of the "functions of the brain." In the earliest literature we meet with terms such as zoonomy, cranioscopy, organology, and craniology. Professor Hufeland reported in 1828 that the Germans commonly spoke of the "skull-doctrine." The term phrenology was first employed by Forster, and thereafter adopted.

The Origins and Nature of Phrenology

Whoever the antecedants, it cannot be denied that the all-important empiricist in this field was Franz Josef Gall. Born in the South German town of Tiefenbronn in 1757 (Fig. 1), he had been intrigued as a boy by the differing talents and traits of his fellow scholars and by their facial and cranial peculiarities. The large, prominent cow-like eyes of two youngsters who shon by reason of their ability to commit to memory long texts constituted the first clue to this correlation. Later he extended his observations more widely. The game became an obsession which he endeavoured to control within scientific channels. He studied medicine in Strasbourg and Vienna, and afterwards he took employment in an Austrian asylum at Baden. His researches now became two-fold in their scope. He went to great lengths to scrutinise the cranio-facial morphology of persons

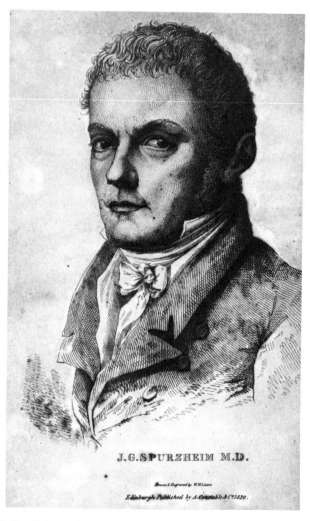

J.G.SPURZHEIM M.D.

FIG. 2. Dr. Johann Gaspar Spurzheim, from an engraving dated 1830.

belonging to every possible class and character—idiots, insane, criminals, peasants, intellectuals, and artists. In addition he scrupulously dissected brains with a method which was all his own. Unlike traditional brain-anatomists, who applied the techniques of a grocer slicing ham, Gall teased out the medullated fibre-tracts and traced their course by means of blunt dissection. Thus he followed the visual fibres back beyond the thalamus to the quadrigeminal body. He made every endeavour to study at autopsy the heads of individuals whose characters and habits he had previously documented. Indeed a visitor to his laboratory has left on record the note "I found people when dying were afraid lest Gall should obtain their skulls, and some left orders in their wills that means should be taken to prevent him."

Gall's doctrine, with its four cardinal tenets, gradually took shape in his mind. His methods of investigation now settled down to a three-fold scheme, whereby he compared extraordinary talent and cranial configuration; unusual localised cranial development with mental characteristics; and deficiencies in development and abnormal mental manifestation.

At first Gall wrote little, but taught by way of lectures. These attracted the interest of a student from Treves, Johann Gaspar Spurzheim, who succeeded Nichlas as his fervent disciple, to become his collaborator and later his evangelist (Fig. 2). But Gall's expositions eventually earned the disapproval of the Church and the interdiction of the Emperor Francis I. In disgust Gall left Vienna, travelled for some years through Europe, and finally settled in Paris residing in the rue Mossilion. His teaching continued at such places as the Athenée Royale, the Hospice de Perfectionnement, and later at the Institution des Jeunes Aveugles. At the same time he acquired a lucrative and fashionable medical practice. It is said that years later the Emperor Francis sought him out in Paris and requested him to return to Austria, but in vain. Between 1810 and 1819 he issued his monograph *Anatomie et Physiologie du Système nerveux en général, et du Cerveau en particulier*, together with an Atlas. Spurzheim collaborated in the first two volumes. The third, which Gall wrote independently, was dedicated to the Prince Clement-Wenceslas-Lothaise de Metternich-Winnebourg-Ochsenhausen, while the last volume was written in honour of Comte Elia Décazes.

Gall by now had isolated 26 organs which purported to correspond with a like number of mental attributes, or "group factors" as we would now say (Fig. 3). These he divided into propensities, sentiments, and intellectual faculties (see Table 1). Note that the faculties have a curious connotation, out of tune with modern thinking. Indeed, according to the phrenological creed, consciousness, will, perception, cognition, memory, abstraction, imagination, and reason were expressly excluded, and intellect was not regarded as a special entity at all. These organs were localised within certain regions of the brain which were demarcated upon the skull

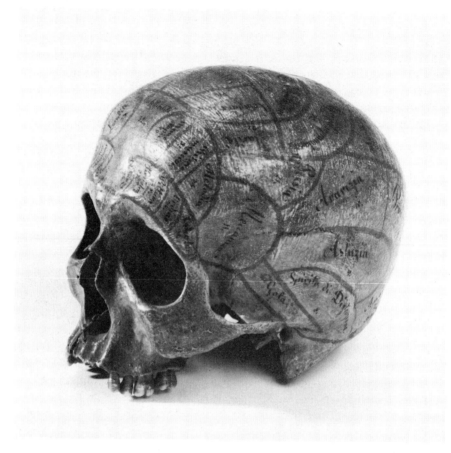

FIG. 3. An actual skull demarcated by Gall himself into 26 organs.

rather than the cortex. It is necessary to add that when speaking of an
underlying "organ", Gall referred to a nervous apparatus or cerebral
region made up both of pulpy and fibrous material, that is, both gray and
white matter. No recognisable macroscopic features demarcated them. The
first to be isolated was the organ of language. As he put it, the manifestation of verbal language depends on a cerebral organ lying on the posterior
part of the superior orbital plate. When hypertrophic, the eye-balls are
rendered prominent and the lower lids baggy. The various cranial areas,
as first identified by Gall, were not necessarily contiguous. Here and there
were gaps, and indeed only about two-thirds of the cerebrum was accounted
for in this manner. Later phrenologists described and located other faculties, e.g., bibativeness, conjugality, vitativeness, sublimity, concentrative-
ness, suavitiveness, and human nature. Spurzheim thus increased Gall's

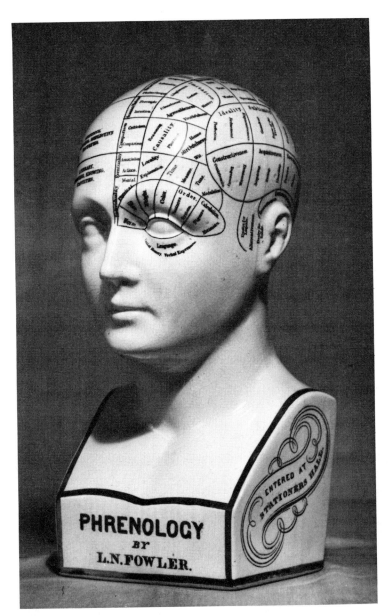

FIG. 4. A porcelain bust 11 inches in height, designed by L. N. Fowler, 337 Strand, London. At the rear of the base is the following inscription: "For thirty years I have studied Crania and living heads from all parts of the world, and have found in every instance that there is a perfect correspondence between the conformation of the healthy skull of an individual and his known characteristics. To make my observations available I have prepared a Bust of superior form and marked the divisions of the Organs in accordance with my researches and varied experience."

TABLE 1. *List of the propensities according to Gall.*
Genus 1.—PROPENSITIES.

1. Amativeness.	6. Destructiveness.
2. Philoprogenitiveness.	7. Secretiveness.
3. Inhabitiveness.	8. Acquisitiveness.
4. Adhesiveness.	9. Constructiveness.
5. Combativeness.	

Genus 2.—SENTIMENTS.

I. *Sentiments common to Man and Animals.*

10. Self-Esteem.	12. Cautiousness.
11. Love of Approbation.	

II. *Sentiments proper to Man.*

13. Benevolence.	18. Marvellousness.
14. Veneration.	19. Ideality.
15. Firmness.	20. Mirthfulness or Gayness.
16. Conscientiousness.	21. Imitation.
17. Hope.	

ORDER II.—INTELLECTUAL FACULTIES.

Genus 1.—PERCEPTIVE.

22. Individuality.	28. Calculation.
23. Configuration.	29. Order.
24. Size.	30. Eventuality.
25. Weight and Resistance.	31. Tune.
26. Coloring.	32. Melody.
27. Locality.	33. Language.

Genus 2.—REFLECTIVE.

34. Comparison.	35. Causality.

original 26 organs to 35, while the Fowler brothers in the States delineated as many as 43 (Fig. 4). It was always admitted that the catalogue of faculties and organs was probably incomplete. Gall realised that the development of basal portions of the brain could not be determined from cranial inspection and he suspected that the organs of hunger, thirst, heat, and cold were probably represented here. Forty years later the Fowlers were discussing the problem of "unascertained organs" and they agreed that certain regions of the brain still constituted a *terra incognita.*

Phrenologists were soon forced to defend their belief that bone-structure correlates with underlying cerebral centres. It was pointed out, for instance, that the cranium might actually conceal hollow structures of great diversity in size and shape, namely the frontal sinus. This structure, which has been dubbed the *opprobrium phrenologicum,* may as a matter of fact overlie no fewer than five of Gall's organs. Phrenologists met this challenge at some length, and insisted that they could ascertain the relative development of all the other organs despite the obstacle of the frontal sinuses. As Combe wrote, "It would be quite as logical to speak of a snow-storm in Norway obstructing the highway from Edinburgh to London, as of a small sinus at the top of the nose concealing the development of Benevolence, Firmness, or Veneration, on the crown of the head."

Although phrenological writings occasionally alluded to the problem of cranial deformities, they never really faced the objections put forward by such pathological conditions as acrocephaly, *Turmschädel,* and scapho-cephaly. Nor did they do more than touch upon the question of artificial deformities of the head. The possible mental repercussions of the flattened crania of the Ashanti and the *déformation couchée* of the peasants in the North of France, were merely glossed over.

To support the contention that the mind was truly made up of a number of discrete mental faculties, phrenologists relied upon a series of arguments. Genius is usually partial; idiocy, too, is incomplete; the various faculties develop and disappear at differing rates; while mental alienation is rarely global in character. To such pieces of evidence the phenomenon of mental dissociation in dreams was quoted.

Another argument which phrenology had to counter at an early date was the objection that mere size of cerebral development did not necessarily indicate functional superiority. The evidence of physiognomy could not be gainsaid, namely that the differing temperaments—sanguine, nervous, bilious, lymphatic—must surely play an important role. This was conceded, and phrenologists inserted a *ceteris paribus* clause into the third article of their dogma, to the effect that "other circumstances besides magnitude being equal, size and vigour of function are in direct correspondence." In discussing the competency of an organ, they drew a subtle distinction between its power, its activity, and its action, the two last properties apparently being expressions of the temperaments.

In retrospect we may consider it odd that Gall, like all his contemporaries of course, had absolutely no conception of asymmetrical brain function. The idea of cerebral dominance did not arise until later, and subsequent phrenologists neglected to incorporate this viewpoint into their own doctrines. To them the cerebral organs were double, being situated in corresponding areas in the two hemispheres. Destruction of an organ on one side would not ablate function provided the opposite organ was preserved. This question was explicitly discussed by Hewett Watson in the ninth volume of the *Phrenological Journal,* in a paper entitled "What is the use of the double brain?" He asserted that perception constituted the active state of either hemisphere, but that the combined activity of the two halves resulted in attention. As he put it "we *see* with either eye but we *look* with both".

The Rise and Fall of Phrenology

The importance of the contributions to anatomy, together with the exciting promise of the philosophical ideas, led to a boom in phrenological doctrines. Perhaps, too, the personality of the protagonists played a part. Gall attracted an enormous clientèle for he was a superb anatomist and demonstrator, intensely devoted to research, dedicated to a search for Truth. Spurzheim, quite a different person, carried the banner abroad and achieved a considerable following in Scotland. At Abernethy's invitation he even lectured to the students at St. Bartholomew's Hospital. He visited Harvard, but died two months after reaching America. Many brain-anatomists, neurophysiologists, and physicians were at first attracted to the novel ideas, though later developments, especially in the direction of prognostics, altered the climate of opinion and caused offence.

At its heyday in Great Britain the cult of phrenology was represented by no fewer than 29 societies. The London Phrenological Society was founded in 1825, met in Buckingham Street, off the Strand, and dined at Barry's Hotel in Princes Street. The conversion of two distinguished professional men in Edinburgh, the brothers Combe, proved an important achievement. While the *Transactions of the Edinburgh Phrenological Society* amounted to but a single volume, the *Phrenological Journal and Miscellany* ran uninterruptedly from 1823 to 1847. In Great Britain other influential men, not all of them medically qualified, joined the ranks of avowed phrenologists. There was Dr. Elliotson of St. Thomas's Hospital, Editor of the *Zoist,* who afterwards became discredited because of his manifold unorthodoxies; he was the first President of the London Phrenological Society. Other important adherents included Sir George Mackenzie; Macnish of Glasgow; Archbishop Watley; Wakly, the uncompromising Editor of the *Lancet;* and Dr. Chevenix. Robert Bentley Todd and John Abernethy gave cautious and qualified approval. Herbert Spencer, who had been present as a boy at Spurzheim's lectures, in his early twenties evinced an interest, contributed papers to the *Zoist,* had his own bumps read, and devised a "cephalograph". In Halle, J. C. Reil took up a characteristic middle course.

Gall's supporters in France included Broussais, the founder of physiological medicine; Blainville; Cloquet; Andral; Geoffrey St. Hilaire; Bouillaud, Dean of the Paris Faculty of Medicine; and the enthusiastic Dr. Vimont of Caen. A local Phrenological Society was formed which included most of the great names in Parisian medicine, and met at the house of the lawyer Appert on the Quai d'Orsay.

Gradually the art of divining character and aptitude came to the fore, and George Combe was summoned to Windsor in 1846 to advise on the educational retardation of the Prince of Wales, and incidentally to examine the heads of his sister and brother, Alice and Alfred. Extravagant appraisals were made. Phrenology was seriously advocated as a system for the proper segregation of convicts, and also as a rational method for the better selection of members of Parliament. Combe proclaimed that Gall's discoveries, if confirmed, would surpass in substantial importance to mankind, those of Harvey, Newton, and Galileo, and that his age would be rendered more illustrious thereby than from the victories of Bonaparte and of Wellington.

But phrenology also excited criticism most acrimonious in character. Among the sterner opponents were Professor Gordon, Lord Jefferey, Lord Brougham, Sir William Hamilton, Professor Ecker, Sir Charles Bell, Sir Benjamin Brodie, Bastian, Barclay, and Roget. More temperate were the strictures of Professor Laycock, teacher of both Hughlings Jackson and of Ferrier. Attacks did not for a moment go unanswered and the controversy was kept up with bitterness. Nor did the popular press remain aloof, and phrenology became the topic or target of very many ballads, broadsides, cartoons, and farces.

Gradually, however, phrenology found its own level in the scheme of things, less as the result of frontal assault than from the steady alteration in physiological thinking. Much of Gall's philosophy ceased to shock, for it was no longer at serious variance with current opinion. As G. H. Lewes put it—"instead of surviving opposition, phrenology has decayed with the declining opposition. It has ceased to be ridiculed, and it has ceased to be declaimed against as immoral and it has ceased to occupy attention." But the activities of some of the peripatetic practitioners and delineators could not be overlooked. Like so many other eccentric cults it lingered on in America long after it had ceased in the United Kingdom to be much more than a vaudeville or seaside memory. But in passing judgement we must make a clear distinction between the attainments of Gall, and the record of phrenology. Even such an avowed disciple as Elliotson long ago made this contrast. The works of Gall were, he said, clear, flowing, full, rigidly philosophical, rich with profound thoughts and glowing illustrations. They spoke for themselves and differed entirely from the writings of Spurzheim which were far better known. But it was Gall's findings that made Spurzheim a phrenologist. Combe and the Edinburgh clique were followers of Spurzheim rather than of Gall.

The Enduring Contributions of Phrenology

We now approach the essential topic of our address. Let us admit at once that the phrenological interlude in the history of science was far from being a sterile one. For many reasons the work of Gall, when stripped of its excrescences, constituted an important landmark in the history of neurology.

Let us, to begin with, recall Gall's immediate neuro-anatomical contributions which have been insensibly absorbed into the corpus of our knowledge. He was one of the first to show that the development of the nervous system was uneven. The cervical and lumbar enlargements of the spinal cord were his discovery. Gall called attention to the essential differences between the gray and the white matter of the nervous system, in structure and in function. Gall was the first to describe the origins of the 2nd, 3rd, 5th, and 6th cranial nerves. He was also the pioneer demonstrator of converging and diverging fibres in the white matter, and he furthermore drew attention to the corpus callosum and to that region which we now speak of as the island of Reil. Such a record of achievement is impressive indeed.

As the result of his researches, no longer could it be maintained that the brain functioned as a whole, like the liver or spleen. The doctrine of holism became seriously disturbed for the first time by Gall's teachings, which led on naturally to the more precise methods of determining local function promulgated by Munk, Hitzig, Fritsch, and Ferrier. That these later studies gave birth to what might be dubbed a "new phrenology" cannot be denied, and some of their more extravagant claims still survive. But already we can see today, in rebuttal as it were, a swing back to a modified holism, of a thoughtful and scientific sort, attuned to modern ideas of brain-function. To say this does not of course deny some measure of cerebral localisation.

When experimental neurophysiologists in the mid 19th century became active, contemporary phrenologists reacted in a highly critical manner. They tilted at "systems based on . . . muscular convulsions of galvanised monkeys" and in an anticipatory vein spoke of "the inability of modern mechanical mutilators and galvanisers to distinguish between the actual motor centres and the mental organs that make use of these centres". Gall had always held in contempt the role of experiment, for he preferred to rely upon observation alone. He had already written an intriguing chapter upon "la Mimique ou la Pantomime" and his disciples drew striking parallels between individual expressive gestures, the specific faculty and its organ, and the effects of electrical stimulation of that self-same cortical area as described by Ferrier and others (Table 2).

Another major contribution of Gall lies in the direction of the more precise anatomy of the brain. Even the highly critical Reil confessed that he had seen in Gall's anatomical demonstrations of the brain more than

TABLE 2. *Correlation of Gall's hypotheses with Ferrier's findings on electrical stimulation of the cortex*

Ferrier		Gall
Electrical stimulation of area	Effects	Corresponding phrenological organ
1	Opposite hind leg advanced, as in walking, thigh being flexed on the pelvis; leg extended; dorsal flexion of foot with spreading or extension of toes.	Love of approbation
2	Flexion, with outward rotation of the thigh; rotation inwards of the thigh, with flexion of the toes.	Pride
2 (dog)	Lateral, or wagging movements of the tail.	Hope
5	Forward extension of the arm and hand, as if to touch something in front.	Benevolence
6 & 7	Clenching of the fist.	Acquisitiveness
9 & 10	Opening of mouth, and retraction of tongue.	Gustativeness
12 (monkeys)	Eyes opened widely; pupils dilated; head and eyes deviated to the opposite side.	Wonder
13	Eyes turn to opposite side; eyelids tend to narrow.	Secretiveness

he had thought that a man could ever discover in his whole life. Flourens too, who was one of Gall's greatest antagonists, was impelled to speak of him as "the profound observer whose genius has opened for us the study of the anatomy and physiology of the brain. I shall never forget the impression I received the first time I saw Gall dissect a brain. It seemed to me as if I had never seen this organ before." His demonstration of the course of the projectional and associational fibres has already been mentioned, and his work led directly on to the techniques of micro-dissection at the hands of Weigert and Marchi. Though Gall, like his contemporaries and those before him, was unaware that the convolutions of the brain possessed not only meaning but also morphological precision, the situation soon began to change. Hitherto the gyri had been regarded as haphazard in their lay-out, rather like the serpentine and random patterns of a dish of spaghetti. A more common analogy was that of coils of intestine as shown by the term "enteroid processes" which Willis had applied to the cortex. Early in the 19th century anatomists were speaking of the gray and white matter of the brain as "cineritious and medullary neurine" and the fissures were termed "anfractuosities". George Combe in 1836 was still describing the appearance of the brain as a mass of "curiously convoluted" matter. Ecker was probably the first adequately to survey and map out the convolutional pattern, facilitated by the earlier observations of Huschke and Gratiolet and Rolando. But the seeds of research had been sown by Gall. Subsequent phrenologists advanced his primary studies by attaching the organ-numerals to various areas of the cortex, rather than the cranium. But the early illustrations still display an arrangement of gyri which is out of harmony with modern views.

Another logical outcome of these doctrines has been the modern science of craniometry. Physical anthropology has gained a good deal from the researches of Gall and his followers. One of the pioneers in this field was Straton who in his *Contributions to the Mathematics of Phrenology* drew attention to certain cranial markers which became known as *Straton's points.* Arising therefrom, N. Morgan in 1871 utilised his *phrenometrical angle* which afforded a ready index of the degree of intellectual development in a particular skull. A wide phrenometrical angle was found in murderers and persons who had committed violent assaults, being much narrower in those of the highest moral type. About the same time came Dr. Cox's measurements based upon the backward projection of the lateral convolutions beyond a plane passing through the organ of causality. F. Bridges invented, and Morgan modified, an instrument for measuring the head in profile which was called the *Phreno-Physiometric Calliper.* This instrument foreshadows many of the devices in later employment, including even the Horsley-Clarke instrument. Such anthropometric constants as the cephalic index, the "German horizontal", Reid's base-line, the linear index, and the facial angle came later. Thus phrenology may be looked upon as an important anticipation of our current use of stereotaxy in neurosurgery.

Nor is it a far cry from Gall's original interest in cranial volume, to the recent precise estimation of the relative figures for brain-volume and extracerebral space, devised by Reichart of Würzburg.

Perhaps, however, the most obvious accomplishment of phrenology has been in the domain of neurological practice. It afforded an important stimulus to the intimate recording and correlation of anatomo-clinical data. The pages of the *Phrenological Journal* contain numerous case-reports where a careful study of signs and symptoms is aligned with a precise description of the nature and extent of the cerebral lesion, in a manner which was quite unusual for the time, and which foreshadowed present-day practice.

Here we may trace the beginnings of our views on cerebral localisation. That our opinions have since then expanded and then later retracted somewhat does not matter. These were necessary stages in knowledge, and we owe much to Gall in setting us off on this adventure.

In this context the subject of aphasia stands in the forefront. Without doubt it was Gall who first focussed attention upon the correlation between the prefrontal lobes and language, as well as between loss of speech and disease of the foremost regions of the brain. Broca has been given too much credit for determining the morbid anatomy of speech-loss, and we are apt to forget the rôle played by Gall and his followers in the first 60 years of the 19th century. The steady stream of Scottish case-reports in the *Phrenological Journal;* the fervent championship by Dean Bouillaud of Gall and his ideas about language; the masterly contribution of his son-in-law Auburtin; all these led up to Broca's shrewd utilisation of a lucky and topical accident of surgical practice. Bouillaud was none too impressed by Broca's good fortune as shown by his description of him as the St. Paul of the new doctrine, and "one of the organisers, subinventors, augmenters, revisers and correctors" of Gall's pioneer and magnificent discoveries.

Later phrenologists were jealous of the credit which had accrued to Broca and to his area which they believed had been discovered and demonstrated 60 years beforehand by Gall. This is perhaps going too far. Gall's organ of language was located more rostrally than the foot of F.3, and moreover it was bilaterally represented. For that matter so was Broca's area to begin with, for he did not realise the greater importance of the left hemisphere until four years later. But nowadays much of this is *vieux jeu,* for a modern aphasiologist cares but little for either Broca's area or that of Gall, and overprecise attempts to localise language are deemed by most of us a rather vain pursuit.

Although the organ of language was the first one to be identified by Gall, and was the initial step leading to the doctrine of phrenology, he was never completely satisfied with it. As he wrote "it will, no doubt, be thought singular that it is precisely on the subject of this faculty and its organ that my works are least complete". His followers did not disagree, and Morgan pointed out the inherent complexity of this faculty of language, embracing so many different talents within the realm of speech. We too may think it odd that Gall should have relegated the accomplishments of reading and writing to the nominative arts, located well away from the organ of language.

If phrenologists were near the target in cases of aphasia, they were sadly astray when it came to the cerebellum. Impressed by the shape of the head of a nymphomaniacal widow of his acquaintance, Gall designated the cerebellum as the seat of the generative instinct, later renamed the organ of amativeness. In this he was not original, for the idea had been put forward a few years previously by Swedenborg. Clinical cases were found which seemed to bear out such a relationship, and a monograph on this subject was published by Gall in collaboration with Vimont and Broussais.

Let us examine the data a little more closely. Gall and his followers believed that disease of this region would bring about an unbridled eroticism, or, less often, an opposite state of sexual apathy and impotency. Furthermore chronic lust could be linked with cerebellar dysfunction, and be witnessed either by an over-development of what we would now call the posterior fossa, or by an objective feeling of heat over the nape of the neck and the occiput.

Some of their case-reports may be quoted:

A woman of ardent temperament, with imperious sexual desires, had often supported, not to say provoked, the embraces of 10, 12, or 15 men in one day. During her stay in the Salpêtrière she frequently experienced *severe pain in the neck,* being then seized by violent sexual desires which she satisfied by masturbating 10 or 12 times a day.

A mulatto boy less than 3 years of age, assaulted little girls and women, attacking them with audacity and determination in order to satisfy his desires. Complaisant young females were always in the offing. Dying from consumption he showed, at autopsy, an extraordinary hypertrophy of the cerebellum.

A man of 32 was taken in coma to the Hotel Dieu having been found on the quayside in the company of prostitutes. During the act of coition with one of them, he had collapsed. At post-mortem a haemorrhagic cavity was found in one of the cerebellar hemispheres.

A robust man of 42, greatly addicted to eating, drinking, and womanising, lost consciousness during a fit of rage when upbraided for passing the night in a house of ill-fame. While still in coma he showed a continual chordee. Autopsy revealed an intracerebellar haemorrhage.

A sempstress of 33 had been very early addicted to venery. In a brothel she had given herself up to every excess of debauchery. Up to the age of 30 she had been fatigued with sexual pleasure, but never satisfied. Finding cohabitation with men failing to assuage her desires, she gave herself passionately to the transports of self-abuse. She sought treatment by cauterisation of the clitoris, and later died of phthisis. Examination showed a tuberculous meningitis in the posterior fossa with cerebellar softenings.

In the collection of the Phrenological Society were a number of casts of skulls some of them with inordinate development of the organ of amativeness. One of them belonged to a man, who at the time of death had been living with his fifth wife. The intervals between the death of a wife and his re-marriage had been less than six weeks in two cases, and in no instance was it more than four months. It is not surprising that in this particular cranial cast the organ of cautiousness was said to have been unduly small. We are told nothing about the organ of hope, nor about that of love of change which ought surely to have been at least as large as that of amativeness. In the monograph on the cerebellum by Gall, Vimont and Broussais we are also informed that the cast of the head of Dr. Gall himself presented a large development of the cerebellum, and that he too was considerably addicted to the indulgence of this propensity.

The notorious crowbar case had come along in 1848 to indicate that extensive destruction of the brain could occur without any obvious loss of mental capacity. But phrenologists hastened to point out the profound change in personality which the victim had undergone, an alteration which accorded well with the doctrines of Gall. Orthodox medicine still nursed the idea that great expanses of the brain were silent areas. Phrenologists would never agree for a moment and rightly asserted that proper testing and enquiry would always uncover considerable modifications in character and comportment. Herein we can trace the beginnings of our current notions of organic brain-change, of highest nervous activity, and of what the Russians term "traumatic nervous debility". Today we neurologists know all too well that appropriate or extended test-procedures at the hands of an expert will bring to light convincing evidence of altered function. Nowadays the so-called silent areas of the brain are eloquent to those who know how to listen. Let us not forget that such doctrines were actually stated first by phrenologists.

Another anticipation of cerebral pathology, and one of the most startling ones, can also be laid to the credit of phrenology. As long ago as 1810 Gall asserted that it was quite possible to determine the sex of any given cerebrum even without inspecting the overlying cranium. Such a claim has been beyond the competency of every orthodox morphologist until the very recent nucleo-cytological researches. I cannot trace however whether this *experimentum crucis,* mooted 150 years ago, was ever specifically substantiated.

The doctrine that the growth and conformation of the brain determines the size and shape of the encompassing cranial box became accepted in the course of time as orthodox teaching. Moreover the belief grew that individual convolutional patterns could be determined by studying the ridges upon the inner table of the skull and this became employed as an index of the morphology of prehistoric cerebra. Perhaps one should add that within the last two decades a contrary wave of scepticism has arisen.

Professor Ackerknecht has proclaimed it a riddle why posterity has not displayed the same indulgence towards Gall that it has shown with regard to the errors and eccentricities of Boerhaave, Haller, Laennec, and Bichat. Doubtless it is because these others never aspired to a scientific philosophy and never became willy-nilly the founders of a cult. Perhaps it was because his anatomical discoveries and his ideas of brain function were keys which unlocked treasuries of vast endeavour that Gall's anatomy still stands secure, even though his physiology is discredited, when not forgotten.

Finally we might refer to Gall as the exponent of a school of philosophy, one which stimulated Spencer and which anticipated the Positivism of August Comte. At first Gall's teachings proved shocking, and were deemed materialistic and opposed to the current romantic *Naturphilosophie,* a type of metaphysics which Gall regarded as speculative. He can, moreover, be numbered among the earliest of scientific criminologists. To him the offender was a medical problem, a victim of his innate disposition. Gall furthermore was a forerunner of the evolutionary philosophy of mid-Victorian biology. He taught that the differences between the brains of animals and man were questions merely of degree. He was a pioneer of comparative anatomy and pointed out the preponderant role of the anterior lobes of the brain, the upper portions being peculiar to man, while the lower parts were but feebly represented in the animal brain. Within these critical regions were represented those noble faculties peculiar to the human species.

Gall's philosophy was materialistic but humane. Being based upon the inherent inequality of man, it was sometimes rated as excessively materialistic. Though in tune with the emancipation of the lower orders, with freethought and the education of the masses, it was nonetheless out of harmony with what we today would call democracy. As he himself wrote . . . "The study of the physiology of the brain shows us the limits and the extent of the moral and intellectual domain of man. It shows us an immense disproportion between the mediocre faculties and the eminent faculties, and it leads us to the conclusion that wherever regulations, decisions and laws are the work of the majority of votes, mediocrity triumphs over genius." As he also asserted . . . "the great majority is formed everywhere by mediocre men who by themselves invent nothing and create nothing."

Summary

The science, art, or philosophy of phrenology started its existence from observation and induction. It is a philosophy founded upon the conception of the inequality of man, promulgated however by pioneers who were endowed with an exalted humanitarian outlook quite foreign to their time.

Enthusiastically acclaimed and also bitterly attacked, it flourished for some decades and then gradually lost ground, so that nowadays it is little more than an interesting memory.

Its ugly side as a system of character-delineation did harm to its prestige. This was scarcely the fault of Gall. Its debasement has been largely responsible for the fact that his very real contributions to medicine have been overlooked.

Even in modern times there have appeared from time to time signs of what we may term a still newer phrenology. Throughout the centuries, brain-maps and blue-prints have exercised a curious fascination. From time to time they gate-crash into our text-books of physiology and of information theory. But most thinking neurologists look askance at all cerebral diagram-makers and cartographers, whether they tell of cortical architectonics, motor homunculi, suppressor bands. or linguistic schemata. Mindful of the fate of phrenology modern neuroscience has but little respect for cerebral mosaics.

How then should we judge Gall today, after we have divorced the accomplishments of the man from the record of his phrenological votaries? Gall represents a "great though misguided and perhaps even slightly ridiculous figure in the rise of a progressive science". This, according to Temkin, was the verdict of the historians of philosophy, Littré and Lewes. Perhaps they were a little too hard. To contemporary neurologists, Gall was a great man.

May I, in conclusion, quote that inspiring anatomist, the mentor of so many of us older medical scientists? "The time has come," he wrote, "for a juster appreciation of the important part played by Gall, and a more adequate recognition of his achievements than has been made in the past. If he was responsible for certain speculations, which in the hands of irresponsible followers have been used for meretricious purposes, it must not be forgotten that Gall's work brought to an end a barren system of philosophy which seriously impeded progress. His contributions to the anatomy of the central nervous system are of far-reaching importance, and to the physiology of the brain and to psychological theory he gave a new orientation and a new inspiration." These were the words of Elliot Grafton Smith, with which you and I might perhaps agree.

Based upon Critchley, M. (1965) : *British Medical Journal*. Vol. 2.

Harveian Oration: "The Divine Banquet of the Brain"

This is the 258th occasion on which Fellows of the College have met in amity to commemorate our generous and perspicacious patron William Harvey "whose sharpenesse of wit and brightnesse of mind, as a light darting from Heaven, has illuminated the whole learned world" to quote my predecessor Dr. Samuel Garth. The circumstance is paramount: the fortuitous choice of spokesman is of minor import, even though it be the supreme dignity which is within the bestowal of our College. One cannot dissemble one's humble gratification for this signal honour, although the task of the Orator grows weightier from year to year. Osler indeed referred to the tribulations of the recipient of the Harveian Oration when it happened to fall to one who, like himself and myself, had lived the life of the arena: in such circumstances one's best efforts bear the stamp of the student rather than the scholar. The political innuendoes in the first of these Orations in 1665 led to the rule that future Orators should submit their manuscript to the President and Censors at least one month beforehand. In imposing this added burden, the College might have been shrewd, but somewhere along the centuries this ordinance became overlooked.

Standing in this new and resplendent auditorium I invite my colleagues to picture the manner in which 350 years ago Harvey, then 37 years of age, ushered in his Lumleian Lecture, being the fourth to hold that distinction. The dates were April 15, 16, and 17, the emplacement being the Great Parlour of the Physitians Colledge overlooking the garden abutting on the city wall. This second dwelling place of ours has never been well documented. Situated at the end of Amen Corner next to the Stationers' Hall it was leased from the Dean and Chapter of St. Paul's in 1614; confiscated in 1649 by the Commonwealth; purchased for £267.10 by Hamey who was ejected by the Churchmen some years later; and it finally perished in the Great Fire just 300 years ago on the night of September the fourth.

Obscurity surrounds much of the Lumleian occasion. We can but surmise who were in attendance. Presumably the reigning President, Henry Atkins, was there—who had been the 22nd and was now the 25th to hold this exalted rank. No doubt the four Censors were present—John Argent, Richard Palmer, Mathew Gwinne, and Theodore Goulston. As to the others there is no record. Surely some of Harvey's colleagues from Padua put in a loyal appearance—Winston, Craige, Fortescue, Willoughby, Darey, Mounsell, Fox, and Lister. No doubt there were also such staunch Fellows and Members as Mayerne, Meverell, Moundeford, Paddy, Reid, Fludd, and perhaps the two Hameys, and almost certainly an innominate contingent of barber surgeons, including Fenton, Mapes, and Kingeman who were colleagues from St. Bartholomew's. We can visualise the lecturer from Aubrey's vivid portrayal ". . . not tall, but of the lowest stature, round faced, olivaster like wainscott in complexion, little eie, round, very black as a Raven. . . ." The notes upon which Harvey's lectures were based were purchased from Sir Hans Sloane in 1754; lost; and then chanced upon in 1876; and published ten years later by the College at the instigation of Sieveking. Recently they have been re-edited with devoted scholarship by Dr. Grace Whitteridge. We are not sure whether Harvey discoursed in Latin or English; he probably resorted to both, even though Aubrey was critical of his Latinity, and the proportion of the vernacular may well have depended upon how many surgeons were present.

To conform to the ordinances of the Lumleian Lectures, Harvey's statements had to be brief and plain, yet nothing visible was to pass unmentioned. On April 15th, Harvey outlined his curriculum to serve in their three courses according to the hour glass. "First, the lower belly, nasty, yet recompensed by admirable variety. Second, the parlour (or thorax), and third, the divine banquet of the brayne."

This engaging phrase is our present concern. Contemporary ideas about the structure and functions of that organ are matters which we do not commonly associate with Harvey. Where, in his philosophy, stood nervous activity, and which side did he favour in the protracted wavering and wrangling as to the relative importance of the heart or the brain in regard to intellectual faculties and emotions? Little more than a stone's throw from Harvey's residence near St. Martin's Church was Puddle Dock, the dwelling-place of William Shakespeare. Though without evidence, we can scarcely doubt that they were acquainted. Twenty-one years earlier the poet had crystallised this very dilemma in his couplet "Tell me where is fancy bred; or in the heart, or in the head?"

Let us today consider first of all Harvey's acquaintance with the morphology of the brain, and then his views as to its functions.

Despite his creative thinking, Harvey was in many matters a traditionalist and a conformist, but little in sympathy with *avant-garde* neoteric philosophers whom he dismissed as "shitt-breeches". When not brooding upon the mysteries of the circulating blood-stream he may well have been content to follow the popular line in philosophy. In the 17th century, medical communication was not easy. Not every anatomical treatise printed before 1616 was necessarily available to Harvey, and we can only hazard a guess as to those upon which he depended. The principal monograph was the *Theatrum Anatomicum* published 11 years earlier by Caspar Bauhin. Harvey must also have relied upon the writings of Fabricius; of Fallopius; of Realdus Columbo; and therefore—more distantly—upon Vesalius, whose *De Fabrica* had appeared in 1542. Most of these anatomists had either studied at Padua or taught there, and must have moulded the ideas of the young Harvey. Nor can we omit the more remote influence of such associates of Vesalius as Guenther, Dryender, Estienne de la Rivière, and Massa.

In 1616 two techniques were in vogue for dissecting the brain: the conventional one employed by Vesalius, Phryesen, Dryender, and Sylvius, whereby the contents of the head were examined from above downwards; and the method of Costanzo Varolio which operated in reverse. Harvey utilised the former. Considerable anatomical detail was familiar to Harvey regarding the coverings of the brain, the ventricles, and many of the smaller basal structures. Odd figures of speech were in common currency, often metaphorically strained, and some of them a trifle robust. Contemporary anatomists referred to the colliculi as testicles and buttocks; the pineal organ was the penis or the pine-cone; close by were the anus and the vulva cerebri. The cerebellum, like a cock's comb, encompassed the vermis, so reminiscent of wood-worms. Nor should we forget the scribe's pen; the drinking cup; and the fisherman's net. In somewhat gentler vein they spoke of the *fleur de lys;* while the septum pellucidum recalled a consecrated wafer.

But in their preoccupation with these minor anatomies, 17th century morphologists had less to say about more important topics such as the distinctions between gray and white substance; the basal ganglia and thalamus; and—in particular—the convolutions. These last-named were dismissed as resembling coils of intestines, or rough sketches of clouds made by incompetent art-students. Vesalius had merely noted that the winding sulci were deeper in man than in animals ". . . that thereby the substance of the brain may be the richer". Willis, like Erasistratus, adopted the analogy of the gut, and spoke of the convolutions of the brain as "enteroid processes". Not until the publication of Gall's *Atlas* in 1810, and the work of Rolando in 1830, Huschke in 1856, Gratiolet in 1856, and particularly Ecker in 1869 was it established that the cerebral convolutions were not haphazard coils, like so much bowel or macaroni, but structures with an established patterning.

Even so fundamental a subject as the decussation of the motor pathways was under dispute. A colleague of Harvey's, Helkiah Crooke, spoke of the notion held by some that the nerves intersected like a Saint Andrew's Crosse ". . . but" said he "the levity of this opinion needeth no confutation". An imagined hegemony of the ventricles over the solid tissues of the brain had long been a veritable dogma. Indeed, since the writings of Herophilus "the butcher", as Tertullian called him, three centuries before Christ, the mediaevalists had regarded the ventricles of the brain as all-important in the processes of thought. There was even a simple cerebro-ventricular localisation of function, the anterior chamber being associated with judgment or commonsense; the middle with cogitation or "phantasie"; and the posterior with memory (Nemesius, Albertus Magnus, Bernard Gordon, Petrus Montagnana, and Lodovico Dolca). Vesalius was perhaps the first to question such views, and was later supported by Caspar Bauhin. Harvey unhesitatingly followed him and irritably rejected the popular belief in the supremacy of the ventricles. Never a very tolerant man, he was out of sympathy with those like Piccolomini who associated the organ of mind with the ventricles and at the same time with certain excretory functions, "and so", he said, "mix up the most divine of faculties with the excrements, and locate the soul in the jakes" (or privy). Half a century later, Malpighi took the argument further ". . . With some religious awe" he wrote ". . . we worshipped its ventricles and the *rete mirabile;* we believed that there were different seats for imagination, memory and other senses. Since eventually, however, the ventricles have been dismissed from this lofty service to become a pair of snuffers, or, so to speak, the sewage drains of excretions, the sinuous white matter of the brain struck our imagination, whose imagined wonderful passages gave fill to our expectations." In cautious vein Malpighi went on: "However I recognise and believe that the structure of the brain is . . . wholly incapable of explaining the phenomena of the senses and of such noble operations."

To discern why the brain became looked upon as the seat of the intellect and of the emotions, we find it necessary to turn back the pages of history some thousand years. So we find the heart emerging first of all as the most important viscus, with the circulating blood and with the liver as alternates.

Among the ancient Egyptians we detect no reference to the head for the heart was deemed to be the all-important centre of spiritual life, of the passions, and of intellectual faculties. The term "ab" signified not only the heart, but also longing, desire, will, wisdom, and courage, while the "hati" or heart-soul referred to the seat of life and every vital function. After death a fantastic ritual occurred whereby the dog-headed Anubis and Horus the hawk-headed carried out a solemn weighing of the heart in the presence of Osiris. In one pan of a huge pair of scales was placed the heart, counterbalanced either by a feather, or by a statuette of Maât, Goddess of truth and justice. Every action of the deceased during life had either augmented or lessened the weight of the heart (the solitary and silent witness throughout this grim ceremony). Thoth, the ibis-headed scribe, was the recorder. If the judgment were favourable, the soul would merge with the divinities throughout eternity; otherwise the crouching Amenait—part lion, part hippopotamus, part crocodile—would pounce and devour the heart of the guilty. Note that in the mythology of the ancient Egyptians, there is no reference to the brain as a medium of thought. Moreover in their medical writings it is with the heart that affective disorders are correlated. "His heart shows weakness. . . . His heart cannot be refreshed by weak remedies" (*Ebers Papyrus*) . . . "His heart is hot, it pulsates . . . . his heart oppressed . . . . he feels his heart" (*Papyrus Berlin*). [The term indicating sorrow (*Zgbgb*) also referred to physical pressure in the region of the heart.] But their later representatives the Copts, and indeed most of the early Christian thinkers, rejected such an eschatology. This pagan notion did not entirely disappear, however, for we find even in the Middle Ages reference to "psychostasis", or the weighing of the soul, so clearly depicted on the 12th century portal of the church of Saint-Trophime, at Arles.

Early Chinese medicine held no place for the brain among the five elements or *Tsangs*, or the six subsidiary organs or *Fus*. The cerebrum encased within the skull was regarded as merely the reservoir of bone-marrow. According to the *Nei Ching* or Canon of Medicine written 2½ millenia B.C. the emotions of anger, happiness, sorrow, and fear were functions of the liver, heart, lung, and kidney respectively. Thought had its seat within the spleen, a viscus possessing a fragrant odour, a sweet taste, and a yellow colour. Never were the cerebral hemispheres the subject of serious comment.

In Hindu mythology a dichotomy existed, with the heart regarded as the essential seat of the soul, consciousness being relegated to the brain. The argument is involved, even fantastic. The *Upanishads* depicted the heart as an inverted lotus with 12 petals, in the centre of which lay the object of meditation, the immortal Personality, and also the domicile of intellect, faith, and truth. But at the moment of death the *Nādīs* of the heart would enter the cranium, the soul being eventually liberated when the summit of the head was pierced. Consciousness was not associated with any physical organ, though it utilised the brain as an instrument. In the work *Serpent Power*, the heart was deemed the abode of the soul, consciousness being disseminated throughout the cerebrospinal system. Six chief centres lay within the spinal cord, each with its particular lotus-flower and its own colour. The heart was symbolised by a 12-petalled lotus red in hue, and meditation upon this region would lead to the lordship of language. Highest and loftiest of all was a luminous thousand-petalled lotus, where supreme beatitude was attained.

Here then we find one of the first indications of a rivalry between the brain and the heart, and the beginnings of the dispute which was to take place during the centuries before Christ, and to some extent throughout the Middle Ages up to the time of William Harvey and even beyond.

Again, in the Semitic-Assyrian civilisation the heart occupied a supreme role though their Babylonian ancestors had for a time paid greater homage to the liver. This latter phase was brief. The heart came to be looked upon as the indispensable organ of bodily life, as well as the centre of all moral, psychological, and inner existence. It did not assume the sole authority over the emotions and sentiments, for the kidneys and liver were still assigned a minor role in the passions. But the heart was suzerain, and in particular it was concerned with intelligence, intuitive thinking, and with calculated thought; it was the podium of memory and attention. To steal one's heart was to practise deceit. We also find in Hebrew texts the earliest references to what we might term the "personality" or "persona" or "ego", which at that time was also localised unequivocally within the heart. The heart becomes the most secret repository of the individual, as well as of conscience, watchful even during sleep. It was also the dwelling-place of the moral or religious life, and the site of fidelity. Note that in the early Semitic philosophy the hemispheres played no role. Indeed there was no exact Hebrew term for the brain, merely a reference to the "marrow of the head".

Among the early beliefs of the Muslims too, the heart was dominant. It was looked upon as the mirror of contemplation, made up of two concentric circles, the outer denoting inspired wisdom, and the inner the witness of unity. The Mohammedan nurtured a spiritual notion of the heart. According to the Qur'an, the heart of the believer is unsheathed like a lighted torch; that of the hypocrite is contorted; while that of the faithless sinner is sleek, insinuating, and devoid of roots.

Disputes arose as soon as the dominion of medical philosophy shifted to Greece. The classical medicine of Hippocrates at Cos was preceded by an interlude in which Cnidus was prominent. Saunders demonstrated clearly that this important inter-regnum was inspired directly by Pharoan medicine. Whatever their theology, the ancient Egyptians were shrewd diagnosticians and therapists, basing their theory of pathology upon putrefaction and the corruptibility of organic matter. This hypothesis was accepted by the men of Cnidus and later became modified by the Hippocratic school in the doctrine of humours. In Cnidan medicine there are few if any references to cerebral or cardiac function, but in classical Greece the situation was quite different. Thus, according to Homer, Sophocles, and Aristophanes, the heart was associated with spiritual life, emotions as well as thought. In this connection the term *phren* was usually employed. Other expressions in common use were *stethos, cardia, hetor* (strictly speaking the lung), *sternon* (or the chest), and *thymos* (which probably related to the air contained within the lung). In metaphorical contexts *thymos* was used in preference to *cardia* and referred to joy, courage, impetuosity, and especially to anger. Somewhat later the Greeks used *nous* and *dianoin* to indicate the seat of intelligence. Philosophers differed in their localisation of the *hegemonikon* or *principatus animi*. Hippocrates, Democrites, and Plato referred this faculty to the brain; Strato to an area between the eyebrows; Erasistratus to the meninges and cerebellum; Horophilus to the ventricles; Parmenides and Epicurus to some region within the thorax; and Empedocles, Diogenes of Babylon, Aristotle, and the School of the Epicurians and Stoics to the heart. Each organ in turn had its heroic age. Some believed that it was not so much the heart, as the blood therein which was all-important. Thus Empedocles localised the *noema* to the pericardial blood, while Philistion narrowed the abode of thought to the left ventricle of the heart.

In most metaphorical contexts *thymos* was preferred to *cardia,* while in the Latin language *cor* survived both in poetic usage and the vernacular. To "recall" was rendered by *recordari,* again implying the location of memory within the heart. Alternative expressions in Latin were *animus* for the emotions and *mens* for the seat of thought, suggesting a certain indecisiveness. Some classical philosophers relegated *animus* to the heart; while others asserted that it dwelt either within the heart or in the brain. Medical thinkers, however, tended to upgrade the heart to a supreme functional role.

This belief in the paramount province of the heart or the blood-stream was shattered by the dogmatic assertion of Alcmaeon, the anatomist of Cretona. He was the first to localise thought-processes to the head, being supported by Aetius, the Byzantine court physician; by Democritus of Thrace; by Hippocrates; by Plato with certain reservations; and by Galen.

The problem once again became complicated, this time by Aristotle, whose doctrines were destined to influence the thinking of many future generations. Aristotle localised within the heart the *sensu commune,* which also comprised memory and imagination. But thought and intelligence (as a rendition of the Greek term *nous*) were not functions of the heart. Indeed they were not localisable at all, being independent of the physical body, and unrelated to any organ.

Thereafter came contention between the schoolmen, with words and figures of speech as weapons. Thus at times the Hebrew words for the heart, *lev* or *levuv,* were translated not as *cardia,* but as *nous,* or *diamoia,* or *psyche.* Semitic references to the heart as signifying intelligence raised peculiar difficulties. Some testaments indeed differed, like the Septuagint and the Vulgate. For example the Hebrew terms *levuv* and *nefish* in the injunction "thou shalt love thy God with all thy *heart,* and with all thy *soul* . . ." were rendered in the Vulgate by *cor* and *anima,* and in the Septuagint by *cardias* and *psyche,* though in a later edition *cardias* became *dianoias.* In the English versions of both the New and Old Testaments, we find over and over again references to the heart in an emotional and also intellectual connotation. The heart is cited as the seat of memory; the source of intellectually directed action; the fount of courage, of envy, and of jealousy. Hardness of the heart denotes incredulity; a double heart means deceit. Differences of opinion, however, may not have been due so much to confusion of thought, as to a question of semantics. It is necessary to enquire how far some of these picturesque phrases employed in the remote past are merely figures of speech. Elaborate metaphor is always a feature of the diction of simple people as well as in the dead languages. Another source of error lies in translation. Even in contemporary experience it is virtually impossible to code and decode information from one linguistic system to another, because of the manifold overtones and associations which become attached to each so-called "full" word. Every message, every word, betrays an "undertext"; that is to say it tells less than it means; while "entropy" or distortion of meaning is almost inevitable.

The early fathers of the Christian Church did not allay the confusion wherein mythophysiology and metaphor had become inextricably entwined. Origen, St. Gregory of Nyssa, and also St. Augustine broke away from precedent, and coming under the influence of neo-Platonic philosophers, more and more used "heart" to indicate intellectual processes. Later came a schism between the Eastern and Western Christian Churches. The former adhered to the rigid letter of the Hebrew scriptures and correlated the heart with intelligence, while the latter associated it with the affective life of man.

In the Roman church the heart gradually became imbued with increasing significance. Based upon the 13th century teachings of St. Bernard and St. Bonaventure, there grew up the cult of the Sacred Heart. This took origin in the mystical experience of St. Gertrude, who dreamed that as she rested her head upon the wounded side of Christ she could feel the pulsation of his heart. This observation became exalted by a progressively theological overlay, to be reinforced by successive Papal decrees into an important doctrinal belief.

Turning to the Latin Americas we find in the mythology of the Aztec civilisation an apotheosis of the heart to a degree paralleled only by the ancient Egyptians. Many rituals might be quoted. After the cremation of a person of high rank, the ashes were preserved in an urn containing a precious stone to symbolise the heart, which was known as "food for the eagle—or divine sun-bird". The most sinister instance of these meso-American rites was the Toxcatl which culminated in the tearing out of the heart with an obsidian knife from the chest of a sacrificial youth, who for a year had been designated viceregent of the sun-god Tezcatlipoca. The still pulsating organ was held up in offering, rubbed upon the lips of an idol, and then placed in a vase and burned. Behind this ghastly ritual lay the desire to revitalise the sun-god and to renew his power.

The Notion of a Soul

In examining the age-old hypotheses regarding the visceral habitat of man's immaterial properties or faculties, we find that the ancients used interchangeably a number of dissimilar concepts. At one time it was a matter of the seat of the emotions; at another of intellectual processes. The idea became insensibly introjected of a *sensu commune,* as well as of a vital principle fundamental to living matter. Two other concepts were also introduced, often as though at the whim of the particular interpreter. I refer to the notion of the soul or spirit; and secondly to the principle of self-awareness. Orphic sects of 6th century Greece believed that within every human being a fallen God was locked up in material form until purged and released. But Socrates seems to have been the first to make serious reference to a psyche—a word which is commonly translated as soul. Originally it meant "breath", but it had come to stand for "courage", as well as "the breath of life" distinguishing animate from inanimate matter. "Psyche" is the ghost which is given up at death to become absorbed into the upper air, or which may quit the body temporarily in syncope. Attic tragedians employed "psyche" instead of heart to refer to the seat of intangible emotions, especially ineffable yearnings or forebodings.

The word "soul" rather than heart was introduced into medical terminology by Plotinus, and for centuries it was applied to vital principle, consciousness, Ego-awareness, reasoning, feeling, and common sensibility. Anatomical terms continued to be used often in a purely figurative sense to indicate notions of a high degree of abstraction. This holopsychosis or lack of specificity led to further errors and misunderstandings when it became a question of rendering Hebrew terms into Greek, thence into Latin, and so on. In strong opposition to the mediaeval ideas of a localisation of a soul within some circumscribed bodily region or organ stood the theologians and most metaphysicians, who, as universalists, denied the soul any localisable habitation. Some medical men, like Stahl and Unzer, were also of this opinion. Kant declared that no experience led him to the belief that his indivisible self could be imprisoned in a microscopical region of the brain, one's soul being everywhere in one's body and in its entirety in each of its parts.

However, the age of scientific materialism was out of harmony with vitalism, and by the mid-19th century the expression "soul" was dropped from the vocabulary of medicine. Possibly its last appearance was in 1877 when Munk spoke of the "soul-blindness" of de-corticated dogs.

But among primitive communities even today, and as far back as records go, there is the concept of Animism, a universal belief in the existence of some immaterial property pervading living creatures, capable of being exterojected into inanimate objects, surviving after death to reappear by dint of reincarnation. To this property the term "soul" is usually applied, though this expression means something entirely different to the cultural anthropologist, to the metaphysician, and to the theologian. Again we must not overlook the source of error introduced by language, for the holophrastic tongues of primitive peoples are not readily interpreted. "Soul" —if we may be permitted to use that word—is conceived in various guises. Sometimes it is looked upon as a miniature mannikin or homunculus. It may be regarded as a single entity or as a multiple one. At the moment of death it escapes the body by the various orifices, especially the mouth and nostrils, provoking elaborate death-bed rituals for trapping the liberated soul and transferring it to the successor. The soul may extend into one's shadow, or to one's reflection in a mirror or surface of a pool; or even into a portrait, making it vulnerable to damage or destruction. It may be associated with certain of the bodily tissues, giving rise to complex taboos and rituals. Among some savage communities the soul is believed to be a property shared by beasts and even plants, and not a human perquisite. Frazer wrote in a cynical vein ". . . The explanation of life by the theory of an indwelling and practically immortal soul is one which the savage does not confine to human beings, but extends to the animate creation in general. In so doing he is more liberal, and perhaps more logical, than the civilised man, who commonly denies to animals the privilege of immortality which he claims for himself. The savage is not so proud; he commonly believes that animals are endowed with feelings and intelligence like those of men, and that, like men, they possess souls which survive the death of their bodies, either to wander about as disembodied spirits or to be born again in animal form."

The "soul" is generally looked upon as made up of the mental endowments characteristic of the individual or of the species. Hence the belief in the assimilation of the soul and its properties by ingestion of the cadaver of an animal or in ceremonial cannibalism. The flesh of a tiger is eaten in order to acquire its peculiar ferocity. Usually the soul is looked upon as occupying a precise anatomical *nidus* which it is important to consume. A common belief is that the circulating blood is the medium encompassing the soul, and ceremonial drinking of the blood imparts the virtues of the dying creature to its captor. (Less often it is a question of drinking the bile or of devouring the liver.) Even more widespread is the cult of eating the heart of a Chieftain or King, or of some animal conspicuous for its courage, in order to inherit the desirable virtues. Such a belief is world-wide in extensity and age-old in antiquity. Thus in the language of the Caribs the very same expression is used to connote the soul, life, and the heart. Scarcely ever is the brain looked upon as the essential organ of the qualities which one seeks to emulate. Maybe the heart owed its predominance over the cerebrum in primitive belief to its greater accessibility. Perhaps the experience of the charnel-house and the battlefield played a part. Life might well have been correlated with the pulsating heart; death with its immobility. The fleeting escape of breath from the dying, and the steaminess arising from the viscera of the recently slaughtered man or creature would suggest the escape of some vaporous vital principle. The brain would not as a rule come under consideration, being encased within its stout and protective cranial box.

The Conception of a Corporeal Awareness

The notion of personal awareness developed much later in the history of philosophy. One of the first to refer to this idea was Fichte with his conception of the Ego. Throughout the 18th and 19th centuries this idea attracted increasing attention. Comar spoke of the "auto-representation of the organism"; the Freudians talked of Ego, Super-Ego, and Id, but without clearly defining these terms; the Würzburg school of psychologists referred to coenesthesia and to the *Ich-Bewusstein;* Bonnier—an otologist —described "schematia"; Jung and his followers an *Animus* and *Anima;* Claparède spoke of *moi-itié* or me-ness; while Oppenheimer's term was "total body experience". Usually, however, credit is given to Henry Head and Gordon Holmes for the beginnings of our ideas of a postural schema, which we now lightly call the body-scheme or body-image.

Today the topic has become too elaborate and the terminology too muddled for clear thinking to prevail. The current terms body-image and body-scheme are made to stand for different notions at different times by different writers. Now it is a perceptual, now a conceptual matter. For this reason the expression "corporeal awareness" is preferable.

Almost insensibly it has become accepted that this process of self-awareness "resides"—if one may be forgiven that term—within the brain rather than any viscus or limb. Expressed differently, corporeal awareness is mediated essentially *via* brain-cells. A victim of the Tudor executioner whose severed head rolled in the dust conceivably may not have undergone an instantaneous oblivion at the moment of decapitation. Were that so, it would not be the bleeding trunk which retained a fleeting awareness, but the disconnected head.

Here then is localisation of a sort. Again here is a tie-up with earlier metaphysical ideas about the existence of a soul, for the terms "body-image" and "soul" have often been used interchangeably. Here too is a hark-back to the disputes as to the precise localisation of the soul and the arguments as to whether the heart or the brain is more significant.

Thus, Van Helmont—an exact contemporary of Harvey—placed the "sensitive soul" or *anima sensitiva motivaque* within the pylorus. "There it sits and there it abides all life long. Not that the sensitive soul dwells in the stomach as in a sack, in a skin, or in a shell. Nor is it confined to that seat after the fashion of things shut up in a purse. In a wholly peculiar manner it is present in a point centrally, . . . it is present in the stomach in some such way as light is present in a burning wick." Voltaire would have no truck with such ideas. "Four thousand volumes of metaphysics" he said "will not teach us what the soul is . . . why do mankind flatter themselves that they alone are gifted with a spiritual and immortal principle? . . . . Perhaps from their inordinate vanity. I am persuaded that if a peacock could speak, he would boast of his soul, and would affirm that it inhabited his magnificent tail."

Even more cynical was that demirep philosopher Diderot, whose writings—perhaps never intended to be taken too seriously—are always entertaining. According to him, the soul ordinarily resides in the head, for it is the head which thinks, imagines, reflects, judges, decides, and ordains; but such was not always so. The first seat of the soul, he said, is in the feet. Since a baby's body, head, and arms are held immobile at the mother's breast, its feet are the only parts which make mobile contact with the outer world. The soul remains in the infant's feet until two or three years, ascending to the legs at four years, and reaching the knees and thighs at 15. "In some persons" said Diderot, "it never gets any higher." He went on to suggest that its location might differ from one person to another, remaining in the feet or legs in the case of a dancer; in the throat in a singer; in the arms of heroes and thugs; within the skulls of learned men; in the card-sharper's two hands; in the champing jaws of a glutton; in the eyes of a coquette; in the "secret jewel" in the case of most women; and with the debauchee in the sole instrument of his passion. Where tender and sensitive persons are concerned, including faithful and constant lovers, the soul dwells in the heart; but in the lazy or stupid it has no habitat at all. In more serious vein Diderot asserted that in a blind person the theatre of the soul is to be found within the finger-tips.

The Attitude of William Harvey

Finally we turn to the rôle played by William Harvey in this intellectual panorama. Although regarded by some of his contemporaries as "an audacious man, a disturber of medical peace, and a seditious citizen of the medical republic" he was actually a conservative in neurological thinking. We can but conclude that with all his genius Harvey had not wholly rejected the tramells of Aristotelean and Galenical superstitions, especially in his belief in a vital spirit and the conveyance of heat to the organs whence it returned cooled to the heart, there to be re-charged with heat. Harvey resorted to the age-old comparison of the vital spirit with the subtile spirit distilled by wine. According to Chauvois this kinship of wine with blood was a mystical idea which had survived from the ancient world into the Middle Ages, and Harvey had not freed himself from this venerable myth. Perhaps Harvey had even indoctrinated his good friend John Donne who three years previously had written ". . . that blood which is the seat of our Souls". This vital spirit passed through the ducts of the peripheral nerve-trunks, and gave rise to movement. That the nerves were hollow was indeed the teaching of most anatomists of that time. Doubts were later raised by Webber, Swammerdam, Willis, and Boerhaave, and this became a topic of virulent controversy. John Locke put his finger upon the linguistic imprecision of his day. At a weary and wordy debate whether the filaments of the nerve-trunks were permeated by a liquor, Locke eventually intervened by suggesting that perhaps the difficulty was merely one of semantics and demanded a clear definition of terms. Taken aback, the learned men acted upon this suggestion, and eventually came to realise that they were more or less in agreement that *some* fluid or subtle matter passed through the conduits of the nerves, but it was not easy to agree whether or not it should be called "liquor"— which they decided was not really worth arguing.

It is true that Harvey exalted the role of the head, speaking of it as the habitation of the soul, the sacristy, the citadel, the richest member of the body, its function being to create fantasy and to recall those which are no longer present, which is "memory". Because of man's faculty of passing judgment on things which are past, he conceives, comprehends, and defines. Harvey was in some doubt as to whether the solid parts or the cavities of the brain were the more important. He remained faithful to Vesalius in ascribing the faculty of memory to the cerebellum. Then in picturesque language Harvey emulated Aristotle in posing questions not all of which he answered. "Should not the heart be regarded as emperor or king?" . . . but a little earlier . . . "should not the brain be considered as king?" And yet Harvey could not get away from the idea that the heart was "the chiefest of all parts of the body" by dint of the quantity of blood and spirits contained therein. In the same context Harvey described the heart as the "inner room, the shrine, where is the fount of heat, the vital spirits, emotion, the passions and respiration".

We must remember however that these views were held by Harvey as a relatively young man. Twelve years after the *Prelectiones* Harvey seems to have abandoned the idea that the heart was the source of heat. He was anticipating the viewpoint of his young colleague Thomas Willis that the heart "is not so noble and principal an organ as it is commonly said to be; but a mere muscle consisting only of flesh and tendons". This was written just 10 years after Nicholas Steno had proclaimed that "the heart is a muscle, that it has all that other muscles possess and nothing but what they possess, so that it is not an organ of innate heat, nor the seat of the soul, neither does it produce vital spirit, nor blood, nor any other humour whatsoever". These forthright conclusions were however not proclaimed until seven years after Harvey's demise.

Harvey did not live to see the upsurge of a materialistic philosophy in medicine. The time was still to come when notions of humours were to be swept aside, and any ideas of a non-material soul were to yield place to hypotheses of electrical activity of the brain, or neuropils and nerve-nets. Starting with the simple observations of Galvani, Volta, Aldini, and du Bois Raymond, there came the electrophysiological applications of Fritsch, Hitzig, Ferrier, and Horsley, and later the work of Caton, Berger, and Adrian. Harvey might have been astonished to learn of modern biophysical speculators who accept the electrical activity of neuronal circuits as adequate to account for all the manifestations of the human mind. But even the term "mind" is outmoded in favour of "neural dispositions". Harvey need not have despaired however. An eloquent school of philosophers of medicine have rebelled against what my colleague Sir Francis Walshe has called the Peter Pan school of science with its "bloodless dance of action potentials" and its "hurrying to-and-fro of molecules". Electrical activity and mental processes may after all be analogues rather than counterparts.

Mr. President, we must admit that the divine banquet of the brain was, and still is, a feast with dishes that remain elusive in their blending, and with sauces whose ingredients are even now a secret. Who, better than Sherrington, has expressed this mystery of cerebral function, using all the prose of a philosopher-poet? . . .

Wonder of wonders, though familiar even to boredom. So much with us that we forget it all our time. The eye sends into the cell-and-fibre forest of the brain throughout the waking day continual rhythmic streams of tiny, individually evanescent, electricalal potentials. This throbbing streaming crowd of electrified shifting points in the spongework of the brain bears no obvious semblance in space-pattern, and even in temporal relation resembles but a little remotely the tiny twodimensional upside-down picture of the outside world which the eyeball paints on the beginnings of its nerve-fibres to the brain. But that little picture sets up an electrical storm. And that electrical storm so set up is one which affects a whole population of brain-cells. Electrical charges have in themselves not the faintest elements of the visual—having, for instance, nothing of "distance", "right-side-upness", nor "vertical", nor "horizontal", nor "colour", nor "brightness", nor "shadow", nor "roundness", nor "squareness", nor "contour", nor "transparency", nor "opacity", nor "near", nor "far", nor visual anything—yet conjure up all these. A shower of little electrical leaks conjures up for me, when I look, the landscape; the castle on the height; or, when I look at him, my friend's face, and how distant he is from me they tell me. Taking their word for it, I go forward and my other senses confirm that he is there.